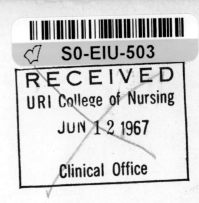

Foundations of
Pediatric Nursing

Foundations of
Pediatric Nursing

VIOLET BROADRIBB, R.N., M.S.
Assistant Professor of Pediatric Nursing,
University of Oregon Medical Center,
Portland, Oregon

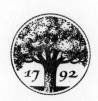

J. B. LIPPINCOTT COMPANY
Philadelphia   Toronto

Distributed in Great Britain by
Pitman Medical Publishing Co., Limited, London

Library of Congress Catalog Card No. 67-17432

Printed in the United States of America

Preface

The pediatric nurse today comes to her assignment with a recognition of responsibilities and goals which differ widely from those of the nurse who worked with children in the past. No longer can she be satisfied with a routine concerned entirely with the bedside care of a sick child. That the physical care of the hospitalized child is of great importance cannot be ignored or slighted; the nurse must never lose sight of the ultimate goal of hospitalization, which is to send a child home in the best possible health, as quickly as possible. As we examine this goal, however, we gradually begin to see the extent of what actually is involved. The child does not exist in a vacuum; he comes from a background unique to this particular individual. It may be a background rich in understanding and love; it may be an emotionally or culturally deprived environment; it may be a totally rejecting one. It is essential that the pediatric nurse learn to see the child as he is; a product of his home environment, but still a *child*, with the same needs, reactions, and developmental tasks as children everywhere. The incident of the child's illness is only a segment of the continuity of his life, albeit an important one. The facts of separation, strangeness, loneliness and discomfort can have severe and lasting consequences in the life of a child. This we recognize and affirm, but we must do more than that. We must learn how to make illness and hospitalization as maturing an experience as it is possible for it to be. We must try to make the experience a period that enables the child to grow a little in strength and security.

We cannot, however, afford to limit our concern to the child in the hospital. The needs of all children, *because* they are children, call for our attention. We must think in the terms given expression at the 1960 White House Conference: to strive "To promote opportunities for children and youth to realize their full potential for a creative life in freedom and dignity."

This book is written with a realization of the nurse's need to develop a broad and deep perspective of the meaning of nursing children. It endeavors to assist the nurse to catch a glimpse of the past in order to enable her to see where we are now, and how we arrived there. Having come this far, what are our present weaknesses, where do we still fail the children presently under our care? Finally, because the student and the young nurse is the policy maker of tomorrow, what is she going to do about it? What are our responsibilities concerning the future of today's child, and how do we see our responsibilities for the children of tomorrow?

No attempt is made in this book to delve deeply into the psychological aspects of child behavior. It is hoped that the student will acquire a working knowledge of them, become motivated to accept the child where he is, and go on from there. In order to do this, however, she will discover that she must understand, at least to some degree, what has happened in this child's life to make him the individual he is. This may well lead her to seek greater understanding of the psychology of childhood: it most certainly will involve her in the study of normal growth and development of infants and children.

As the title implies, the major function of this text is to provide a *foundation;* to help the student lay a groundwork on which she can build to the depth and breadth she needs and desires. The emphasis is on getting started. If she can learn to adjust to the child by putting herself in his place for a short time, to think his thoughts and feel his needs, to understand his limitations—and his possibilities—she will be well on her way toward becoming a successful worker with children.

The author believes that the student needs practical help as well as broad guidelines. Included in the text are suggestions concerning the day-by-day care for the child in health and sickness. Some background concerning the effect of illness on the child is given, in the belief that the nurse who understands the nature of the condition is better able to give the child the support and physical care necessary for his recovery. Emotional support for the hospitalized child is extremely important: of equal importance is the physical care the child receives. Frequently, the physical care given the child *is* the means by which emotional support is given.

The bibliography has been chosen mainly for the purpose of acquainting the student with the variety and richness of the available resources. Again, the purpose is to help motivate the student to search further and dig deeper. As she begins to realize the extent of research, of the horizons which are opening before her eyes, the very fascination of the search may lead her on, and on.

Included in the appendix are outlines of the more common procedures used in pediatric nursing. While the author realizes that procedures differ in detail in the various children's hospitals, the principles on which procedures are built remain the same. The student should have no difficulty applying the modifications which may be necessary to fit any given situation.

Also included in the appendix are the normal blood values at different ages and normal rate of heart beat and respiration. The necessary preparation for certain tests, such as Addis count, or glucose tolerance, is outlined. Other pertinent information, such as the conversion of fahrenheit to centigrade and abbreviations commonly used, is also included.

Violet Broadribb

Acknowledgements

Grateful appreciation is expressed to the many persons who freely gave of their time and their energy to make this book possible. Among those who read it, and who made many suggestions are Doctors Richard Olmstead, Robert Campbell, Julia Grach, Ralph Robertson, Clifton Way, Ralph Kamm, Edwin Kayser and Lawrence Wolff—all of the University of Oregon Medical School. Appreciation is also expressed to Dr. Carl Ashley of the Oregon Health Bureau.

Sincere appreciation is expressed to Mrs. Sylvia McSkimming, Miss Sarah Rich, Miss Peggy Cooke, and to Mrs. Helen Kataguri, who, as pediatric head nurses, showed wonderful patience and cooperation while patients were photographed and parents were interviewed. A warm "thank you" is also given to the staff members who helped so much.

Sincerest appreciation is expressed to Mr. David T. Miller, editor, of the J. B. Lippincott Company for his guidance and support; to Mr. Paul Miller for his excellent photography, and to Mrs. Clarice Francone for her fine drawings. Appreciation is also expressed to the publishers and to the companies who generously granted permission for the use of quotations and illustrations.

Acknowledgement and gratitude is expressed to Mrs. Isabel Lawrence for her very considerable clerical assistance.

Contents

UNIT ONE: INTRODUCTION TO PEDIATRIC NURSING

1. HISTORY OF CHILD CARE 3
   Child Care in Primitive Societies 4
   Child Care in Ancient Civilizations 5
   Former Child Care Practices 7

2. PIONEERS IN MODERN THINKING 12
   The Development of Institutional Care 12
   The Modern Hospital 15

3. PRESENT-DAY CONCEPTS OF CHILD CARE IN HOSPITALS 20
   Visiting 21
   Other Present-Day Concepts 25

4. THE PLAY PROGRAM IN THE PEDIATRIC AREA 28
   Importance of Play for All Children 28
   Children with Limited Opportunities for Play 34
   Therapeutic Characteristics of Play 40

5. OBSERVATION OF THE SICK CHILD 45
   Section 1. The Hospitalized Child 45
   The Importance of Knowing about the Child 46
   Section 2. Communicating with Children 51

UNIT TWO: THE PRENATAL AND POSTNATAL PERIODS

6. LIFE BEFORE BIRTH 57
   Introduction 57
   Prenatal Environment 58
   Prenatal Physical Development 60
   Education for Parenthood 62

7. NEONATAL GROWTH AND DEVELOPMENT 64
   The Birth Experience 64
   Hospital Care of the Newborn 72

7. NEONATAL GROWTH AND DEVELOPMENT (*Continued*)
  Parent Teaching 76
  The New Infant at Home 76

8. NURSING CARE OF THE NEWBORN WITH ILLNESS OR ABNORMALITY   86
  Neonatal Hazards 86
  The Premature Infant 87
  Care of the Newborn Infant with Congenital Anomalies . . 95
  Congenital Metabolic Defects 107
  Galactosemia 109
  Congenital Rubella 110

UNIT THREE: THE INFANT

9. AGE FOUR WEEKS TO ONE YEAR 117
  Maturation and Development 119
  Infant Nutrition 125
  Maintenance of Health 130
  Daily Living 132
  Hospital Care of the Infant 137

10. NURSING IN SPECIFIC CONDITIONS OF INFANCY 155
  Congenital Anomalies 155
  Conditions of the Gastrointestinal System 169
  Congenital Hypertrophic Pyloric Stenosis 173
  Conditions of the Respiratory Tract 180

11. ORTHOPEDIC CONDITIONS OF INFANCY 188
  Congenital Talipes Equinovarus (Congenital Clubfoot) . . 188
  Congenital Dislocation of the Hip 191

UNIT FOUR: NURSING THE TODDLER

12. NORMAL GROWTH AND DEVELOPMENT FROM 1 TO 3 197
  Physical Development 197
  Milestones in Normal Growth and Development
    During the Toddler Years 198
  Personality Development 202
  The Toddler in the Hospital 203
  Caring for the Burned Child 211

13. ACCIDENTS AND ACCIDENTAL POISONING 218
    Accidents 218
    Accidental Poisoning 222
    The Nurse in the Hospital 228
    Aspiration of Foreign Bodies 229
    Fractures in Childhood 230
    Abused Children: the Battered-Child Syndrome 236

14. ILLNESS IN THE TODDLER AGE GROUP 258
    Conditions of the Respiratory Tract 258
    Conditions of Metabolic Imbalance 271
    Eye Conditions of Infancy and Childhood 280

UNIT FIVE: THE PRESCHOOL CHILD

15. NORMAL GROWTH AND DEVELOPMENT 293
    Average Developmental Level of the Preschool Child . . . 294
    The Preschool Child in the Hospital 297

16. THE MENTALLY RETARDED CHILD 305
    Norms of Intellectual Ability and Adaptive Behavior . . . 306
    Terms Used for Measuring Extent of Mental Impairment . 306
    Etiological Factors in Mental Retardation 307
    Meeting the Needs of the Mentally Handicapped Child . . 308
    Teaching Self-Help to the Child 310
    Discipline for the Retarded Child 314
    The Other Members of the Family 315
    Home Care vs. Institutional Care 315
    Continuing Care 316
    Specific Conditions of Mental Disability 317

17. PROBLEMS OF EVERYDAY LIVING 325
    The Chronically Ill Child 325
    The Child with a Fatal Illness 331
    Blood Dyscrasias 337
    Leukemia in Children 341
    Hemophilia 343

18. OTHER DISORDERS OF CHILDHOOD 353
    Communicable Diseases of Childhood 353
    Care of the Child with a Communicable Disease
        (Isolation Practices in the Hospital) 361

18. OTHER DISORDERS OF CHILDHOOD (*Continued*)

Convulsive Disorders 363
Acute Glomerulonephritis 368
Childhood Nephrosis (Lipoid Nephrosis;
    Nephrotic Syndrome) 368

UNIT SIX: THE SCHOOL AGE CHILD

19. NORMAL GROWTH AND DEVELOPMENT 375
The Health of a School Age Child 375
Characteristics of a Six- to Seven-Year-Old 378
Characteristics of a Seven- to Ten-Year-Old 379
School Days 379
Emotional Support for the Child 380
Developmental Tasks 381
Providing Sex Education 382
The Deprived Child 383
The Child in the Hospital Environment 383

20. THE CHILD WITH DIABETES MELLITUS 389
The Classification of Diabetes 389
Incidence and Etiology 389
Presenting Symptoms 390
Definitive Diagnosis 391
Treatment and Family Teaching 391
Adolescence 399
Future Health 400
Babies of Diabetic Mothers 400

21. THE CHILD WITH HEART DISEASE 402
Early Indications of Cardiac Difficulty 403
Surgical Correction 404
Diagnostic Tests 407
An Outline of the Common Types of
    Congenital Heart Disease 408

22. RHEUMATIC FEVER AND RHEUMATIC CARDITIS 423
Clinical Aspects 423
Nursing Care 428
What is the Meaning of this Type of Illness to a Child? . . 430

23. HANDICAPPED CHILDREN 433
        Hearing Problems in the Child 433
        The Child with a Visual Defect 441
        Cerebral Palsy 445

UNIT SEVEN: THE ADOLESCENT

24. NORMAL GROWTH AND DEVELOPMENT 457

25. EMOTIONAL DEVELOPMENT OF THE ADOLESCENT—
     CONDITIONS OF ADOLESCENCE 467
        Acne Vulgaris 467
        The Handicapped Adolescent 469
        Emotional Problems 470
        Problems of Unwed Teenage Mothers 472
        Normal, Adjusted Teenagers 474

UNIT EIGHT: CHILDREN OF THE NATION
AND OF THE WORLD

26. CHILDREN OF THE NATION 479
        Child Care Outside the Home 483
        Children of Migrant Workers 488
        Children of the American Indians 489
        Pledge to Children 490

27. CHILDREN OF THE WORLD 493
        Conditions of Malnutrition 493
        Communicable Diseases 496
        The World's Children 497
        Intercountry Adoptions 499

28. THE ROLE OF THE NURSE IN THE COMMUNITY 502

     APPENDIX 507

     INDEX 557

UNIT 1

INTRODUCTION TO PEDIATRIC NURSING

1

History of Child Care

A baby is a precious thing, whether it is a kitten, a puppy, or an infant. Certainly we can all agree that a mother has some instinct to love and protect her baby under the greatest stress and danger. In all ages of recorded history, we read about mothers who have connived, plotted, broken laws and defied customs to safeguard their children and to provide for their well-being.

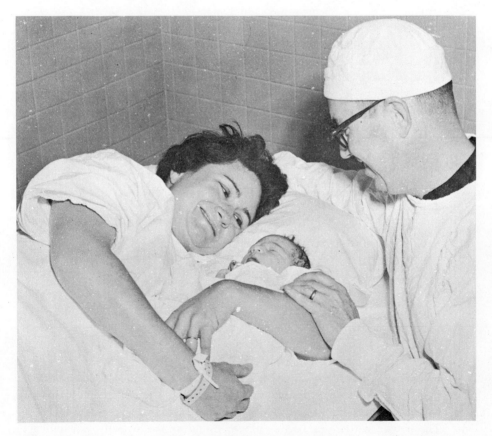

Fig. 1. A new family.

CHILD CARE IN PRIMITIVE SOCIETIES

When we speak about primitive peoples and their concept of the worth of the child, we should remember that we are thinking of the customs and mores of a society as a whole, and not necessarily of the individual members of that society.

For instance, when a culture decreed that no malformed infant could be permitted to live, we need not believe that all mothers accepted this verdict without question. We have evidence that they did not, in fact. We need to keep in mind that societies are made up of individuals, with their own private desires and codes of conduct.

People in general are conformists, however, who find it easier to go along with the prevailing customs and to believe as they are told to believe without much question. It is easier to adjust thinking according to custom than to risk censure and disapproval from society.

Keeping in mind that we can speak only of cultures and societies as groups, and not of their individual members, it is interesting to trace some of the thinking about children throughout past history. In addition to making fascinating reading, it may help us to understand better our own beliefs and feelings. It may even stimulate us as nurses to re-examine some of our present-day concepts. How many of the rituals and routines that we follow in the hospital do we accept without question because this is the way we have always done?

We know that primitive peoples were nomads moving from place to place in search of the essentials of life. As edible roots, berries and plants were used up, the people sought new fields, so that it was necessary to move frequently. Protection from wild animals and from adverse weather conditions was also essential. It often became necessary to move very quickly.

Any impediment to rapid action could have serious consequences for the entire tribe. Difficulties did not allow feelings of tenderness or pity to endanger the lives of the group as a whole. It was natural, perhaps essential, to look with favor only on the strong, hardy individual who could stand the rigors of such a life. Times called for an heroic people.

Children who tired easily, who needed much care and attention, were a distinct hazard to the tribe. It was simple to favor the strong, healthy child and to formulate justifiable occasions for the destruction of puny, sickly, or malformed infants.

As the art of fire-making became known and tribes learned to domesticate the wild animals for their use, to cultivate the ground, to plant and to hunt, they tended to settle down in areas that were familiar to them. Those who settled in barren places found unproductivity a handicap. Children were still valued in terms of their potential for future contributions to society, rather than enjoyed for their own sake. They were thought of as future farmers, warriors, or hunters. Infanticide was still a common practice whenever the child was sickly, malformed or, frequently, whenever the child had the misfortune to be born a female.

Perhaps we are not as far removed from this kind of thinking as we would like to believe. What are we taught in disaster nursing? To whom would the precious life-giving blood or medicine go in times of stress: to the weak and feeble, or to the strong, the most likely to survive? The one who would be of most value to the group, or the one who perhaps needed it most? In times of security, it is easy to consider and help the weak or handicapped. When the threat is to an entire community or to a way of life, our values are apt to change.

In primitive thinking, superstition and ignorance also had much influence on practices. We tend to fear that which we do not understand. We can find ability to cope with events only as we see meaning in them.

What could be more natural than to believe that the awesome display of thunder and lightning with its destructive potential was a voice of displeasure from a superior being? Or that a deformed child was the result of wrong doing and therefore must be destroyed? Even today, the first reaction of a parent on seeing a disfigured newborn infant is usually "What did I do wrong?"

The practice of abandoning infants to die of exposure did not seem as inhuman in many cultures as it does in ours. Even in recent times, among some primitive peoples, it has been believed that a child is not really a human being until he has formally been given a name and presented to the spirits and to the people (around the eighth day of life). This ritual is thought to give a soul to the infant.

CHILD CARE IN ANCIENT CIVILIZATIONS

The people who settled in fertile, well-watered lands developed a different concept of the worth of the child. He was no longer a hazard to the tribe; therefore, society could afford to protect him. We read that in the fertile Nile valley children were highly valued and that infanticide was forbidden by law. When the son of a slave woman, condemned to death by the decree of a cruel king, was rescued from the river, because of the love and pity of the king's own daughter to become the deliverer of his people, it was his mother's defiance as well as the pity of the princess that saved his life.

The people of the Nile valley developed a fairly enlightened concept of the care and treatment of children. Children lived mostly out of doors, and they indulged in lively games. Their clothing allowed freedom of movement: in fact they wore none before the age of five. They were sent to school to learn to read and to write, to figure, and to participate in athletics.

In another culture, that of Babylon, the Code of Hammurabi (2250 B.C.) outlined very clearly the civil, religious and medical justice due women and children.

The Egyptians had some concept of the idea that the child has specific ailments, distinguishable from those of adults. The Papyrus Ebers, which was found in an Egyptian tomb (dating from about 1500 B.C.) is a sort of encyclopedia of medical knowledge consisting of a collection from many sources, mostly from an earlier era. Although it is a compendium of forklore and medical practices, it has one section devoted to children's diseases.

In India also there appear at an early date references and data regarding diseases peculiar to children. A clear, rational doctrine of pediatric medicine appears during the first and second centuries B.C.

In general, however, children were considered to be small adults and were treated as such. Also, even in Egypt and Greece, cruel practices prevailed. Superstition and fear of the gods influenced their daily lives just as it did among their neighbors. Defective children in Greece were exposed to die, and there is evidence that in Egypt children were sometimes killed and buried with their parents to keep them company in the afterworld. Infanticide, however, though forbidden in Egypt was common in India.

Effect of the Great Religions

The great religions of the world, Judaism, Mohammedanism and Christianity, have played a large part in the development of the philosophy regarding the sanctity of life. For instance, in the Old Testament of the Bible, we find an advance in thinking from the time of Abraham, who thought that God had asked him to offer his son as a burnt offering as other peoples did to their gods, to the prophet Jeremiah, many generations later, who declared that this was an abominable practice and never demanded by the Hebrew God.

However, the people of Israel from the beginning of history have in general valued their children highly. The greatest reproach a Hebrew woman could have was to be childless.

Later, in the course of European history, children were valued for reasons of expediency. Wars and epidemics decimated whole countries, to the extent that they could have been wiped out without a large new population to replace them. Great plagues spread over Europe during the 18th century. Records show that 43,000 children died of whooping cough in Sweden during the years between 1749 and 1761, and that over 140,000 died of small-pox during the same period.

FORMER CHILD CARE PRACTICES

It is now rather amusing to read about former practices of child care. In older times, it was the custom in many societies to wash the new born child and then rub salt into the skin to make it tough and thick. Infants were wrapped in long bands of cloth (swaddling clothes) to keep their bodies straight. In India, the head was tightly bandaged in order to mould its shape and to close the fontanelles. Here again the Egyptians were exceptional, dressing their infants in loose clothing and advocating breast feeding. (Figs. 2 and 3)

The use of wet nurses is an old institution. A wet nurse is a woman who has recently given birth to an infant and is able to nurse another woman's child along with her own, or sometimes in place of her own. This practice became quite fashionable in Europe, although certain characteristics were often demanded of wet nurses. It was believed that behavior traits, among other things, could be transmitted in the milk; so the wet nurse had to be a model of virtue. After weaning, the child was sometimes given goat's milk rather than cow's milk; the goat being taught to straddle the crib to allow the child to suck directly. However,

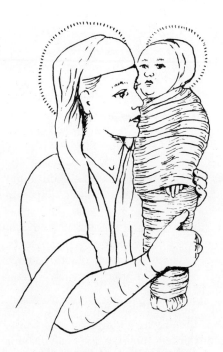

Fig. 2. Infant swaddling—from a painting of Madonna and child. (Andrea Mantegna, 1431–1506.)

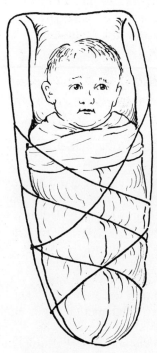

Fig. 3. Infant swaddling—an Indian child on a cradle board.

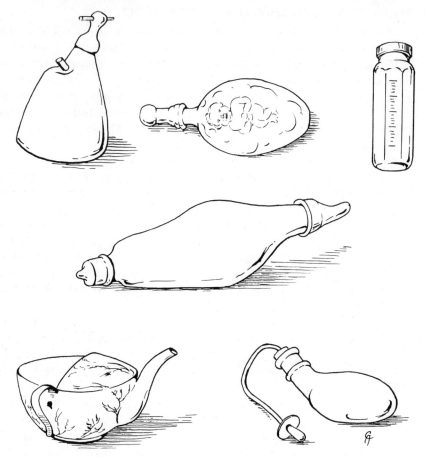

Fig. 4. Bottles and feeding equipment, ancient and modern.

animal milk was often in disfavor as it was thought that the child might imbibe animal behavior. Pap was often used in place of milk. Pap consisted of bread boiled in water, or sometimes in beer or wine, with sugar added. It was fed to the infant by allowing him to suck it from the adult's finger, or it was thinned and fed from bottles or pap-boats.

Bottles were curiously shaped and difficult to clean. Cloth, sponge and wood were among the materials used for nipples, because rubber nipples were not perfected before 1816. (Fig. 4)

The abandonment of infants, either those of illegitimate birth or those born into families who could not keep them, was widespread. As Christianity spread over Europe, the religious orders took the responsibility for the care of the sick and the helpless, and this care was expanded to include abandoned infants. The first infant asylum on record was established by the Archbishop of Milan in 787.

Effect of the Industrial Revolution

The industrial revolution brought great changes in Great Britain and other parts of Europe early in the 1800's. The population of Europe was largely rural until the invention of machinery. Then a mass migration into the cities occurred, especially in Great Britain. A book written in 1833 (now a part of the Ford Collection in the New York Public Library) gives some interesting light on the conditions that existed at that time. Written in the interest of social reform, it quotes facts and figures. A description of the typical day in the life of the mill worker of that time is given in some detail.

The worker rose between 4 and 5 A.M., went to the mill and worked until 8 A.M., when a breakfast of milk and porridge was brought to him. He was allowed to take a half-hour for this meal eaten at his machine. From 8:30, he worked without a break until 12 noon, when he had one hour to go home for dinner. At 1 P.M. he started work again and worked without interruption, except for 20 minutes for tea and bread, until 9 P.M. Then he went home for supper. The staple diet consisted of potatoes, wheat bread, a very small amount of animal food, some eggs and fish, and tea or coffee.

Since the first machines used for spinning were simple and small, they could be tended by small children. A large number of the workers were between the ages of 6 and 12 years. They were apprentices taken chiefly from workhouses and foundling homes. One company employed 1,000 such children.

There was little ventilation or temperature regulation. The work day (or night) was 12 hours long. As late as 1816, out of 10,000 employees in a certain 10 mills, 415 were under 10 years of age, and 4,404 were under 18 years of age. Figures given for 1833 showed very nearly the same conditions.

A report given before a board of inquiry contained this statement: "The fingers of children at an early age are very supple, and they are more easily led into habits of performing the duties of their station." Also, "the work is full as well done by children, is better done by children."

Another crime against children that existed in Great Britain, and many other countries as well, was a wide-spread practice called "baby-farming." This consisted of taking children into boarding homes, with no questions asked. As the children were mainly of illegitimate birth, and no money was forthcoming after the initial sum, it was to the advantage of the baby farmer to hasten the child's death. The abuse was so widespread that a committee was appointed in Great Britain to "inquire as to the best means of preventing the destruction of lives of infants put out to hire by their parents." Eventually, various laws were passed for inspection of boarding homes.

Period of Gradual Reform

As the public conscience became aroused to the plight of dependent children, orphan asylums came into being. Although we now shudder over the description of orphan homes and foundling homes of the 19th century, they certainly were an improvement over the workhouses and baby farms. Charles Dickens, who was interested in social reform, gives us some graphic pictures of workhouses and boarding schools in *Oliver Twist* and *David Copperfield*.

In America, where much the same conditions existed, Charles Brace was instrumental in forming the Children's Aid Society in 1853, which had as its purpose the removal of thousands of homeless children from the streets of New York City and into foster homes.

Children's courts, as distinguished from common courts where both children and all types of criminals appeared together, came into being in the United States in 1899, although some attempt had been made earlier to hear child prisoners separately from adults.

Child labor laws had a long, hard struggle. As early as 1819, the minimum age of 9 years was set up as law in England, but there was no enforcement. It took reformers such as Dickens and others to arouse public attention and concern to the point at which remedial legislation would be demanded. In the United States, boys under 10 worked in mines, and little girls worked long hours in factories. A federal labor law passed in 1917 was declared unconstitutional after 9 months, and it was not until 1941 that any federal law was successful in regard to regulation of child labor.

Even those who had an interest in bettering the lot of children however, thought of them as miniature adults, and so treated them. The first hospital for children in America admitted both women and children. The following year (1855) the first hospital in America for sick children only, opened in Philadelphia. Eventually, many children's hospitals in the United States and throughout the world came into being. Although many children's hospitals in the United States at one time maintained schools of nursing, the only one continuing to do so is the Boston Children's Hospital.

BIBLIOGRAPHY

Abt, A.: History of Pediatrics. *In* Abt, A., and Garrison, F.: History of Pediatrics. Chap. 1. Philadelphia, W. B. Saunders, 1964.

Abt, I.: History of Pediatrics. *In* Brenneman, J.: Practice of Pediatrics. Vol. 1, chap. 1. Hagerstown, Prior, 1945.

Bradbury, D. E., and Oetinger, K.: Five Decades of Action for Children. A History of the Children's Bureau. Washington, D. C., United States Department of Health, Education and Welfare, Children's Bureau, 1962.

Drake, T. G. H.: Infant Feeding in England and France from 1750 to 1800. Am. J. Dis. Child., 39:1049, 1930.

Garrison, F.: An Introduction to the History of Medicine. 4th ed. Philadelphia, W. B. Saunders, 1929.

————: History of Pediatrics. *In* Abt, I.: Pediatrics. vol. 1, chap. 1. Philadelphia, W. B. Saunders, 1923.

Gaskell, P.: The Manufacturing Population of England. London, Baldwin and Cradock, 1833.

Halford, J.: Baby Farming. vol 2, p. 840. Chicago, Encyclopedia Britannica, 1945.

Hoebel, E. A.: Man in the Primitive World. 2nd ed., pp. 374, 376, New York, McGraw-Hill, 1958.

Lipton, E. L., *et al.*: Swaddling, A Child Care Practice: Historical, Cultural and Experimental Observations. Pediat. (supplement) 35:521, 1965.

Old Testament: Genesis, 22:1–14, Exodus, 2:1–10, Jeremiah, 7:30–32.

2

Pioneers in Modern Thinking

The previous chapter dealt with the gradual growth among the peoples of the world of compassion for children and the increasing awareness of their problems. As knowledge of sanitation and infant nutrition grew, it became increasingly evident that the children of the poor benefited little from this knowledge.

THE DEVELOPMENT OF INSTITUTIONAL CARE

Especially affected were those who had been abandoned because of poverty or illegitimate birth and were being cared for in institutions. Their condition was appalling. A great step had been taken, however, when religious orders began to take abandoned infants within their shelter. The first such asylum on record was established by the Archbishop of Milan in 787, and thereafter asylums under the care of the Catholic church continued to appear in Rome and in France. Some of the most noteworthy were established by St. Vincent de Paul in the early 17th century.

From the 17th through the 19th centuries, children's institutions were established in Germany, England, Ireland, Russia and South America. Many were founded by religious orders and later taken over by municipal authorities. These were not hospitals, but shelters for abandoned children and infants born out of wedlock. For a time, it was common practice to hang baskets outside the doors of these shelters so that infants might be left without any mark of identification.

Unsanitary conditions, ignorance and neglect, as well as lack of knowledge of proper infant nutrition, became characteristic of these institutions. Even into the 19th century, mortality rates were 50 percent to 100 percent. In fact, Malthus (a British economist of the early 1800's) is said to have expressed the view that the most effective way to arrest the growth of population would be to multiply institutions for receiving newborn infants.

Many of the asylums were converted into children's hospitals for both the sick and the well. St. Vincent de Paul reorganized an asylum into what is believed to have been the first children's hospital, the Hospice des Enfants Trouvés, in 1670.

Hospitalism. Eventually, medical men throughout western Europe became concerned about the conditions in these asylums and hospitals. Although many instances of efforts to improve these conditions are on record, one outstanding example can be quoted. The Infant Asylum of Berlin had an extremely poor record prior to 1900. New administrators put into effect the practice of isolating children with septic conditions, and are said to be among the first to cut infant mortality sharply by the simple practice of boiling their milk. They tried to improve the nutrition of the children, and put forth the idea that a nurse should not have more than eight or nine children under her care during the daytime, as well as the then novel idea that well infants should be protected from *hospitalism.*

The term *hospitalism* is used frequently throughout the writings on institutionalization of children. Spitz defined hospitalism as "a vitiated condition of the body due to long confinement in the hospital," but said that it had come to be used almost entirely to denote the evil effects of institutional care on infants.

American Association for the Study and Prevention of Infant Mortality. Conditions in general, however, both in Europe and in America, showed little or no improvement. Many physicians appeared to recognize that institutionalization of children had extremely bad results. This was brought forth in a spectacular manner in the United States in 1914 at a meeting of the American Association for the Study and Prevention of Infant Mortality. The subject considered was "Mortality in So-Called Foundling Homes." Although foundling homes were numerous through-out the nation, few records were kept. One of the very few reports (made by the New York State Department of Charities on 11 institutions in that state) was appalling. It indicated an average death rate of infants under 2 years of age at 422.5 per 1000 as against a rate of 87.4 per 1000 infants in the general population during a 4-year period.

The many comments on these findings included one made by a physician who told of an institution in which no infant lived to be 2 years old. Another told of an institution in which all babies on admission were categorized as being in "hopeless" condition, in order to cover all eventualities.

Dr. Dwight Chapin became known as one of the foremost pioneers in the fight against these conditions in the United States. Believing that insanitation and ignorance were mainly responsible for the appalling death rate, he pleaded for accurate data in order to help in the formula-tion of a plan of attack. Few records were kept of the age or condition of the child on admission, his growth or progress during his stay, or what became of him on discharge. Dr. Chapin believed that only when these were known could measures be taken in prevention.

Period of Improvement

It was known that the major cause of death in children's institutions was the intractable diarrhea that the majority of these children developed. As early as 1901, the simple practice of boiling milk at the Berlin Asylum had resulted in a sharp reduction in mortality rates. The same results were obtained in San Francisco. When the Associated Charities in San Francisco became concerned over a mortality rate of 59 per cent in the foundling homes under their care and supervision, they decided to board the babies out in foster homes. Soon, a weekly baby clinic was organized. Visiting nurses supervised the homes and encouraged the foster mothers to attend the clinic, where safe milk was dispensed and information given on sanitation and infant feeding. Early in the experiment, the mortality rate dropped to 12 per cent, and eventually the sphere of the clinic was widened to include the care of children in their own homes.

Asepsis and Isolation. A new era now began in the institutional care of children, for the sick, as well as for the healthy. A period of asepsis and isolation began. Babies were placed in individual cubicles and the staff strictly forbidden to pick up the children unless absolutely necessary. Crib sides were usually draped with clean sheets so that the infant had nothing to do but stare at the ceiling. The importance of toys in the infant's development was completely ignored or not understood.

The incidence of diarrhea declined, but the high mortality rate continued. Dr. Joseph Brenneman (of the Children's Memorial Hospital in Chicago) was one of the first to suspect that the infants suffered from a lack of stimulation. Writing about the management of the infant ward in his hospital in 1932, he related the rule that every infant must be picked up, carried around and "mothered" several times a day. Other measures in effect dictated that no infant was to be admitted who could be cared for at home or in a foster home, and that every infant was to be discharged as soon as possible. Such thinking was indeed unusual.

Recent Advances. During the 1940's and 1950's many social scientists, psychiatrists and pediatricians began the study of the adverse effects of institutionalization on children. Anna Freud and her associates studied children who had been removed from their families and placed in residential nurseries in the country during the bombing of London in World War II. There were many other well-known names among those who conducted studies to support the hypothesis that emotional deprivation caused potential physical damage as well as irreversible psychological harm.

In 1946, René Spitz gave the results of studies in which he believed he had proved that deprivation of maternal care caused a state of dazed stupor in an infant. This condition could become irreversible, he believed, if the love-object was not returned to the infant within a reasonable length of time. He coined the term *anaclitic depression* to describe this state.

Spitz's findings were widely accepted, as were similar studies made by Bakwin in 1949. Bakwin found that small infants hospitalized for a long period of time actually developed physical symptoms, which he attributed to a lack of emotional stimulation and a lack of feeding satisfaction.

It remained for Dr. John Bowlby of the Tavistock Clinic in London to explore the subject of maternal deprivation thoroughly, working under the auspices of the World Health Organization. His report in 1951 received world-wide attention. He discussed the short-term and long-term effects of maternal deprivation, especially on the child between the ages of 1 and 3 or 4 years.

At this age, the child has been able to establish a separate identity from his mother, but he is still wholly dependent on her for ego support. Separation from her is therefore intolerable to the child and regression results.

Much of Dr. Bowlby's study was geared to the separation of the child through hospitalization. As one result of his findings, he inaugurated the practice, in the Tavistock Clinic, of allowing the mother to be admitted to the hospital with her child and to participate in the child's care. This practice has been followed in some other hospitals, in both Europe and America.

A documentary film made by Robertson (an associate of Dr. Bowlby) during the 6-day stay of a 2-year-old girl in the hospital gives strong support to the theory of regression, withdrawal and lack of interest, despite the fact that her mother and father were allowed to visit her daily. Bowlby and his associates were also concerned that the effects of separation might become irreversible and show up as psychological damage in later years.

Many changes were brought about by these and similar studies. Foundling homes and orphanages slowly gave way to foster homes. At the present time foster-home placement is yielding to the idea of keeping the child in his own home, if this is feasible, by giving financial and emotional support.

THE MODERN HOSPITAL

Hospital 'policies have become liberalized. A relaxation of strict isolation practices for all children has not resulted in cross-contamination as had been feared. Children play happily together in playrooms and in wards. Parents visit freely, hold their children, and are frequently allowed to participate in their care. Some hospitals have opened their doors to parents without restriction. When a child does not have anyone to visit him, volunteer mothers take up the slack. Some hospitals, having insufficient space to allow all mothers to stay with their child throughout

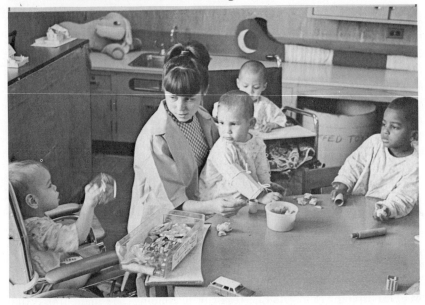

Fig. 5. Children play happily together.

the length of their stay, have made provision for this volunteer-mother care for children between the critical ages of 2½ and 3 years. (Figs. 5 and 6)

No one disputes that deprivation of emotional support, especially during the early ego-forming years, has disastrous results. It is understood that a small child needs a mother figure to sustain him, and the

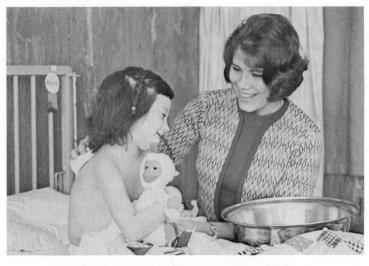

Fig. 6. Parents can participate in their child's care.

ever-changing shifts in the hospital situation make a mother figure hard to come by, for mothers usually do not stay on duty in 8-hour shifts for 5-day weeks.

It is not clear, however, whether a mother who rejects her child is better than a foster mother, or even a warm mother figure in an institution. Many, perhaps most, normal mothers may have periods of partial rejection when the memory of past independence seems particularly desirable. The child can stand considerable turmoil in his family setting if he feels that security and love are present. Whether he can stand rejection from his love-object without permanent harm is another matter. Present-day thinking seems to be that a substitute mother figure can contribute more to the child's security than a rejecting mother, although more study of this question is needed.

One of the beneficial results of the past studies, however, has been to make doctors and nurses more conscious of the child's need for emotional satisfaction and stimulation. Infants and children who have received love and security in their homes seem to suffer most when removed from their families. These are the children who scream when

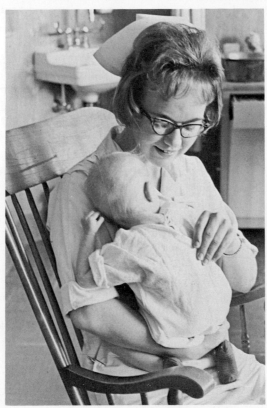

Fig. 7. Nursing is cuddling.

their parents leave them and refuse to be consoled by anyone. They are the ones about whom we say "They are spoiled, and would be much better off if their parents' visiting were restricted." In this manner, we would remove any small measure of security the child has left and reduce him to dull despair. Is that what we want?

However, the child who has already suffered rejection—to the extent that he fears to put his confidence in anyone—is apt to be even more rejected in the hospital. The child who has a warm home relationship may employ wiles and blandishments to get what he wants, but the rejected child knows better. So, he withdraws and refuses to respond to anyone. He is the one who is going to be further rejected in the hospital until all of his previous beliefs are confirmed completely.

Nursing is as much rocking, cuddling, and loving a child as it is giving physical care. The prescription for T.L.C.—tender loving care— still applies to all children; the sullen, rejecting one as well as the cute little blond with curly hair and winning ways. (Fig. 7)

Recently, some doubt has been cast on the inevitable and irreversible effects of deprivation, especially with respect to its effects in future years. It is generally well known that not everyone deprived as a child grows up to be delinquent or develops an unloving personality.

An interesting report reassessing the long-term effects of maternal deprivation was published in 1962 by the World Health Organization. This report, by Prugh, consists of several thoughtful papers written by today's psychologists and social scientists. They review the extensive research made since Bowlby's monograph of 1951 and weigh much of the evidence used by him and by Spitz and others at the time. The report presents many fascinating areas for additional research. It builds on the work done previously and acknowledges a great debt to those who pointed out the way. No one belittles the work done already, but the need for further research is shown, particularly in the light of the possibility of the reversing effects of environment as well as the results of the effort put forth by the individual himself.

BIBLIOGRAPHY

Abt, A.: History of Pediatrics. *In* Abt, A., and Garrison, F.: History of Pediatrics. Chap. 1. Philadelphia, W. B. Saunders, 1964.

Abt, I.: History of Pediatrics. *In* Brenneman, J.: Practice of Pediatrics. Vol. 1, chap. 1, Hagerstown, W. F. Prior, 1945.

Bakwin, H.: Emotional deprivation in infants. J. Pediat., 35:512, 1949.

Bowlby, J.: Maternal Care and Mental Health. Geneva, World Health Organization, 1951.

Burlingame, D., and Freud, A.: Young Children in Wartime. London, George Allen & Unwin, 1942.

Chapin, H. D.: A plea for accurate statistics in infant's institutions. Arch. Pediat., 32:724, 1915.

———: Are institutions for infants really necessary? J.A.M.A., 64:1, 1915.

Freud, A., and Burlingame, D.: Infants Without Families. New York, International Universities Press, 1944.

————: War and Children. Part 1. New York, International Universities Press, 1944.

Garrison, F.: An Introduction to the History of Medicine. 4th ed. Philadelphia, W. B. Saunders, 1929.

Holsclaw, F., and Rude, A.: Morbidity and mortality of the associated charities feeding clinic—San Francisco. Arch. Pediat., *32:*181, 1915.

Provence, S., and Lipton, R.: Infants in Institutions. New York, International Universities Press, 1963.

Prugh, D., *et al.*: Deprivation of Maternal Care—a Reassessment of its Effects. Geneva, World Health Organization, 1962.

Robertson, J.: A Two-Year-Old goes to the Hospital. Film, 16 mm., sound 45 min. London, Tavistock Clinic, 1958.

Senn, M.: A relook at the effects of maternal deprivation. Children, *9:*237, 1962.

Spitz, R.: Anaclitic depression. Psychoanal. Stud. Child., *2:*313, 1946.

————: Hospitalism. Psychoanal. Stud. Child., *1:*53, 1945.

3

Present Day Concepts
of Child Care in Hospitals

Most children in our culture experience at least one period of hospitalization before they reach adulthood. This may be short term or long, pleasant or disturbing, a single experience or repeated periods. If we realize this, we need to be very sure that we understand what we are doing to the children when they are with us. It has been said that a hospital experience can be either disturbing enough to cause personality changes, or an advantageous, maturing experience for the child. Can we discover any factors involved in the hospital situation that help to bring about either of these results?

Present-day children's units in the hospital vary so widely in their scope and their practices that it is difficult to discuss accurately any common practice. The nurse may read of many present-day practices which, although they seem desirable to her, do not exist in her hospital, her school or her community. There are many reasons for this; the physical facilities may not lend themselves to new ideas, or economic resources may be limited. Community thinking may not accept the new ideas. There are many considerations that may enter into local practices.

The nurse, however, becomes increasingly aware of certain needs. It is quite possible that she will have an opportunity to help with the planning and the inauguration of new methods for the care of the whole child. In any event, it is essential for her to be aware of present-day studies, research projects, and the application of modern ideas. As a member of the health team, the nurse has an important role to play. As a future administrator or educator, the young nurse needs to investigate, to understand, and to accept or reject modern trends in child care.

Much of our present thinking is the result of the work of the pioneers in child care whom we have previously discussed. Some of their ideas have been accepted whole-heartedly. Some studies are suspect as being poorly controlled, so that results may not necessarily be valid. At times, we suspect, opinion entered in, with the result that research was slanted toward previously formulated concepts.

Obviously, it is impossible to prove that certain childhood experiences have life-long effects. We believe this to be true, however, and certainly evidence points in this direction. Nevertheless, uncontrollable variables also enter into consideration. The child's hereditary endowment, his environment, his culture, his place in the family and in the community, to mention a few things, must all be considered. Not every rejected child grows up to be delinquent. A child from a broken home, deeming himself unwanted, may determine that his future home and family will be stable and loving.

However, we do know enough to be confident in saying that a child needs to be secure before he can accept insecurity, that he needs acceptance to enable him to accept, that he needs love to be able to love. He may, by his own inner strength, be able to move toward these goals during life, but why put unnecessary obstacles in his path? He will find enough of them without our help. Yet so often, in the hospital, we do just that.

VISITING

Some of the newer practices that have been tried and proved to be effective should be discussed. One of the most important has been the liberalization of visiting hours. Bowlby and others have furnished enough evidence about the adverse effect of separation during hospitalization to convince the majority of administrators.

Hospitals for acute illnesses generally changed rules long ago from visiting hours of once weekly, or even twice monthly, to daily. Gradually, the rule of "2 to 4 P.M.," or other rigidly defined periods of 1 or 2 hours for parent visiting, are being replaced with "2 to 8 P.M.," or even sometimes with a rule including some morning hours.

Free Visiting

The plan for free visiting throughout the day has been more difficult to accept. Even in centers in which one would expect understanding permissiveness, one is often greatly disappointed. It is still not uncommon for a distracted parent to receive assurance from her doctor that she may spend as much time as she wishes with her sick child, only to find that this is not the case, and that the child would have to be put on the critical list before she can do so. She feels that the situation *is* critical—and so does the child.

Some personnel, who believe that the child needs his mother, ignore infractions of the rules and look the other way if mothers come early or stay late. This makes the situation difficult for those who believe that hospital rules are made to be kept, or for those parents who encounter a permissive nurse one day, only to be put out in righteous indignation by someone else the next day.

Dane Prugh makes the observation that "Of obviously greater importance than the permissive techniques themselves (in avoiding emotional trauma) are the attitudes and quality of the ward personnel who apply them."

Mrs. W. had only been persuaded to bring her son into the hospital for surgery with the understanding that she could be with him most of the time. Billy had a serious heart defect that might shortly end his life unless repaired, yet surgery held a high potential risk for him.

In addition to her mental conflict as to whether she had taken the right course, and the feelings of guilt whenever his condition appeared to worsen, Mrs. W. had domestic and economic problems. To the casual observer on the ward, she was, frankly, a plain nuisance. She was hyper-critical of Billy's care, insisted on carrying out much of it herself, and yet refused to accept the importance of some of the procedures. The staff believed that she made the child too dependent on her, and they were quite openly resentful of her interference and criticism.

The students became thoroughly imbued with the attitude that "We could give Billy much better care if his mother would stay at home and not interfere."

Yet, when they sat down in conference to discuss this problem, they could present forth little evidence that Mrs. W. had actually hindered her son's recovery. True, she was apt to say "No use offering him fluids; he won't drink, never would," or "He's always had a poor appetite; been a finicky eater all his life."

Had anyone spent any time really trying to get to know Mrs. W., or trying to establish any friendly relations with her? Well, no: she was too disagreeable. Had anyone explained to her not only the importance of fluids, but the "whys and wherefores?" No, no one knew her that well. "But she gets in our way, and we could do more for Billy if she wasn't here."

Then was it for Billy's sake that they wished her gone, or because of their own feelings? This was harder to answer. No one could honestly say that Billy's care was significantly neglected, or that by spending a little time with his mother they might not have established better rela-tions and a greater understanding between them. They reluctantly con-cluded that she bothered the staff with her attitude.

Billy was a very frightened little boy who desperately needed his mother's presence. Did not the fact that he recovered against such enor-mous odds prove anything? It might even have been possible that his mother's presence compensated for those extra ounces of fluid that he might have taken had she not been so certain that he wouldn't.

We let our own feelings get in the way of thinking so often that we confuse them with the patient's welfare. That the child cries when his mother leaves should indicate that he still reacts in a normal manner. It ought not to mean to us that his mother should not be allowed to visit because she "upsets" him. When he reaches the point when he can let her go without showing any emotion, we will have real cause for worry. Do we really believe that a child is better off when, in despair, he believes that his mother has deserted him? Do we believe that when he has assumed an attitude of indifference in order to live with his despair that he has *adjusted* to the situation?

Some mothers, it is true, are too anxious or too guilt ridden to be comfortable in the hospital. No one should require a mother to stay, or should make her feel neglectful, if she chooses not to stay. However, neither should she be denied the right to be with her child as much as she wishes, nor should she ever be made to feel that she is interfering with her child's care when she is present.

It would seem that a little thought and understanding could open the doors to mothers whenever they desire to come. Mothers usually are anxious to participate in their children's care. This can do wonders for both their own and their children's security. After all, these are their children, they were theirs before they came to the hospital, and they will return to their mothers when they leave. Why separate them now, when they need her as they will never again? It does not make good sense.

The mother should not, however, be expected to do more than she desires to do. It costs a great deal to be a patient in the hospital, and the patient is entitled to all of the care he needs from the hospital staff. Some parents are so conscious of the cost that they resent being asked to do anything themselves. If they know that they are not required to help, but are free to do so if they desire, they can then relax and consider the needs of their children.

The nurse needs to think for herself, especially if she still encounters the old stubborn way of thinking that parents are nuisances and get in the way. She needs to wonder why we, as nurses, are so arrogant as to assume our great superiority over others. Have we proved that we can give the child greater love and more perceptive understanding than the parent?

Can we honestly say that most parents are ignorant of their own children's needs, either physically, emotionally—or any other way? Perhaps much of the feeling one encounters against parents goes back to the days when principles of hygiene and sanitation were not as well known as they are at present. Most certainly it was necessary to guard the child against superimposed infection. Perhaps, with typical American enthusiasm, we overdid things. We think that if a certain practice is good, more of the same would be better.

We completely lost sight of the fact that the child belongs to his parents and will go back to them. If the home lacks certain health practices, how is anyone going to make improvements if he has no example to follow? The majority of parents have the welfare of their children at heart, and are especially interested in learning effective ways of bringing them up. If sound, effective health practices are followed in the hospital, parents quickly pick up new understanding and skill. We often hear "This is the way they did it in the hospital," but how often can we continue to hear it if parents are not allowed to see what goes on? The practice of doing all treatment and nursing care before visiting hours does not help at all.

Unfortunately, as nurses, we are sometimes apt to be careless in our health practice in the hospital. A child may have learned to bush his teeth and to wash his hands before meals. Yet time and again, one can open a bedside stand and search in vain for a toothbrush. Or the child uses a bedpan or urinal, with never an opportunity to wash his hands. What sort of health teaching is this? Here is a ready-made opportunity for sound teaching. Perhaps it is no wonder that we do not want parents to see our own poor habits. It seems incredible that a profession dedicated to the promotion of health deliberately undoes the parent's patient teaching of months. We need to take a long, hard look at ourselves as health teachers. (Fig. 8)

Living In

An interesting practice has been inaugurated in some areas—that of allowing the parent or parents to live in with the child. Some hospitals find that limited space seems to make this provision difficult, and they limit the rooming-in to parents of children between the ages of 1 and 3 or 4 years, the period of separation believed to be the most traumatic to the majority of children. Others allow this practice only if the child has a private room. If an imaginative 4-year-old can people his own room at home with strange and horrible night monsters, what can he not do in a

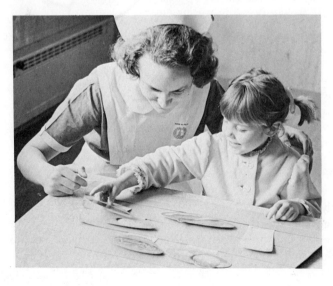

Fig. 8. Learning principles of nutrition.

ward or room in totally new and different surroundings? Few things can be more frightening then than to be alone in a strange place in the middle of the night.

In hospitals where parents are admitted along with their children, folding cots or convertible lounge chairs are provided. Some fortunate units have lounges in which parents can relax, visit with each other or enjoy a coffee break. Some provide an opportunity for the parent to eat with the child, and still others have cafeteria services available.

If this service is not provided, free visiting hours have proved to be definite adjuncts to parent education and have been helpful in fulfilling the hospital's function as a public health leader and teacher. If the parents can observe sound health practices being carried out, they have an opportunity to present problems about which they themselves have been puzzled. Furthermore, they do not have to go home and wonder about what secret and dreadful procedures are being carried out on their children in their absence.

Visiting in Long-term Care Facilities

The question of free visiting hours has been discussed here in relation to the children's units in hospitals for acute illnesses. There are numerous hospitals for children requiring long-term care, and those require separate consideration. Many of these still limit visiting rather drastically, although some are beginning to examine their practices more thoughtfully. Arguments are apt to be that the child adjusts more easily to a long-term hospitalization if he is not disturbed by frequent visits from his parents. This premise cannot be taken seriously, as a child left in an institution for months—or even years—denied even the right to the limited security that daily visits from his parents could bring, is surely the most lonely and desolate of human beings.

An argument with somewhat more validity is that these children come from widespread areas, and many are too far away from home to allow frequent visiting. This seems a poor reason for limiting those who could come. Volunteer mothers from the community can help fill this gap, and could easily be recruited. At its very best, an institution is an extremely poor substitute for a home.

OTHER PRESENT DAY CONCEPTS

Early Ambulation. Short-term hospitals can learn one thing from long-term residences however, and many have. The children are generally ambulated early; even children in casts are helped out of bed and into chairs, or especially constructed carts, unless definitely contraindicated. The children put on daytime clothes and wear regular shoes. One cannot but be puzzled as to why little cotton dresses and suits are not as easy to make and to launder as hospital nightgowns. Certainly it is a morale booster to get dressed in the daytime and to wear shoes.

Volunteer Mothers. There are other areas in which we see the need for changes. Volunteer mothers to come in to mother the child or infant who has known nothing but rejection, or through no fault of his own has no one to come to visit him, fill a real need.

Play and Teaching Activities. The playroom with a planned program is a well established fact in many areas. Certainly the need is recognized. An exciting program is the provision of regular school teachers in the short-term children's units. Convalescent hospitals, and those for crippled children, have had this service for some time; and "home-bound" teachers have occasionally come in to the individual child in regular hospitals. However, the idea of teachers regularly employed by the school system and working in the children's unit of a general hospital is rather new. One such plan consists of three regularly employed school teachers for a unit of about 30 children. As this hospital unfortunately does not have an adolescent unit, two additional teachers teach high school subjects to teenagers throughout the hospital. All children do regular schoolwork unless too ill. At 9 A.M., the teachers come around to each ward, bring the child's school bag to him, and get him started on his work for the

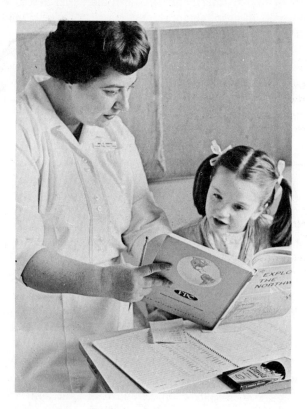

Fig. 9. School continues in the hospital.

day. Because of the diversity of ages and grades, individual study is the rule. Every effort is made to furnish the child with the same books and the same kind of instruction he has been receiving in school. Many children bring their school books with them. The school teachers go from child to child, moving on quietly when treatments are due. At noon, materials are collected, then after a rest period, the afternoon is given over to schoolwork and crafts. Excellent rapport is established between nursing and educational personnel. The teachers are employed by the school system, thus school hours and holidays are observed. This makes a long, idle summer for the children however, which needs to be filled. This is where volunteers can be a great help. High school students, or young women contemplating nursing as a career should welcome the opportunity, as it fills a great need. (Figs. 9 and 10)

BIBLIOGRAPHY

Blake, F.: The Child, His Parents and The Nurse. Philadelphia, J. B. Lippincott, 1954.
Bowlby, J.: Child Care and the Growth of Love. Baltimore, Penguin, 1953.
Dimock, H. G.: The Child in Hospital. Philadelphia, F. A. Davis, 1960.
Doernbecher Hospital, University of Oregon Medical School Hospital: Public School Program.
Prugh, D., et al.: A Study of the emotional reactions of children and families to hospitalization and illness. Am. J. Orthopsychiat., 23:70, 1953.
Robertson, J.: Hospitals and Children: A Parent's-Eye View. New York, International Universities Press, 1963.
————: Young Children in Hospitals. New York, Basic Books, 1958.
Ross Laboratories: Family-Centered Pediatric Nursing Care. Ross Laboratories, 1964.

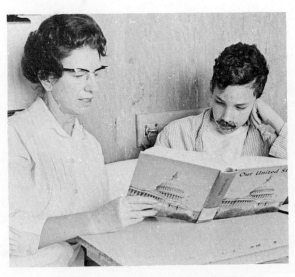

Fig. 10. Keeping up with his studies.

4

The Play Program in the Pediatric Area

Playing with children is important and as a therapy is a concept new to some nurses. Some nurses still believe that the only function of the hospital is to get the patient well. This, of course, is the prime objective of all pediatric departments, but what these nurses fail to see is that physical care is only one aspect of the entire nursing plan. One cannot consider as separate the child's physical, emotional, mental and social needs. Each one is a part of the others in such a way that it would be impossible to care for one without having considerable effect on the others as well.

It has been said that a child does not stop growing and developing when he enters the hospital. This is something to think about. Without meaning to, nurses are apt to think of the child patient as being somehow different from the children they see on the street, in the bus, or in the neighborhood. Actually, the only difference is that the child patient is restrained by his illness, or by hospital rules, from carrying out his developmental tasks in a satisfactory manner. To present for discharge a child who is healthy in mind and body is the objective of all nursing care.

IMPORTANCE OF PLAY FOR ALL CHILDREN

Play is the business of children. It is only by practice, by imitation of the adult world, by trial and error, that the child learns. The apparently aimless movements of the infant are actually purposeful. His incessant postural activity is his work, and a tremendous amount of energy is needed for it. In this way, he strengthens his muscles, perfects his coordination, and keeps abreast of his rapidly maturing nerve cells.

As the infant matures, every stage of development calls for the learning of new skills. This learning is physical as well as mental and emotional. The muscles must be used, and will ache if forcibly kept still for any length of time. The mind must interpret and learn, but there cannot be any significant mental or physical stimulation in an emotionally deprived atmosphere. The infant needs approval, love, and praise to stimulate him, and to provide the all-important background of security.

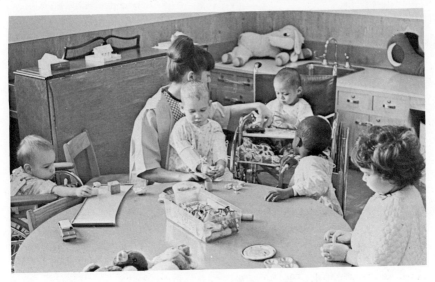

Fig. 11. Children in a playroom.

Hospital Play Programs

The hospitalization of children has changed markedly in the last few years. Newer treatments have shortened the need for bed rest in many instances. There are, of course, still many conditions that prohibit activity, either temporarily, or on a long-term basis. A visit to the pediatric wards today, however, shows many beds empty during the daytime hours.

Hospitals have met the challenge of the child's needs in various ways. Ideally, a spacious playroom, well equipped for the particular age group, and well attended, is the answer. Newly built or remodeled hospitals can plan for these playrooms as an essential part of the children's wing. Some hospitals have met the challenge in other ways, sometimes by taking over some other room for a playroom. Naturally, these rooms are not always ideal for this purpose, but can be made to serve. (Fig. 11)

Other pediatric departments, unable to find a spare room, have used ingenuity and imagination in planning play experience. In large wards, toys, tables and chairs are provided. Toy carts, which are circulated from bed to bed, are easily made.

Sometimes, when a central playroom is used, it is very easy to forget the child who is confined to his bed back in the room. Actually, keeping a number of playroom children occupied in a constructive manner requires total concentration. Although some playrooms are large enough to allow a few cribs to be brought in, not all children on bed rest are able to tolerate the busy pace of the playroom.

There may even be some advantages in having to use the ward for

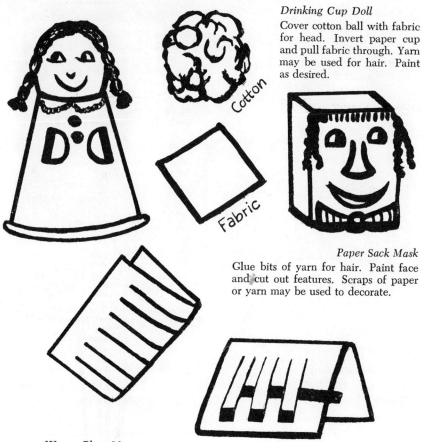

Drinking Cup Doll
Cover cotton ball with fabric for head. Invert paper cup and pull fabric through. Yarn may be used for hair. Paint as desired.

Paper Sack Mask
Glue bits of yarn for hair. Paint face and cut out features. Scraps of paper or yarn may be used to decorate.

Woven Place Mats
Construction paper cut as shown. Contrast with strips as shown.

Bird Cage
Make perch out of two pieces of string and cut-off straw. Bird may be drawn out of construction paper or purchased. Attach perch strings to bottom of plastic berry basket and invert. Attach second basket and tie together with ribbon.

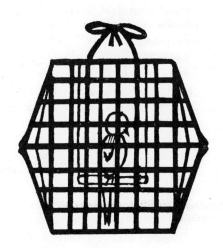

Simple homemade toys are easily constructed.

Diorama

Shoe box colored paper background figures from drinking cups, pipe cleaners, clothespins. Trees from pipe cleaners or heavy paper with spools for standards.

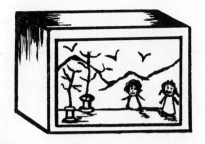

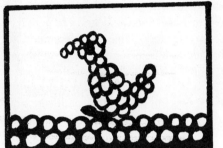

Clothespin doll

Yarn hair
Pipecleaner arms
Dress or paint as desired

Bean Mosaic

Assorted beans and peas glued on with cement. Construction paper or cardboard for background.

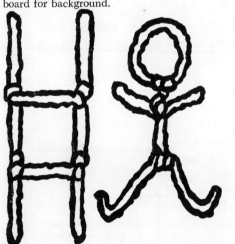

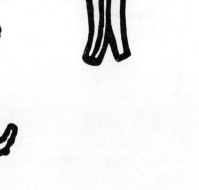

Pipe Cleaners

Twist pipe cleaners into various shapes.

Colored Straw Beads

Cut up drinking straws into various sizes and string. Straws may be colored or painted.

play activities. The children on bed rest may participate in the same activities as the ambulatory children, and this may be quite a morale booster for them. Children on bed rest can have their beds protected by sheets of plastic and join in the finger painting, water play, or other messy activities. They can have their beds rearranged so that they feel they belong to the group.

The mobile child who can roam at will can find some diversion for himself. True, this may take the form of some unacceptable activity, but he will find something if he is unrestricted. The child confined to his bed has a serious problem. If his nurse has any interest in children, she talks to him as she bathes him, but all too often personal contact ends there. The child may be too sick to be interested in play, and clutching his favorite toy may be enough activity for him. Most children who are confined to their beds, however, need something to occupy their minds and to provide stimulus.

Play Experience in Nursing

It is now a commonly accepted practice to include play experience in each student nurse's educational background. This is excellent for a number of reasons, but there is one danger to guard against. The student nurse may feel that because she is not play nurse for the day, she has no obligation toward directing the child's activities. This feeling stems largely from the student's attitude toward her pediatric experience. If she has an enthusiasm for her work with children, and a genuine interest in their welfare, she not only sees this as an obligation, but as a challenge to her ingenuity and to her imagination. To rescue a child from apathy and withdrawal provides one of the greatest satisfactions known to a nurse.

One frequently sees the student nurse out at the desk after her morning cares are done. Certainly, she needs to read her patient's chart, and to get all the information she can about the patients in the department, but it sometimes is an indication that she feels insecure and inadequate with the child after his physical care is completed. She is apt to take refuge in some activity that takes her away from him. She feels sorry for the child, but she does not know what to do for him, and so she frequently finds herself busy elsewhere. She is also apt to feel guilty because of her withdrawal from the child, and the pediatric experience becomes less of a fulfillment for her.

One student made the remark that she disliked playroom experience. "It takes imagination to play with children," she said, "and I just don't have any."

Many young nurses, perhaps a majority of them, have been baby sitters during high school; either as a means of making money, or as older sisters in the family, or as an adoring aunt. Perhaps they have also had experience as camp counselors, Sunday school teachers, vacation-school teachers and helpers. Why, then, are they so unsure of themselves in the hospital situation?

Perhaps this panic stems from the nurse's conception of her role, as well as her mental image of the hospitalized child. She must again remind herself that these are *children*, quite similar to her brothers and sisters, her neighbors and friends. Illness and strangeness may cause them to put on a front of apathy, indifference, or even dullness. Down underneath is still a person with all of the instincts, capabilities, longings and potential of any child at that particular level of development. Who will bring out this hidden child for all to see? Can the nurse? What a challenge! (Fig. 12)

Below is described an incident that brings into sharp focus the possibilities for the nurse's understanding of the child. It is one of the highlights in pediatric nursing.

Play in Pediatric Nursing: An Example

Merrilee was a tot just under 3 years of age who had been through a ghastly experience. She and an older sister had been temporarily alone

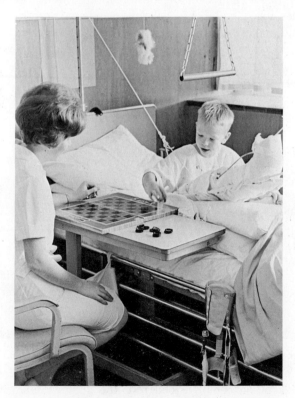

Fig. 12. This is nursing too.

in their house when the whole building burned down. Merrilee was rescued, but she suffered extensive second and third degree burns on her face and on her body. Weeks of isolation in the hospital, painful procedures, and difficult, agonizing movements, had taken their toll of this little one's emotional state. She had come to prefer to be alone, showing no interest in anyone. After all, why should she? Usually, the entrance of a nurse or doctor only meant more pain.

Eventually, the time came when the urgency of physical care subsided, and concern was felt over this child's uniformly negative responses. She was encouraged to sit up in a chair and look out into the corridor, but she cried whenever she was placed facing in that direction.

Day by day, quiet, persistent effort on the part of the staff brought a slight response, but one day the breakthrough really came. A student nurse, noticing that the only unburned areas were Merrilee's feet and lower legs, thought that some play activity involving her feet would be painless and might stimulate interest. She asked the recreational leader for a hand puppet, and was given a brightly colored duck. She placed this on Merrilee's foot, and the child was entranced. She made the duck open his mouth, quack, and soon Duckie was biting the toes of the other foot.

Merrilee forgot to be shy. All day, people came to her door to see a proud child make Duckie bite her toes. She chatted excitedly and freely. Other students, not to be outdone, invented other games, and soon Merrilee was running about her room. She just naturally shrugged off any discomfort and commenced using other parts of her body. Soon she was transferred to the ward, and here one had difficulty recognizing the child who had rejected everyone. As a leader in mischief, she became unsurpassed. She related lovingly and trustingly to everyone, and was soon well on the way toward being spoiled.

Certainly it is true that one does not know instinctively how to be at ease with children simply because one is a nurse, or because one has had previous experience with children. If a recreational leader needs training, why shouldn't the student nurse have some guidance as well? It certainly is not realistic to send her into the playroom with nothing more than a "Today you are play nurse."

Suggestions for crafts, games and just "things to do" are abundant and easily found. Anyone with a little persistence can find plenty of help in pamphlets, books, magazines and newspapers. Here, it may be helpful to suggest some specific activities for various situations.

CHILDREN WITH LIMITED OPPORTUNITIES FOR PLAY

The Child on Complete Bed Rest

First, consider the child on complete bed rest. Very few children today are kept on complete bed rest, the greatest single reason being the presence of rheumatic fever, either with or without heart involvement. Sydenham's chorea is generally accepted as a manifestation of rheumatic fever, and is treated in the same manner.

Before any discussion of complete or strict bed rest can be attempted, it is necessary to define the term. This is somewhat difficult when dealing with children. One is much more confident when speaking of adults. An interpretation of complete bed rest should mean that the patient does nothing for himself; he is bathed, fed and turned, and encouraged to avoid excitement and strain.

How does one go about keeping a child on such strict bed rest? He lacks the experience for understanding the issues involved. He lives for the here-and-now, not for a vague and shadowy future. Do we restrain him? If so, will his resistance and resentment prove a greater strain on his heart than free movement about his bed?

It is necessary to find out how much restriction is actually meant by this term. It could mean that the child is kept in bed but is allowed to feed himself, and also allowed some quiet activities. It could simply mean that the child is not allowed to have bathroom privileges. It could *also* mean just what it says; the child is kept quietly in bed, is fed, bathed, allowed to do no schoolwork or anything involving the use of his arms. His visitors and his television are restricted. In such a case, he probably would be receiving some sedation to help control his restlessness. Doctors vary the meaning of the term when they use it as a prescription for different children.

After ascertaining just how much activity the child is allowed, the nurse can make her plans. At the moment, we are speaking about the child who feels physically well enough to chafe against his enforced inactivity. For the child in acute distress or pain, the condition itself limits activity. The normally active, fun-loving boy or girl who is so sharply restricted finds this a great trial, and it is one for those caring for him; yet he needs mental stimulation to prevent him from suffering considerable psychological damage. This aspect of his care is at least as important as his physical handling, and requires even more thought and planning. Frequently, it is helpful to pool the thinking and planning of all concerned in a ward or staff conference.

Suggestions for activities. The American Heart Association has suggestions available for the asking. Most of them do not take the expenditure of money but utilize common everyday materials. Many suggestions to help the child occupy his mind during the long hours of enforced idleness are available in other publications.

Fast growing plants are fun to watch. One can almost see them grow. The nurse can take an eggshell, fill it with water or dirt, and dropping a seed into it, find that it soon starts to grow. She can take an egg carton and stand the eggshells upright in it, first coloring the shells if she wishes. In water, large seeds such as melon, squash, grapefruit, grow pretty vines. Nearly any flower seed grows in dirt. A sweet-potato vine is very pretty, with heart-shaped leaves, and grows from a slice of sweet potato kept in water, or in dirt. A carrot or a beet makes a vine. For even more fun, take a large carrot, scoop out the inside, make two holes in the sides near the top for a cord or ribbon to hang it by. Fill the hollowed-out portion with water, and hang it. The carrot must be kept filled with water, however, so choose as large a carrot as you can find, because it dries out quickly.

An herb garden is fun to watch grow. Parsley grows quickly and profusely. Garlic, dill, chive and other herbs can be grown in pots or planters. There is great satisfaction for a child in being able to give mother a sprig of parsley or rosemary to dress up her dinner.

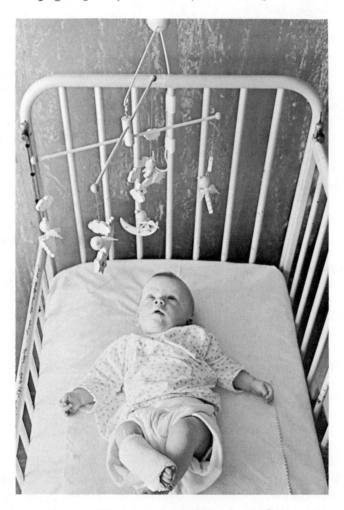

Fig. 13. Mobiles are fun to watch.

Pets, of course, are a great source of satisfaction. These require care and are not always allowed. However, a small fish in a fish bowl at the child's bedside may be a great comfort to him and require practically no care on the part of the staff. One boy kept a goldfish at his bedside, and they became great friends. Eventually, when he went home after some months in a convalescent hospital, he held the bowl up to the car window all the way home so that "Jimmy" could see the scenery too. He was sure that after many months of confinement Jimmy would be as anxious to see the outside world as he was himself.

Mobiles are great fun to watch. They can be made with cellophane straws in various shapes and sizes such as stars, triangles or other forms, using paper figures such as butterflies, birds or angels, to flutter gaily about. (Fig. 13)

If you live in an area where colored plastic baskets are used for marketing berries, ask people to save them for you. They make beautiful bird cages. Place one for top and one for bottom, lace them together with ribbon and hang a small paper or plastic bird inside. Hang from a hook with a gay ribbon and bow. Of course, live birds in real cages are wonderful diversions if anyone is available to care for them.

Record players and television are both fine for children's wards, but may prove too stimulating for some children. If television is provided, make sure that someone supervises the program and the reception. Too often, one walks into a room where the television is either out of focus, or the program is an adult one, totally unsuited to the audience.

Greeting cards that are sent to the child make a cheerful wall decoration, and can be put up with masking tape. If cards do not come, this may be an opportunity to use some of the greeting cards that people are always anxious to donate to the children's ward. Naturally, the cards from family and friends are more welcome, and the suggestion to schoolmates or fellow Scouts that Jimmy does not want to be left out of things may inspire short letters and cards.

Surprise boxes are an excellent tonic for the person confined to bed. A shoe box filled with small packages, one to be opened each day, gives a little spice to life, and helps the person look forward to tomorrow. If there is no family to make such a box, is there any reason why nurses cannot include making one of these boxes as a part of nursing care? The child with little stimulation from friends or family is the child needing this type of care more than the others.

The Child on Simple Bed Rest

The child on bed rest without other limitations, can have more active occupations. There are, of course, many children whose condition makes bed rest advisable or mandatory. The child may move about his bed freely, may feel well, but because of some condition may not be allowed

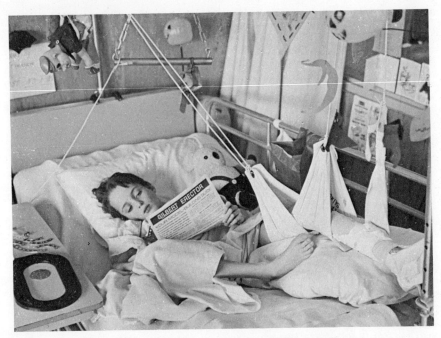

Fig. 14. An absorbing interest for a child on bed rest.

to get up. Perhaps he has a cast that limits his ability to move about. Perhaps he has a slight fever, or a slight cold, or a condition that may necessitate bed rest but does not restrict his activity while in bed. He feels fine, but he must stay in bed as he sees the others troop off gaily to the playroom. Such children suffer from boredom, and may lose interest in life in general if some stimulus is not provided for them.

It should not be too difficult to find occupation for these children. Most of the crafts can be carried out on a sturdy table. For the school-age child of perhaps 5 to 8 years of age, crafts are interesting and may become absorbing. (Fig. 14)

A child's problem is solved. A good example of this was Bobby—a patient in a school-age ward—who, because of an infection, was placed in a room alone. He was apathetic, listless, whiny, and disagreeable. It was just before Christmas, and the whole ward was busy making decorations, but the report was that Bobby was not interested in doing anything, and was a thoroughly disagreeable little boy.

One of the nurses decided that Bobby should be brought into the activities somehow, but she found it difficult to arouse any enthusiasm in this 6-year-old boy. Finally, she took some paper medicine cups, water paint, and plain string into his room. She painted the outside of the cup red, punched a hole in the bottom and hung it up. Bobby was interested and soon had a row of Christmas bells—red, green and gold—strung across his room. Next he made paper chains, and finally engaged in a really big project. Stencils of Christmas scenes were available, so he traced, colored, and gave pictures to his favorite people, after liberally decorating his own room with them. This was much more satisfying than putting up just any old pictures.

These activities seemed to bring back much of his old interest in life. His appetite improved, and he became much more lively. He was discharged to return shortly after Christmas, and this time he was in the ward with the other boys. He became a thoroughly typical boy, lively and full of mischief; so it seemed that he had learned that the hospital could be fun after all.

For the toddler who must have his activity restricted, a special kind of toy must be provided. Everything goes into his mouth (with potentially dangerous results) as you may discover the first time you rescue a small car, marble, or coin from starting down a small child's throat. Crayons are colorful, and to a toddler, meant to be eaten. Paper is to be torn and perhaps to be eaten as well.

Cloth books are safe, as well as stuffed animals, although even here the nurse must make sure that there are no ripped seams, because stuffing is great fun to pull out, or any button eyes to remove. Large, sturdy cars, trucks, and planes are fun.

The older child, who can be trusted with crayons, finger paints, coloring books, or with blunt scissors, can find a great deal of satisfaction and diversion, even though he must stay in bed.

Suggestions for the Child With Limited Mental Ability

Mention must be made of the child whose mental abilities are limited. He is in need of recreation as much as the normal child, perhaps more so. Try to discover the kind of toy that satisfies him, even though it is at a very low level for his chronological age. Even the child who appears to be functioning at an extremely low level may have his attention caught by a bright object hanging within his field of vision. (See also section on mental retardation.)

The nurse must consider the limitations imposed by any disease, such as the desirable amount of activity and the amount of restriction of movement. It would seem to be as important for the nurse to plan the child's recreational activity as to plan his individual nursing care. All ages, as well as all conditions, must be considered.

The Infant

The infant can of course benefit greatly from stimulation. There is seldom an occasion when the nurse should leave the infant without some type of play material suitable for his age. A cradle gym takes only a minute to fasten across the crib, and more than once an apathetic infant, having accidentally batted one of the toys with his hand or foot, has found stimulation and interest in trying again. Sturdy rattles and soft, cuddly animals are a part of the picture. If the child is at the age when he derives his greatest pleasure from throwing his toys out, it is profitable to tie them to the crib sides. (Fig. 14)

Babies can often be put in playpens, perhaps more frequently than nurses realize. This may well provide a change of scene as well as give an opportunity to stretch those developing muscles.

THERAPEUTIC CHARACTERISTICS OF PLAY

We must not forget the *therapeutic value of play* that is frequently important. The incident of the burned child who learned to manipulate a puppet with her feet is one example. Another one could be the manipulation of various kinds of toys for the purpose of strengthening weak muscles.

If the nurse is uncertain about what kind of toy to use, or needs to have her imagination stimulated, a visit to the occupational therapist is helpful. Nurses can make a real contribution to the sick child's well-being and ultimate recovery. The nurse must understand the importance of a relaxed, happy atmosphere in the total picture of nursing care.

Some children have very little contact with the outside world through visitors or mail. Such children look on wistfully as a more fortunate roommate opens his cards or letters. It takes but little time or imagination to drop a card in the mail, or even a cheery note. To be valuable, these should come through the mail, so that Johnny will get real mail, just like the others. That someone cares enough to send a card is excellent medicine.

We do not do *play therapy* as such, of course. That is not our purpose, nor are we justified in trying to make it so. However, we are in one sense using therapy for the children. The time the child spends in the hospital should not remain empty. He does not live in a vacuum, but continues to grow and to develop. We can help or hinder this growth by the opportunities that we provide for him. A play program needs thought and planning if it is to be anything more than a means of keeping the children quiet. A trained recreation leader appears to be an essential part of the pediatric staff, and the nurse can learn much from her. The "play lady" is only one person however, and is not in as close and personal contact with the individual child as is the nurse caring for him.

Group play can be of great value in helping the sick child overcome boredom or homesickness. If the ward is a noisy one, or the children appear to be over stimulated, quiet games are frequently calming. Games like "I packed my suitcase" may be effective, or the continuous story, going from child to child. One student introduced a story telling hour while giving morning baths. One child started an adventure story that was followed by fantastic adventures from the next bed, each child trying to outdo the others in imagination and fantasy. Even the shy, unhappy child found himself drawn into the company. Another time, the charge nurse was puzzled to find the ward door closed, but on opening it she discovered the reason. The nurse was bathing one child while leading a vigorous chorus of *Old MacDonald Had a Farm*. Material benefits from such thoughtfulness are apparent; the child sleeps better, eats better, and has less tendency to think about himself.

Mention has been made of *television*. Certainly it has a place in the picture, but it should be used intelligently. It has also been demonstrated that a child given something interesting or constructive to do, spends far less time as a mere observer of television.

When There Is No Existing Play Program

Much of the previous discussion has been concerned with hospitals at which a play program has been initiated. The nurse may very well find herself in a situation where no such program exists, and may find that the initiative for starting such a program must be her own. A well organized program is in effect in many hospitals, and the nurse easily becomes a part of it. There are still many hospitals without such a program.

There seems to be no real reason why a nurse cannot work toward such a program if she is convinced of the necessity for it. It certainly is not difficult, and need not be expensive. Play materials are easily improvised from the simplest articles. Pretty pictures have been made by pasting lima beans, green or yellow split peas, and red beans onto a cardboard plate in a flower design. Some of the happiest children were scaring the nurses with horrendous masks made from paper bags pulled over their heads, with eyes, nose and mouth cut out.

Socks or stockings make excellent hand puppets, or can make delightful stuffed dolls. Soap can be carved into animals by the child who can be trusted with the necessary tools. Finger paint, paste and modeling clay can be made very simply at home. Spools, cardboard, craft paper, milk bottle caps, discs from round boxes, can all be put to use to make delightful dioramas enclosed in deep shoe boxes.

Cellophane and macaroni straws make necklaces, and pointed drinking cups make fine doll bodies. It takes more imagination than money to stock a play cupboard. (See pp. 30–31)

There are so many *booklets and pamphlets* available for suggestions that the nurse need not feel at a loss as to where or how to start. Some references are listed at the end of the chapter. Many of these, or others equally as valuable, can be found in the public library. Recipes for making play dough, finger paint and *papier mâche* are also given at the end of this chapter. When the nurse has discovered for herself the fun for both patient and nurse, she quickly finds ideas of her own.

TABLE 3–1. TOYS SUITABLE FOR VARIOUS AGE GROUPS.

INFANTS

Cradle gym
Rattles (doughnut, dumbell, plastic keys)
Soft balls

Soft washable dolls and animals
Floating bath toys
Pots and pans
Small plastic or wooden blocks

TODDLERS—AGE 1-2 YEARS

Cloth, plastic books (illustrations of familiar objects, preferably one to a page)
Nested blocks of soft plastic or wood

Push toys and pull toys
Telephone
Dolls
Musical top

PRESCHOOLERS

Record player, nursery rhymes
Large wooden beads for stringing
Housekeeping toys
Transportation toys (tricycle, trucks, cars, wagon)
Blocks
Hammer and peg bench

Floor trains
Blackboard and chalk
Easel and brushes
Clay, crayons and finger paint
Outdoor toys, sand box, swing, small slide
Books (short stories, action stories)
Drum

KINDERGARTNERS AND FIRST GRADERS

Blocks
Dolls
Housekeeping toys
Dress-up clothes, tea parties
Outdoor toys
Easels, blackboards, paint

Blunt scissors, simple sewing sets, paste and colored paper
Doll house
Simple puzzles
Books, records
Matching card games

OLDER CHILDREN

Paper dolls
Table games
Books for self-reading
Electric trains

Bicycles
Work benches, good tools and materials
Puppets and marionettes
Crafts

THOSE IN MIDDLE CHILDHOOD—9-12 YEARS

Hobby collections
Telegraph sets, short-wave radio*
Model car, boat and plane sets

Table games
Outdoor sports

These are but a few suggestions for appropriate toys and games for various age groups.

* Electrical appliances in the hospital (such as X-ray) may interfere with reception.

A place to keep these materials is frequently a problem. A consultation with the nurse in charge may reveal a cupboard or closet that could be used. The nurse needs to decide whether she wishes to have the materials available to the children, or whether she puts someone in charge to hand out the materials as they are needed. In any case, she should

TABLE 3–2. RECIPES FOR HOMEMADE PLAY SUPPLIES.

FINGER PAINT

Mix ½ cup starch with ½ cup water, add 1½ cups boiling water, cook until clear. Mix with ½ cup soap flakes to desired thickness. When cool, pour into small jars with tight lids. Add vegetable coloring as desired. Glazed shelf paper may be used for canvas, wet paper with sponge or cloth before using.

MODELING DOUGH

Mix 1 cup salt and 2 cups flour, add enough water to make a dough. Use enough flour so that dough is not sticky. Children like to use cooky cutters and rolling pin with this. Vegetable colors can be kneaded into the dough.

PASTE

Old-fashioned paste is made with flour and water, cooked until clear. Oil of cloves and powdered alum may be used to keep paste from spoiling.

PAPIER MÂCHE

Tear up old newspapers into small pieces and cover with boiling water. Soak overnight. Add flour in the proportion of 1 part flour to 4 parts of the paper mixture, and 1 part salt to ¼ of the flour. Mix with hands (the children will love to do this) until pulpy. Add oil of cloves and powdered alum for preserving, and colors as desired. Use for figures, puppets, relief maps.

---

remember that the children are still in the hospital when she has left them at the end of her day. One sometimes sees all play materials put away under lock and key after 3:30 or 4 P.M. and totally inaccessible over the weekends.

Books, of course, play a large part in children's entertainment. If your hospital does not have a children's library, why not start one? One group of students started a drive among their friends and families for used books suitable for children, and soon acquired a very respectable library. A word of caution is needed. The books must be carefully screened against trash or unsuitable material. Some people see a book drive as a chance to get rid of all the old books that they have been saving for years. The children's librarian at the public library would be glad to help choose the books. A great deal of tact is necessary in dealing with donors whose generosity exceeds their judgement. Nevertheless, a children's library is a profitable venture.

Toys can be collected in the same manner. They must be sturdy, durable and suitable. At one school, the student nurses had fun with "dorm" parties, at which they mended and repainted toys. Making doll wardrobes, knitting dollhouse rugs, crocheting drapes and curtains—all were fun. In fact, one group had several sessions in which they papered rooms in a homemade dollhouse, made fixtures, rugs, curtains, and finally painted the outside of the house. When finished, it was put on a portable table and used in the ward, mainly for the children who had to stay in bed. A family was provided with the dollhouse, and the children were encouraged to make clothes for them if they wished. This proved to be a great morale booster, especially for the homesick child. The house took quite a beating however, and required frequent refurnishing and repainting. The furniture can be made from sturdy cardboard and replaced frequently, or may be made from heavier material that can withstand rather rough use.

BIBLIOGRAPHY

Blake, F. G.: The Child, His Parents and the Nurse. Philadelphia, J. B. Lippincott, 1954.
Brooks, M. M.: Hospital play has a purpose. J. Nat. Assn. Nursery Education, 1959.
Diversions for the Sick: Boston, John Hancock Mutual Life Insurance Co., 1959.
Plank, E. N.: Working with Children in Hospitals. Cleveland, Western Reserve University Press, 1962.
Play School Association: Why—Play in a Hospital How—. New York, Play Schools Association.

SUGGESTED READINGS FOR FURTHER STUDY

Benz, G. S.: Pediatric Nursing. 5th ed., pp. 282-296. St. Louis, C. V. Mosby, 1964.
Dodds, M.: Have Fun—Get Well! 9th ed. New York, American Heart Association, 1962.
Horwich, F.: The Ding Dong School Book. New York, Rand, McNally & Co., 1953.
Johnson, J.: Home Play for the Preschool Child. New York, Harper & Bros., 1957.
Keiser, A.: Here's How and When. New York, Friendship Press, 1957.
United States Department of Health, Education and Welfare, Children's Bureau: Handbook for Recreation. Washington, U. S. Government Printing Office, 1960.
———: Home Play and Play Equipment. Washington, U. S. Government Printing Office, 1965.

5

Observation of the Sick Child

SECTION 1. THE HOSPITALIZED CHILD

No one questions that a sick child comes to the hospital to be healed of his physical illness, if that is possible, or that the task of the nurse is to help in that process. It is equally true that we, as nurses, cannot function adequately in that capacity unless we understand the child's emotional needs—according to his age level, and in relation to him as an individual. This understanding is of considerable importance, for we know that healing takes place most readily in a positive, accepting environment. Security, acceptance and warm human relationships are the most potent of all medicines.

The fact still remains, however, that the child has come to be treated for his physical disability, with the goal seen clearly as a return to his family. We must not neglect the physical care while offering emotional support. In actual practice, it is difficult to give one without giving the other; certainly emotional support may be manifested through the kind of physical care the nurse gives.

The nurse has learned that in order to give good nursing care, she must see the child as a person in his own right, as well as a member of his family. This means many things. It means that she should know certain things about him before she enters his room. She should know his name, his nickname, and his age. She needs to know the special words he uses to make his needs and his desires understood. It is helpful to know something about his family, whether he is an only child, or whether he is the oldest, youngest, or in-between, and whether both parents are living with him at home. This kind of information changes the "patient in for eye surgery" to "Bobby, a 4-year-old boy."

In most children's departments, the parents are asked to fill out a form giving this information on admission. It may also include items pertinent to the child's age: if a toddler, information concerning toilet training, "security blanket" or favorite cuddly toy, ability to feed self, and similar things. This sheet is then placed on the child's chart, with necessary items copied onto the Kardex file.

THE IMPORTANCE OF KNOWING ABOUT THE CHILD

The nurse also needs to have a firm background knowledge of normal growth and development if she is to give competent care. Here is a 2-year-old under her care. What should she expect of him in the way of motor skills? Should he be able to feed himself entirely, cut up his food and open his milk carton, or should she offer to help? What is the average weight of a child at this age, and how does he compare? What are normal skills for a 2-year-old boy? If it is important to know that 98.6°F is a normal body temperature, it is also important to know what is normal behavior for various age groups. No one expects the nurse to remember all the details of normal growth and development, nor should she expect this child to be like all other 2-year-olds, but her assignment to this particular child gives her the opportunity to check her general knowledge from the texts, and to apply that knowledge. For instance, she does not hold a drinking straw to the lips of a year old baby and expect him to understand how to use it.

Some nurses have found it helpful to start a card index growth and development file. This is a quick and convenient reference source, with the advantage of space for added details as they are encountered in daily life. Frequently one encounters some particular act or reaction in a child, with the immediate thought, "But that is typical for a 2-, or 4-, or 6-year-old."

The nurse is able to give better care if she knows something of the child's physical history. Has he been a healthy child, with this his first hospital admission, or has he had repeated illnesses with many admissions? One may expect him to react differently to his present admission in response to previous experience. The child experiencing his first hospitalization may be frightened, shy, bewildered. The old-timer may take it in stride, or may be very angry and resentful.

The nurse needs to know the child's admitting diagnosis. Although certain techniques and skills are called for simply because this is an ill child, the type of illness may call for specialized knowledge and skill.

Finally, the nurse would do well to put together all the knowledge she has acquired and form it into a pattern. She should find it helpful to write it down as a composite picture of the child. As she studies this picture, what needs and problems does she expect to emerge, to be coped with when she starts caring for him? Here is a child at a certain level of development, with a specific background, both modified by a certain disease. Mix these with his own distinctive personality, and what is likely to happen? After the nurse has become involved, she has no time to try out various approaches; she needs an immediate plan of action. Perhaps it does not fit the situation entirely, perhaps she has misjudged the child. She expected the child to respond to her loving manner, but all she received was rejection. She had devised a way to help him through an unpleasant experience, and he would have none of it. At the end of the day, she evaluates the situation, discards certain techniques and adopts a new approach for the next day. She modifies, changes, or follows through as her day's experience has taught her.

The Nursing Care Plan

Some nurses have found that making a nursing care plan, using pocket-size index cards that they can carry with them, has proved helpful. One such plan is illustrated here.

FIRST CARDS

Name Bobby S.	Age 2	Diagnosis Malnutrition
Pertinent Background	*Development*	*Comparison to Average*
1. place in family	present weight	% weight for age
2. type of home	present height	% height for age
3. birth weight	motor development	
4. birth height	speech	
5. pertinent	adaptive	
background	behavior	
material	etc.	

Add symptoms of disease that the child exhibits, comparison with textbook picture; medications ordered with effects desired and toxic reactions; treatments and procedures scheduled, as indicated.

WORK CARDS (SAMPLE) FIRST AND SECOND DAY

Objective	Anticipated Problems	Anticipated Solution	Evaluation
1. to foster security	1. expect him to be shy, may not relate to me	1. kindness, but let him make advances	1. worked well, tomorrow will try . . .
2.	2. may rebel against bed rest	2. divert him by (suggest according to age)	2. cried, would not be diverted will try . . .
3.	3. may refuse food and drink	3. plan a tea party	3. no problem N.P.O. today

At the end of the first day, the nurse reviews and evaluates, notes new problems, discards those solved or that did not appear, and makes her work card for the next day.

FOLLOW-UP CARDS
Evaluation, Teaching, Long Term Planning

1. evaluation of results
2. planning for future needs
3. plans for parent, child, nurse teaching
4. long-term home care
5. community resource
6. bibliography

This kind of care plan has proved valuable to the nurse. It is also taken to clinical conferences and serves as a basis for discussion. The nurse presents the knowledge and understanding she has acquired, shares her findings with the staff, and gains added insight through the discussion centered around her preliminary study.

This certainly is not an inflexible form, to be used as it is, but a plan of some sort is very helpful. The nurse no longer thinks of this child-patient as "the patient in room 415" or as "the child with malnutrition." Rather, she thinks of him as 2-year-old Bobby who has been taken from his home and put under her care.

The nurse can now care for him with some definite ideas about his needs and about how to meet them. In the course of the day, she may discover that he does not entirely conform to her expectations, and that perhaps her solutions were not entirely satisfactory, so she goes on from there. She has provided a measure of security for herself, however, before caring for Bobby, and her own confidence should provide strength for the child.

Some nurses fail to see the importance of planning before they know the child. They find themselves, however, much more at ease if they have anticipated some of the problems that can be expected to develop when they are caring for the child of this age, who comes from a specific background and has a specific disease.

The Importance of Meaningful Observation

Caring for 2-year-old Bobby means more than this, however. He has not learned many words, and his background experience is decidedly limited. His mother has thought for him, anticipated and met his problems before he even knew that he had any. Here in the hospital, he may feel miserable, be nauseated or have a headache, or any number of other symptoms may be manifested. He cannot express them, perhaps cannot even localize them. The nurse must be the one alert enough to read the signs and to interpret them. Above all, she must remember to record them.

The doctor makes rounds at 9 A.M., and sees Bobby crying, or sleeping, or lying in an apathetic manner. He seeks information from the nurse's notes and reads, "Bed bath and A.M. care, ate poorly, sleeping." The doctor does not particularly care whether Bobby had a bed bath, he looks clean enough. "Ate poorly," what does that mean? "Sleeping," he saw that for himself. Of what use were these notes to him, telling about the child's condition, his symptoms, state of well-being?

As the nurse is the only person with the opportunity to observe the child over any period of time, the pediatrician would like to be able to rely heavily on her observations. She may not always know the significance of certain signs, but if they are different, if the child acts in any manner other than the way he has been observed to act, she should note this. Perhaps it has no significance: that is fine. Perhaps it signifies a need to wait and see. It may be, however, a clue to the child's condition, and this no one can afford to miss.

Aspects of Child Observation

Probably the most important role the nurse can play in her care is to be constantly observant. This means being cognizant of the child's behavior, being aware of the factors influencing that behavior, and being aware of the constancy of that behavior. These statements need to be broken down and considered separately.

Awareness of Child's Behavior

  a. Observe how he behaves in all respects.
    1. physical behavior
    2. emotional response
    3. intellectual response
  b. Be aware of factors influencing your observations.
    1. Child's age; correlate this behavior with expected behavior for his age.
    2. His environment; be aware that he is in an abnormal environment.
    3. His previous experience; how much separation from his parents has he previously experienced? Has he ever been hospitalized before?
  c. Be aware of the constancy of his behavior.
    1. Does he constantly manifest the same behavior, or is his reaction today different from that of yesterday?
    2. If his reaction is inconsistent, are there any reasons you can discover for the change? For example, does he seem sad and moody when ordinarily he is sunny and cheerful?

These general observations become more meaningful when considered from the various age levels.

The Infant

State of activity. A healthy infant is constantly active. Some are more intense and curious than others, but all are absorbed in this developmental task of their age. Illness modifies this level of activity. An important measure of the severity of the illness is the degree of impairment of activity in the infant. Does he lie quietly and manifest little or no interest in his surroundings? Do you find him in the same position every time you look at him?

State of muscular tension. The muscular state of an infant is tense, his grasp is tight, he raises his head when prone, and he kicks with vigor.

When lying supine, there is a space between the mattress and his back. How does this infant compare? Does he lie relaxed, with arms and legs straight and lax? Does he make any attempt to turn his head or raise it if placed in a prone position? Does he move about his crib?

Constancy of reaction. A healthy infant shows a relative constancy of response and does not regress in his development. Was this child peppy and vigorous yesterday, but less so today? Did he respond to discomfort and painful procedures in an apathetic manner? Was he formerly interested in food, but now turns away? Does he respond to your presence or voice with his usual interest, or does he now turn his head and cry?

Behavior indicating pain.

1. A healthy baby appreciates being loved and picked up. Does this child cry or protest when handled, and seem to prefer being left alone? Perhaps he cries when picked up, but stills after being held quietly for a time, thus indicating that something hurts when he is moved.

2. A healthy baby shows activity as distinguished from restlessness. Does this baby turn his head fretfully from side to side? Perhaps he pulls his ear or rubs his head. Perhaps he turns and rolls constantly, seeming to try to get away from pain. Is he indicating by these actions the discomfort that he cannot put into words?

3. A healthy baby shows activity in every part of his body. This infant guards an arm or leg, or portion of his body, because it hurts to move it.

Physical signs of illness. Babies normally have a strong, vigorous cry. A weak, feeble cry, or a whimper indicate trouble. Nerve involvement may show in a high pitched, shrill cry. Perhaps he cries for long periods of time, refusing to be soothed. Sometimes, if the infant appears to cry excessively, a cry chart is helpful to determine just how much he actually does cry. Observe the infant every half hour, and fill in the time period with various shadings of color for his activity at the time, such as sleeping, feeding, lying quietly awake or crying. This makes your observations less subjective.

THE INFANT'S COLOR. A healthy infant has a rosy tinge to his skin. His fingertips and toes are pink, his mucous membranes are pink-tinged. Is this child pale, with shadows under his eyes, or does his skin appear mottled? Does he show unusual pallor or blueness around his eyes and nose, or in his fingertips? Are his mucous membranes pale?

THE INFANT'S APPETITE OR FEEDING PATTERN. A healthy infant has an interest in food. He exhibits an eagerness and impatience for satisfaction of his hunger. The sick infant may show an indifference toward his formula, or suck half-heartedly. He may vomit his feeding or habitually regurgitate. He may take his feeding and subsequently exhibit discomfort.

BIZARRE BEHAVIOR. Any kind of behavior that differs from that expected for the level of development should be noted. Is this child overly good, or passive, in the face of strange surroundings? Does he, on the other hand, respond with rejection to every overture, friendly or otherwise? Is he overly clinging, never seeming satisfied with the amount of attention he receives?

It cannot be stressed too strongly that any *one* manifestation in itself may not be significant. The important thing is whether this behavior is consistent with this particular child, or whether it is a change from previous behavior. Perhaps he has always been pale or passive, or fussy in his feeding. Any such behavior needs to be noted, of course, but much of the significance depends greatly on the constancy of such behavior. As a nurse, can you tactfully, without alarming the parent, try to discover if he has always been a finicky eater, or been overactive, or an unusually quiet child? Of course, you have been observing and recording changes since admission to the hospital.

The Older Child

All of the previous observations are valid for the older child as well. In addition, there are a few somewhat different, or more mature reactions that may indicate an unhealthy state.

a. *Covering up for pain or discomfort.* A child seldom sees any enjoyment in illness or hospitalization. His burning desire is to get home again, and he will often go to great lengths to cover up any discomfort. Watch him sometime when he does not know that you are. Is he limping, or holding one side of his abdomen, or showing any other sign of pain? If so, what does he do when he sees you watching him? Does he straighten up and say that he was just playing? Do you take his word for this, or do you report the behavior?

b. *Extremes of aggression or passivity.* How does this child behave? Does he resist any and all advances, and strike out against playmates or adults? Perhaps instead, he accepts everything. Even more important, is this a change in behavior? How can you know unless you have been consistently observant and have recorded behavior?

c. *Reaction with parents.* Get a feeling of how a child reacts to his parents and they to him. How he reacts on the ward may be a reflection of his feelings toward his parents, or theirs to him. It may also reflect the parent's attitude to the situation of illness and hospitalization, or to the care that he now receives.

SECTION 2. COMMUNICATING WITH CHILDREN

The nurse must realize that she is always communicating with her child patients regardless of whether they are able to understand her words or to answer her. The infant attaches his own meaning to her actions and thus forms his own evaluation of her. His background is too limited for him to realize that she is rushed or insecure when she picks him up abruptly or handles him in a hurried, impersonal manner. What she is telling him is that she is a potentially frightening person, that she does not love him. He relies entirely on his senses for information about his environment. Everyone knows that an infant can be called a rascal or any harsh name, and that he coos with delight if the tone is soothing, warm and loving.

The child who has reached the age when he can begin to differentiate between persons tends to be frightened of strangers. Anything unknown is potentially dangerous even to the adult. This phase usually begins sometime after the sixth month of life. Previously, an infant who has a background of security responds favorably to any warm, accepting person. Now, however, he has learned to recognize persons, and if he does not know them, he has no inner experience to tell him that they are friends. If you make sudden, abrupt, or loud approaches to him he is pretty sure to think that you are up to no good. If you let him stay secure in his mother's arms while he looks you over, this is helpful. You need to stay rather aloof as he makes his appraisal, and let him initiate the relationship. If his past experience with people has been good, it will not be long before he is making the advances and wanting you to respond.

This distrust of strangers may carry on through three or four years of life. If this is your first day to care for Johnny and he does not appear ready to accept you, try to be casual. Do not give him the feeling that you reject him, but let him see by your interested and warm manner with all the children that every one of them means something to you. Go slowly and gently, and do not reject him or his behavior. If he is showing rejecting or aggressive behavior, or being a "bad boy" he may be putting up a defense against his own fears. You should overlook as much of this behavior as possible. If it is such that it cannot be overlooked, either for his own or other's safety or well-being, be firm, and do whatever is necessary without showing anger or disgust.

Some young nurses have considerable difficulty in accepting their own feelings while working with children. Miss Green came to her advisor greatly troubled because she felt anger and hostility toward the children when they misbehaved. Another young nurse was disturbed because she could not accept the child who did not obey immediately when she spoke. The nurse needs to understand that she brings her own feelings, fears and conflicts to a new situation. Persons often feel a great inadequacy when they first have relationships with children. Perhaps they secretly feel that they are not the all-knowing, all-powerful persons the child thinks they are, and are afraid that they are going to be found out, so they in turn use aggressive feelings to cover their own insecurity. The nurse needs to understand this and be willing to accept the fact that she, too, is very human. She can still consciously accept the child, and she will find that as she grows more secure, she can learn to understand him.

A good nurse must be self-accepting and self-confident, it is true, but she does not necessarily begin that way. She usually has to grow in maturity and insight.

After the nurse has honestly faced and accepted herself, she is free to turn to the child. She is no longer preoccupied with her own inner inadequacies and fears. Perhaps she does have the impulse to command and demand instant and complete obedience. She can accept this as a result of unfortunate experiences in her earlier life, but she does not need to stop there. Now she must consider the child's environment, his background and his stage of development, and will try to discover why he behaves as he does. Is it a result of his own inconsistent handling at home, or is it the urge to try toward independence that his nature demands? Perhaps it might even be a response to her own authoritarian attitude. Careful consideration should help her modify her expectations. If a child senses the nurse's genuine interest, he eventually puts forth some effort to respond.

BIBLIOGRAPHY

Bird, B.: Talking with Patients. Part 2. Philadelphia, J. B. Lippincott, 1955.
Juberg, R. C.: Heredity counseling. Nurs. Outlook, *14*:28, (Jan.) 1966.
Peplau, H.: Talking with patients. Amer. J. Nurs., *60*:964, 1960.
Rose, M. H.: Communicating with children. Nurs. Outlook, *9*:428, 1961.

SUGGESTED READING FOR FURTHER STUDY

Dittmann, L.: A child's sense of trust. Amer. J. Nurs., *66*:91, 1966.
Jacobson, H., and Reid, D.: High-risk pregnancy, ii. A pattern of comprehensive maternal and child care. New Eng. J. Med., *271*:302, 1964.
Stone, A. R.: Cues to interpersonal stress due to pregnancy. Amer. J. Nurs., *65*:88, (Nov.) 1965.

UNIT 2

THE PRENATAL AND POSTNATAL PERIODS

6

Life Before Birth

INTRODUCTION

Miss Black, a student nurse, was both pleased and excited when her rotation to the obstetrics department approached, because she was looking forward to her own future as a wife and as a mother. This experience, she thought, would have much personal significance for her. In this, she was not disappointed; in addition, she found the newborn nursery particularly fascinating. "When I first went into the newborn nursery," she said, "I thought—here are rows of babies all alike—and I wondered how I would ever be able to tell them apart. Now I am surprised that I ever had such a thought, they are so individual, so different."

And individual they are. Anyone trained to observe the newborn infant can clearly distinguish personality traits as well as physical differences.

It is a mistake to think of life beginning only at birth. We should think instead of growth and development proceeding in a continuum, with conception at one end and maturity at the other. We must go back much further than conception, of course, to look for clues to the child's personality and physical being. We certainly should expect development, at least with respect to personality, to proceed beyond adolescence.

For present purposes, however, we are considering life between these two landmarks. There are highlights along the way, and for purposes of clarity, we break down this period of life into smaller periods. We use the terms prenatal, neonatal, infancy, preschool, childhood and adoles-

TABLE 6-1. CLASSIFICATION OF DEVELOPMENT PERIODS

Period	Age
1. prenatal	0 – 10 lunar months
2. neonatal (or postnatal)	birth – 4 weeks
3. infancy	4 weeks – 12 months
4. toddler	1 – 3 years
5. preschool	3 – 6 years
6. school years	6 – 10 years (approximately)
7. preadolescence	10 – 13 years (approximately)
8. adolescence	13 – adulthood

cence. Even then, these are only general terms, and are more easily handled if separated into still smaller units.

We know that there is an orderly progression of growth and development, and we know that the healthy individual, living in a fairly normal and constant environment, progresses in this orderly manner. He does not walk before he creeps, nor does he run before he walks. We know that much of his mental and emotional development depends on his physical maturation.

There are, however, countless possibilities inherent in individuals for variation within this sequence. Each child follows his own course. We need to keep this in mind as we follow the several stages of infancy and childhood.

PRENATAL ENVIRONMENT

Not too long ago, it was believed that a mother could strongly influence her child during the prenatal period. If she wanted him to appreciate music and art, she would attend concerts and visit art galleries. She was encouraged to think in a positive, cheerful manner, and to avoid traumatic experiences. She could "mark" her unborn child both physically and emotionally.

Superstitions. Superstitions regarding physical markings were prevalent, and to a considerable extent, still are. The frequently observed congenital hemangioma known as a "strawberry mark," for example, was once thought to be caused by the mother having eaten strawberries during her pregnancy.

As more knowledge of intrauterine life was acquired, the fallacy of such thinking became apparent. The fetus was seen to have a safe, comfortable, protected life in utero. His only contact with his mother was strictly a physical one. He was safely cushioned by a layer of water that prevented injury. His only contact with his mother's metabolism was by the umbilical cord, which carried his own blood to the placenta where it absorbed nutrients and discarded waste. Therefore, it became obvious that nervous shocks, impressions, or any functions of the maternal central nervous system could not affect him.

This, as far as it goes, is perfectly true. The maternal blood supply to the placenta can, however, carry things other than nutrients, and these can pass through the placental barrier as well.

Drugs, viruses, and hormones. These have a direct effect on the fetus. Whether endocrine secretions play any part in influencing postnatal behavior is an interesting speculation, but research at present has not effectively demonstrated any such effect.

In another sense, however, *maternal attitudes* and *traits* can affect the child's postnatal life. This sense is the manner in which they affect the mother's own personality and her attitude toward the child. That this is extremely important to the child (as well as to the mother) is obvious.

This does not mean that the mother should feel guilty about every feeling of rejection or of "less-than-joy" that she may have over the forthcoming birth. She certainly is going to have these—regardless of how ardently she desires a child.

Motherhood today certainly does not produce the profound changes in living that it once did. Most young women can continue employment outside of the home during at least part of the pregnancy, perhaps even with plans for a maternity leave with later return to employment.

Even under the most favorable conditions, however, pregnancy can be disrupting. A first pregnancy naturally brings some doubts and, with them, a sense of insecurity. There may be times when the mother-to-be deplores her ungainly figure and mourns the curtailment of her freedom. Certainly she is not always on "cloud nine," no matter how happy she is about the pregnancy. Most of the time, life goes on in a matter-of-fact way, and may become extremely boring at times. Fortunately, today's young woman has plenty to occupy her time and attention during this period.

The woman anticipating her third or fourth child may sometimes have feelings of inadequacy and doubt, regardless of the pregnancy having been planned.

The nurse can help the mother understand that these feelings are usual and normal. Certainly the child needs to come into a home where security and love are abundant, but he needs human parents too. A mother who strives to be perfect, and worries unduly about her shortcomings, does not provide as much security for her child and for herself as the mother who accepts both her child and herself for what they are, and has a good time doing so.

This, however, is quite different from the profound rejection a mother may feel for her pregnancy, and which may carry over to the postnatal period.

A very young adolescent cannot normally be expected to accept pregnancy willingly. She still has far too much growing and maturing of her own to do. If this is complicated by an unmarried status, she almost certainly is going to be dismayed and resentful.

No two children are ever born into the same environment. The first-born comes into a home in which the parents are inexperienced, and in which both child and parents must learn together.

The young parents may experience considerable anxiety and try to raise their baby "by the book." When the second or third child arrives, they probably trust their own judgment, provide a more relaxed environment, and prepare to enjoy their child thoroughly for what he is.

Another infant may come into the home of *adolescent parents,* especially today in this era of early marriages. These parents are still making their own adjustments to life and are trying to grow up. A baby may find his adjustment somewhat more difficult.

The child born to an *unmarried mother* is apt to have the worst problems. As an infant, he is no different from any other human being, but society treats him as if he were. Even though his mother may give him up at birth in order that he can have a normal home, his prenatal environment has not been normal. Because of society's attitude, his mother frequently fails to obtain the adequate care and advice necessary for a normal birth and a healthy development. Her ignorance and immaturity, may just scare her, and again she fails to obtain help.

PRENATAL PHYSICAL DEVELOPMENT

We have been discussing the unborn child's emotional environment. His physical growth needs to be reviewed briefly.

Gestation period. The period of nine calendar months (or ten lunar months) is the normal prenatal period. A baby born before the sixth month has little chance for survival. Deviations in the age of newborn babies are normal, but it is perfectly clear that the closer the infant comes to the normal age for birth, the greater his chances are for a healthy neonatal period.

Organogenesis. This commences shortly after conception and is nearly complete at the end of the third prenatal month, thus any insult to the fetus during the first trimester may easily have an effect on the developing organs.

The heart begins to beat about the third week of fetal life. All reflexes are present by the end of the fourth month except for functional respiration and vocal response. Nerve cells are all present by the fifth month, although not functionally mature.

During the third trimester the child has developed to the extent that he is viable if circumstances cause an early birth, although, if born, he needs expert and constant care. During this period, he lays down subcutaneous fat, stores iron for postnatal use, and develops additional ability to begin independent life.

Hazards to Normal Development

Maternal infections. A mother's infections provide distinct hazards to the embryo. Evidence of the harm caused by the rubella virus has been well authenticated. Rubella is generally a mild disease, causing no particular harm or complications to healthy persons. When a woman contracts rubella during the first trimester of pregnancy, however, the virus is capable of penetrating the placental barrier and of damaging the developing embryonic tissues.

Rubella. Not all cases of maternal rubella during the first trimester of pregnancy result in injury to the developing child, but the percentage is high. The danger is so real that preventive measures have been suggested. It is to the advantage of every young woman to have developed immunity before she reaches child-bearing age. The only manner known at present to develop immunity is to have had the disease. "Measles parties" for young women have been popular, but indiscriminate exposure to the virus has at times resulted in the virus being carried to others, who because of some physical condition, may be particularly harmed by this infection. Individual planned exposure is probably more sensible.

Although one attack of rubella usually gives life-long immunity, the pregnant woman should still avoid exposure during the first trimester if at all possible. Various rashes are often mistaken for rubella, and it cannot be entirely certain that she will not contract the disease. There also appears to be some evidence that she could transmit the virus to the embryo, even though she does not show any clinical signs herself.

Other viral infections, such as those caused by Coxsackie or Echo viruses, do not appear to harm the embryo, but further study is indicated.

Syphilis. The spirochetes causing syphilis can be transmitted to the fetus from an infected mother, so that the infant is born with the disease. Adequate treatment of the infected mother with penicillin is imperative to prevent the child from being born with this disease.

Drug toxicity. Much has been made of the toxic effect of drugs on the developing fetus since the tragedy of the "thalidomide" babies during the early 1960's. Although the damage done was spectacular, we know that many drugs are capable of injuring the embryo. The best advice to give a pregnant woman is that she should take only those medications prescribed by her doctor. This applies even to such common drugs as aspirin, sedatives and laxatives.

Abdominal irradiations. Irradiation of the abdomen of a pregnant woman may arrest embryonic development and cause malformations. The most sensitive period of organogenesis begins within a week or so after conception, when pregnancy is still unsuspected. Therefore, X-ray examination of the abdomen of any married woman of child-bearing age should be carried out only during the first two weeks following a regular menstrual period.

Genetic factors. These factors have, of course, a profound influence on a new baby. Within a relatively short period of time, the science of human genetics has made tremendous strides toward explaining some of the mysteries of human development. Now it is possible to understand the mechanism underlying many abnormal conditions that follow a genetic pattern. In some instances, prediction of the likelihood of defective offspring can be made with a fair degree of accuracy.

Genetic counseling. Such counseling is important to many young married couples concerned about the advisability of having children. One does not give advice as such, but rather one helps them understand as fully as possible all factors involved. This kind of help must be given only by a well qualified genetic specialist. Much harm can be done by those with inadequate understanding and information.

The Prenatal Effects of Maternal Nutrition

The unborn child has a comfortable nutritional arrangement with his mother. Generally speaking, a prospective mother who follows a sensible diet, and augments it correctly to fit the needs of the child, provides adequately for both herself and her child.

Maternal dietary allowances of protein, iron, riboflavin and ascorbic acid need to be increased, as well as vitamin D and calcium. The infant needs access to sufficient iron to build up his store for postnatal living during the first few months. All of his nutritional needs will be met, as nearly as possible, to the detriment of his mother's health if her own nutrition is inadequate.

The adolescent mother-to-be has additional problems. Her own nutritive requirements are high because of her own continuing growth, and pregnancy adds considerably to those requirements.

Unfortunately, many adolescents have poor eating habits, and it is not easy to change them suddenly during pregnancy. In fact, to be effective, proper nutrition should be provided long before pregnancy occurs. The problem is a difficult one. The adolescent is concerned with her own efforts toward independence and maturity, and dietary concern is not often evident. If, as it often happens, the pregnancy is unwanted, the girl has even less motivation toward health care.

EDUCATION FOR PARENTHOOD

Education for parenthood is one of our prime needs. We are becoming increasingly disturbed over the breakdowns in our "affluent" society. Some of our concern is about our high infant mortality rate with the unsolved problem of prematurity; the large number of mentally retarded; social problems, such as the breakdown in family structure, neglect or abuse of children, illegitimate pregnancies, juvenile delinquency and culturally deprived families.

National attention has been directed toward the importance of locating and assisting women in the "high-risk" pregnancy group. These are women in particular need of prenatal care because of socioeconomic factors, poor health, history of previous difficulties in childbirth, lack of knowledge of prenatal hygiene, just to mention a few reasons.

Particular attention has been focused on providing adequate prenatal clinics. A prenatal clinic is inadequate if it cannot serve the population for which it is intended.

An adequate prenatal clinic should be located in the area where it is needed. The amount of money and time involved in reaching a clinic some distance away discourages early and regular attendance.

A clinic is inadequate if it is too small or deficient in personnel. Women are not encouraged to attend if they need to wait hours for attention, an attention too often routine, impersonal and inadequate.

Successful clinics need adequately trained personnel representing the various disciplines involved in healthy childbearing. One expects to find competent obstetricians and registered nurses. Are there nutritionists, social workers, family counselors as well? Is there a human, personal atmosphere, a genuine interest in people?

Necessary instruction concerning prenatal care and hygiene, including an understanding of fetal development and the mechanics of childbirth, is provided in classes for prospective parents under varying sponsorship. Too often, those in greatest need of this service, who have the least opportunity to learn elsewhere, are the ones who know little about their availability, or are not encouraged to attend.

Our awakening concern is encouraging, but education for parenthood, if it is to be at all effective, must begin long before pregnancy; indeed, it must begin before marriage. Particularly in view of the increasing number of early marriages, greater attempts must be made in the schools, churches, and youth organizations, to provide opportunities for discussion and instruction in a realistic approach to proper nutrition, sex education, family relationships and social problems.

It would seem that every nurse has some responsibility, whether she is in public health, institutional nursing, or is just a plain member of society. She must inform herself about the availability of adequate resources in her neighborhood, her city, her state. Are the schools, the churches and the PTA, taking their share of responsibility? Are local public health facilities adequate? How does she see her own role in the community? Perhaps she ought to fill in some of the gaps in her own knowledge as well as to accept her share of responsibility toward a better community.

BIBLIOGRAPHY

Fishbein, M., (ed.): Birth Defects. pp. 156–163. Philadelphia, J. B. Lippincott, 1963.

Juberg, R. C.: Heredity counseling. Nurs. Outlook, *14:*28, (Jan.) 1966.

National Foundation—March of Dimes: Birth Defects—Reprint Series. *(selected readings.)* Philadelphia, National Foundation—March of Dimes, 1964.

Nelson, W., (ed): Textbook of Pediatrics. 8th ed. Philadelphia, W. B. Saunders, 1964.

Proudfit, F. T., and Robinson, C. H.: Normal and Therapeutic Nutrition. 12th ed. New York, Macmillan, 1961.

SUGGESTED READINGS FOR FURTHER STUDY

Jacobson, H., and Reid, D.: High risk pregnancy, a pattern of comprehensive maternal and child care. New Engl. J. Med., *271:*302, 1964.

Stone, A. R.: Cues to interpersonal stress due to pregnancy. Amer. J. Nurs., *65:*88, (Nov.) 1965.

7

Neonatal Growth and Development

THE BIRTH EXPERIENCE

The prenatal infant is difficult to visualize as a person, except, perhaps, to his mother. His distinct personality can be appreciated only as he becomes a baby whom we can see and fondle. What do we expect of the average newborn? Suppose we take Johnny (an average baby) as our model.

Johnny is ready to be born after a prenatal existence of 10 lunar months. We know that the birth experience will be physically traumatic to him, and we wonder if it may be emotionally traumatic as well. He has been growing in a warm, dark place, securely held and cushioned against injury by a surrounding layer of water. His needs have been met without any awareness on his part that he has had any. He has been gently rocked by his mother's movements, and supported by her body.

He has now reached the point in his development at which he can function outside his mother's body. He is far from being a finished product, but the systems of his body that he needs in order to maintain his own existence are now in working order.

At the time of birth, Johnny experienced considerable physical buffeting. Uterine contractions propelled him down the birth canal with his own head acting as the dilator. His head pounded against his mother's perineum in a rhythmic manner for some time. Eventually, as he emerged into this bright noisy world, the shock of birth brought a cry from him that fulfilled a physical need. He drew air into his lungs with the first breath and initiated the breathing process, and thus he became responsible for the first time for the maintenance of his own life.

Some like to imagine that this first cry has additional significance. It does sound remarkably like a loud, angry protest against expulsion from a protected, close, warm atmosphere into a drafty, noisy place that is utterly strange and confusing. His cry seems to indicate his need for warm, loving protective care.

Our Johnny has come safely through this traumatic experience of birth, and is ready to begin the big adventure of independent living.

Those organs of his body that are essential for maintenance of life are developed to the point at which they can function adequately if—and only if—someone is at hand to meet his needs—Completely.

It is indeed impossible to separate his physical *needs* from his *emotional needs* during the neonatal period, which constitutes the first four weeks of life. At this period of his development, his emotional needs are met only by prompt, efficient attention to his physical necessities. Here is a stranger in a completely new and strange country. He knows nothing of the language, or the customs; the prohibitions, or indeed, of the rewards.

Where he came from, we really do not know. The mechanics of his making we can understand. The study of embryology is fascinating, with the frontiers of science being pushed ever further back. However, no one as yet has been able to answer the question "Who am I?," or "Where did I come from?" Seeing the miracle of birth brings an acute consciousness of these questions, and we do well to ponder them. At the moment, however, we must concern ourselves with the newborn's own tasks, which he must master if he is to enter our world.

Neonatal tasks. The first, and the most important task for the newborn is to *oxygenate* his own red blood cells, and this he starts to do with his first cry. During his protected existence within his mother's body, he received enough oxygen for his limited needs from his mother's blood. Now, he must acquire his own, and he needs practice. He made occasional tentative tries before he left his protected home, but it was not really important to him then. Now his existence depends on his ability to breathe. Having entered this interesting life, the urge to stay is the strongest of all. He uses every possible means to which he has access in order to stay alive.

His breathing is of the abdominal type, and is irregular and uneven. Normal respirations during this period may vary from 20 (during sleep) to over 100 per minute (when crying). The average rate is 40 to 60 per minute.

His urge to live is so strong that if placed on his abdomen, he raises his head to clear his airway. At birth, the muscles at the back of his neck are strong enough to allow him to raise his head momentarily from a prone position. He cannot do this if he is lying on a soft pillow, or if there are loose articles of clothing to cling to his nose or mouth, or if he is weak and listless. A healthy, vigorous baby does not smother easily without strong protest.

His heart has been beating since early fetal life. The newborn's heartbeat ranges between 90 and 180, with 130 beats per minute as the average rate.

Adjustments in circulation must be made at birth. During fetal life, the lungs were inactive, requiring only a small amount of blood to nourish their tissues. Blood was circulated through the umbilical artery to the placenta, where waste products and carbon dioxide were exchanged for oxygen and nutrients. The blood was then returned to the fetus through the umbilical vein.

At birth, the umbilical cord is cut, and the infant establishes his own independent system. *Certain circulatory bypasses,* such as the *ductus arteriosus,* the *foramen ovale,* the *ductus venosus* are no longer necessary.

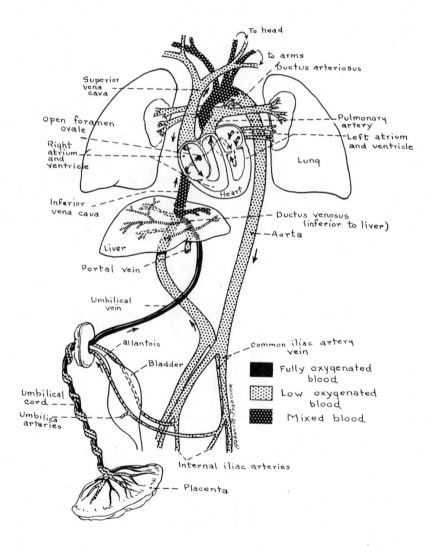

Fig. 15. Fetal circulation.

They close and atrophy after birth, although probably more gradually than had formerly been supposed. (Figs. 15 and 16)

The intestinal tract is functional, with meconium normally passed from 8 to 24 hours after birth. Meconium is a sticky, greenish-black substance, composed of intestinal secretions that have accumulated during fetal life. Meconium persists for two to three days, changing through the first postnatal week to a pasty yellow stool as food enters the intestinal tract.

The kidneys are also functional, although they have not entirely developed their complex structure. The nurse must watch for the first voiding as well as for the first bowel movement, to determine the normal functioning of the systems, as well as the patency of the outlets.

Physical development. As the newborn assumes control over his own activities, his brain is relatively well developed. It is so well developed, in fact, that he looks rather grotesque to us; his head is very large in proportion to his body. His head is one-fourth as long as his body, and

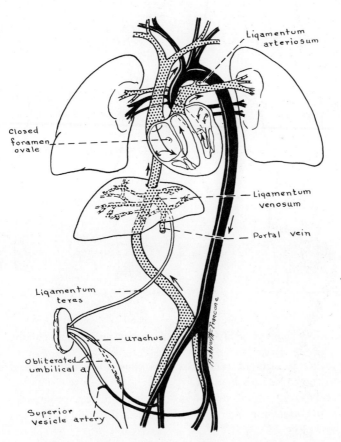

Fig. 16. Normal blood circulation after birth.

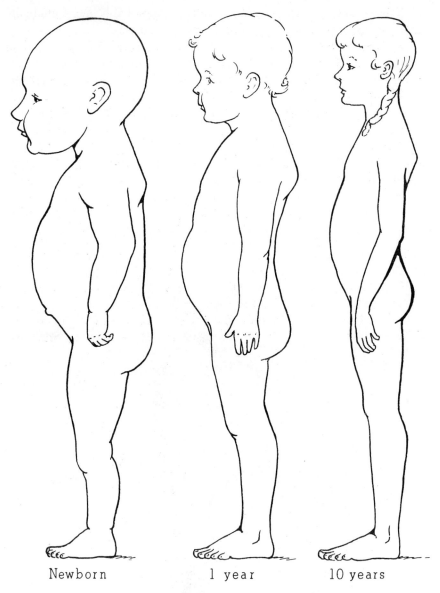

Newborn   1 year   10 years

Fig. 17. Changes in body proportions during infancy and childhood.

slightly larger in circumference than his chest. His skull is large in proportion to the rest of his head. (Fig. 17)

Prenatal development proceeds in a head-to-feet progression, called
the *cephalocaudal* progression, which persists throughout the early period
of infancy. (Fig. 18)

Muscular development proceeds from the center outwards, in a *proximal-distal sequence.* Development also goes from the *general* to the *specific,* the gross muscles being brought under control before the finer muscles. The baby demonstrates this when he pushes forward with his whole body in his eagerness for food.

Neonatal Needs

Immediately after birth, the newborn needs rest, warmth and security. His need for food can wait for a few hours. He needs to be wrapped securely and warmly, watched carefully, and allowed to sleep. Many nurses are confused at times as to the meaning of nursing care. They find it difficult to realize that continuous observation of the newborn infant is the best nursing care they can give him.

A newborn infant is able to take advantage of opportunities for survival, but he cannot initiate them. He can breathe and assimilate oxygen if his airways are kept open. He can suck, swallow, and metabolize milk if it is offered to him; he cannot go after it. He can only signal his need to relieve his hunger pains by crying, loudly and persistently.

He quickly acquires the ability to regulate his body heat, but again he needs help, for he cannot control his environment.

In areas less important to immediate survival, he is less well developed. His legs are short, his bones not yet calcified. His feet are only promises

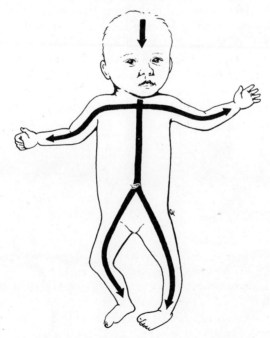

Fig. 18. The cephalocaudal and proximal-
distal sequences of development.

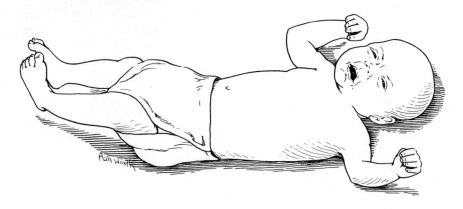

Fig. 19. Moro or startle reflex.

of things to come; but he does not need them at present for walking or standing.

Neonatal Reflexes

The newborn infant's behavior is governed by reflexes triggered by his immature nervous system. He *startles* easily when his equilibrium is disturbed. Put him down suddenly on a flat surface and he will tense, throw his arms out in an embracing motion and usually cry. This is the *Moro* reflex, also called the startle reflex. (Fig. 19)

The infant also tends to assume the position that was most comfortable for him in utero. If placed on his back, he turns his head sharply to one side, extends the arm on the same side and flexes the opposite arm in a sort of fencing position. (Fig. 20) This is known as the *tonic neck* posi-

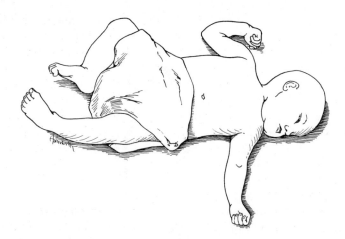

Fig. 20. Tonic neck reflex.

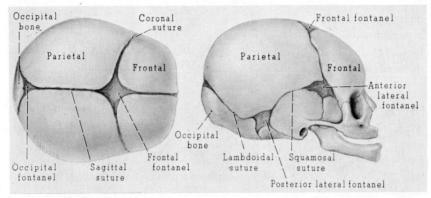

Fig. 21. Infant skull showing fontanelles and cranial sutures.

tion, assumed by all normal newborns much of the time. This positional reflex disappears in about 16 weeks, as the infant matures.

Other reflexes are present: the infant has a sucking as well as a swallowing reflex; he makes "rooting" movements with his face as he seeks food; he makes walking movements when supported upright. These walking movements are only reflex and will soon disappear.

Fontanelles

In order to facilitate the passage of the large head of the newborn infant through the birth canal, the skull bones are not united but can mold and overlap. The seven bones of the skull are divided by narrow spaces called sutures. At the point of juncture of these bones, triangular spaces called fontanelles are present. The two palpable fontanelles at birth are the anterior, at the juncture of the frontal and parietal bones, and the posterior, at the juncture of the parietal and occipital bones. (Fig. 21)

The brain is covered with a tough membrane, making it difficult to injure the child at the fontanelles, with ordinary handling. Mothers need to be assured that the baby's scalp can be washed over these points without harm, and ordinary cleansing can be helpful in preventing the frequent accumulation of crusts composed of oil, serum and dirt popularly known as *cradle-cap*.

During the first few months of life, the sections of bony skull calcify and join together; the posterior fontanelle disappearing after four to six weeks, and the anterior fontanelle closing between the end of the first year and the 18th month.

Developmental Tasks

The infant immediately commences, or rather, continues, his developmental task of *exercising* his *muscles*. His arms and legs are moving constantly when he is awake, and even in sleep he frequently moves to change a position or to stretch a muscle. His muscles are maintained in a tensed state as though for ready action, his legs are drawn up, and his fists are clinched. A newborn infant who habitually lies in a relaxed manner, with supple, soft musculature, needs to be watched closely for central nervous system inadequacy.

Picture of Johnny

A picture of our infant, Johnny, looks somewhat like this. He weighs on an average of 7 to 7½ pounds, and is approximately 21 to 22 inches long. He has a head circumference of about 35 cm. His eyes are gray, not yet having received pigmentation, and they move with a lack of coordination that gives him the appearance of being cross-eyed at times.

His head is large, his arms and legs short, his muscles tense and firm, and his lower jaw recedes a little. He lies in a position that suggests instant readiness for action, even in sleep—his state for about 20 of the 24 hours. When awake, he stares and blinks at a strong light, but apparently he sees nothing clearly.

He *startles* at a loud noise, and he ceases his crying or postural activity momentarily if spoken to in a soft soothing voice, indicating that his *hearing* is quite acute once the pressure in his ears is equalized. He is acutely aware of *touch*, quieting even immediately after birth if held closely. A light touch on the lips elicits the sucking response, and he will turn his head to seek the source of nourishment. He has a less acute sense of *pain*, however, struggling more against restraints on the circumcision board than against the surgery itself. Indeed, he may become absorbed in sucking glucose water and ignore the whole affair.

HOSPITAL CARE OF THE NEWBORN

Care in the Delivery Room

Immediately after birth, the newborn infant must *establish respiration* in order to live. He will be held head down to allow amniotic fluid, blood and mucus to drain from his pharynx. At this time, gentle suction with a soft rubber bulb syringe may be applied to his nose and mouth.

Sixty seconds after birth, a scoring system is used to evaluate his condition. This evaluation is called the Apgar scoring chart.* The infant is given a score of 0, 1 or 2 for each of five signs. A score of 10 indicates an infant in the best possible condition. Infants with scores under 5 need prompt diagnosis and treatment.

The Apgar score, attached to the infant's chart, furnishes a reliable guide for subsequent care, and gives a reliable index of his condition.

If the infant has not started breathing within one minute of birth, some method of resuscitation must be used. Gentle physical stimulation such as snapping the soles of the feet or passing a nasal catheter may be all that is needed. Swinging, compressing the chest, tubbing and other

TABLE NO. 7–1. APGAR SCORING CHART

SIGN	APGAR SCORE		
	0	1	2
Heart rate	absent	below 100	above 100
Respiratory rate	absent	slow, irregular	good, crying
Muscle tone	limp	some flexion of extremities	active motion
Reflex irritability	no response	grimace	cough or sneeze
Color	blue, pale	body pink, extremities blue	completely pink

(Developed by Dr. Virginia Apgar)

manipulations may do harm, and only delay the application of proper therapy. (Fig. 22)

For infants in poor condition, oxygen inhalation may be helpful, after it has been determined that the infant's tongue is not obstructing the airway. A small pharyngeal airway properly placed, keeps the tongue from falling back against the posterior pharyngeal wall. Oxygen administered under proper supervision may be given by mask under either steady or controlled intermittent pressure.

Any instrumentation such as laryngoscopy, or use of oxygen under high pressure, must be done by an experienced person, usually the anesthetist. In an emergency, mouth-to-mouth breathing may be attempted, with short puffs of air from the operator's mouth (not lungs). The danger here is from alveolar rupture if force is used. There is also some danger of infection, necessitating the prophylactic use of antibiotics.

Care of the cord. The cord is clamped and cut and left without

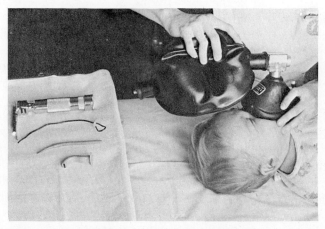

Fig. 22. Using resuscitation apparatus; Ambu bag being used on infant. The tray contains a laryngoscope, a wire stylet, an endotracheal catheter, and an airway.

dressing. The cord stump is inspected daily; in many nurseries it is painted daily with a bactericidal dye to help prevent infection.

Identification. The infant must be identified in some manner before leaving the delivery room. The American Academy of Pediatrics recommends two identical bands being placed on the infant's wrists or ankles, showing the mother's full name, admission number, sex of infant, and date and time of birth. The infant's foot, palm and fingers should be printed as well as the mother's fingers.

Care of the eyes. The eyes must be treated as a prophylactic measure against gonorrheal infection. Silver nitrate 1 per cent, is a requirement in most states and many other countries. Other forms of prophylaxis, such as the use of penicillin ophthalmic solution, is allowed in some states, but some form of prophylaxis is mandatory.

Silver nitrate has a tendency to irritate the eyes, therefore the instillation must be followed in one or two minutes with an irrigation of warm sterile saline solution.

The infant has been in a *warm, stable environment* before birth, with no need to provide his own heat regulation. Until he can adjust to the outside environment, he must be kept warm, examined on a warm table, and warmly wrapped and placed in a heated crib.

The mother should be shown her baby promptly, if she is awake, while still in the delivery room. Some hospitals now allow the father to be present at the birth of the baby, a practice that provides great satisfaction to many new parents.

Care in the Newborn Nursery

The infant can now be transported to the nursery, either warmly wrapped and carried in the nurse's arms, or in a movable heated crib, depending on his condition and on hospital policy.

On acceptance in the nursery, he is identified, weighed, and checked over carefully; he also has his temperature taken. The foot of his bassinet is elevated at an angle of 15 to 20° for the first 24 hours because of the possibility of respiratory distress. The infant should be turned from side to side every 2 or 3 hours.

Temperature of the newborn. If a rectal temperature is taken, care must be used not to insert the thermometer for more than 2 cm. Instances of bowel perforations from rectal thermometers and infant rectal tubes or catheters are on record. Many nurseries make a practice of taking axillary temperatures. This is done by placing the bulb of the thermometer in the infant's axilla, holding his arm to his side, and keeping the thermometer in place for 1½ to 2 minutes.

Maintenance of a stable temperature in the newborn is important. An axillary temperature of 96° to 99° is considered within normal limits. Means employed for stabilization of the infant's temperature are warm clothing, a nursery temperature of approximately 75° and, if necessary, a heated crib.

Bathing and dressing the infant. Today's thinking about cleansing the newborn infant's skin favors use of a soap or solution containing hexachlorophene to lower incidence of skin infections.

The infant should be dressed in a diaper, a shirt or a gown, wrapped in a blanket, and positioned on his side. The newborn appears to feel more secure if wrapped rather closely in a light blanket during the period of adjustment to extra-uterine living.

Rooming-in

The practice of rooming-in has much in it to be commended. In this plan, the infant's crib is placed beside the mother's bed in order to permit mother and child to be cared for together. It is interesting to note that many of the so-called "under-developed" countries have followed this practice throughout history, and that many more sophisticated countries use it without question.

The American Academy of Pediatrics, in setting standards for hospital care for newborn infants, presents the following special features of rooming-in:

Special features of rooming-in are that it (1) provides the mother and infant with a natural mother-child experience beginning as soon after delivery as the mother is capable of assuming the care of her baby; (2) fosters infant feeding on a permissive plan; (3) facilitates instruction of mothers and fathers in infant care, and (4) reduces the incidence of cross-infection among infants.

Types of plans. Rooming-in plans have been worked out in various ways. Some nurseries permit baby to stay at the mother's bedside throughout the day, returning him to the nursery at night. Others provide continuous rooming-in, but nearly all make some provision for the baby to be taken into the nursery when necessary for the mother's comfort.

Rooming-in has done much for mothers who are unhappy with the rigid schedule and enforced separation that a nursery fosters. There are many good mothers, however, who, for various reasons, do not wish to use the rooming-in plan. A mother with several small children may appreciate the short period of rest, quiet, and absence of responsibility that the hospital can provide.

Another mother, having her first child, may be overwhelmed at the prospect of great responsibility this soon, and prefer to accept it gradually. The point to remember is that no mother should be over-persuaded, or made to feel in any way that she is something other than a good mother if she is not enthusiastic about rooming-in.

A nurse, herself in good health and normal emotional adjustment, may fail to appreciate the adjustments the new mother is making. Usually the patient is over-sensitive, and can easily read meanings into carelessly spoken words. The nurse must cultivate sensitivity in all areas, but perhaps this is especially necessary when she responds to the emotions and reactions of a new mother.

When rooming-in is not used, it is important that the mother be given a chance to hold and examine her baby as soon as possible. If she is weak or still sleepy, she may desire nothing more than an opportunity to see him and to be assured of his soundness, with more leisurely acquaintance later. She should, however, be shown a completely unclothed baby in order to see for herself that he is completely normal as well as to assure herself of the infant's sex.

When the newborn has a visible defect, a frank and informative discussion with both parents is appreciated. Usually, the obstetrician or the pediatrician wishes to give the initial information, followed by—or with—further tactful and understanding discussions with the nurse caring for mother and child.

PARENT TEACHING

The practice of holding classes for mothers, while they are still in the hospital, in bathing and feeding the new baby, formula preparation, and general care, is well established. The majority of mothers are happy to take advantage of these classes; even mothers who have raised other children. "It gives me a chance to keep up with newer ideas," is often heard.

When demonstrating or lecturing, the nurse must remember to use simple, everyday language, and to be explicit. The advice to use "one to one" of a formula preparation was intended to mean one measure of formula powder to one ounce of water, but to the new mother, it meant equal proportions. In this case, a demonstration rather than an explanation would have prevented such an error.

The nurse should realize that an experienced mother may have much to offer. Classes are at their best when they become discussion groups. This technique may be difficult for the young, inexperienced nurse or nursing student who feels inadequate in the presence of the mothers. Often, her only defense is an authoritarian, rigid manner. With experience, however, she can soon learn to relax and to enjoy the give and take.

THE NEW INFANT AT HOME

There can be no question that the new infant creates considerable change in the home, whether he is the first child, or the fifth. Certainly the parents of a first child have a great deal of adjustment to make and are inclined to depend on "the book" as the ultimate authority. Dr. Spock gives excellent advice when he tells young parents "Don't be afraid to trust your own common sense. . . . take it easy, trust you own instincts, and follow the directions that your doctor gives you."

In homes where the previous baby is being displaced by the newcomer, some preparation is necessary. It is well to move the older child to his larger crib some time before the new baby appears so that he can take pride in being "a big boy now." Preparation of the toddler for a new brother or sister is helpful, but should not be very intense until just before the expected birth.

Probably the greatest help in preparing the child of any age to accept the new baby is to make him feel that this is "our baby," not just "Mommie's baby." If he can help care for the baby according to his ability, this contributes to his feeling that he is still important in the family.

The displaced toddler almost certainly feels some jealousy. With careful planning, mother can reserve some time for cuddling and playing with the toddler just as she did before. Perhaps he may profit from a little extra attention for a time. Anything to make him realize that his mother loves him just as much as ever, and that there is plenty of room in her life for both children would be helpful.

The small child should not be made to grow up too soon. He may regress and go back to some of his babyish behavior. He should not be shamed or reproved, but understood and given a bit more love and attention. Perhaps the father could occasionally take over care of the new baby while mother devotes herself to the older child.

Older children in the home may at times also feel resentful of the time and attention the new baby requires, especially if they are required to give too much of their time in caring for the younger ones. This needs consideration too. With care and understanding, the experience of having a new baby in the home can become a rewarding one for all.

Nutrition of the Newborn Infant

The timing of the newborn child's first feeding depends partly on his condition and partly on the philosophy of those responsible for him. Some physicians would prefer to allow the infant a period of rest immediately following birth, bringing the child to the breast after a period of 6 to 12 hours. Others advocate putting the child to breast when he shows a definite readiness, and the mother has recovered sufficiently.

Breast Feeding

Breast feeding appears to be coming back into favor in the United States after a period during which many women rejected it in favor of artificial feeding. Even the woman who returns to employment outside the home after a month and a half or two may feel that there are advantages to breast feeding during this short period.

That there are advantages is true. Breast milk is easily digested, needs no preparation and is available as needed. It does not sour or become contaminated in a healthy mother.

There are few contraindications to breast feeding. Certain maternal illnesses such as tuberculosis or severe malnutrition are reasons against breast feeding. An infant's inability to nurse due to physical causes such as prematurity or cleft lip defect makes special feeding measures necessary. Another pregnancy will make breast feeding too much of a drain on the mother.

The healthy mother must be entirely free to make her own decisions in this matter. If she does not desire to breast feed her infant, she must not be made to feel guilty or inadequate as a mother. The advantages of breast feeding may be enumerated if she is undecided: the lack of milk contamination, its availability, and the ease of formula preparation. (Fig. 23)

The infant who is loved, and held for his feedings, who experiences the same kind of closeness that the breast-fed infant receives, probably does not suffer emotionally because he is bottle-fed. A certain number of infants, however, do appear to have allergic reactions to cow's milk, which

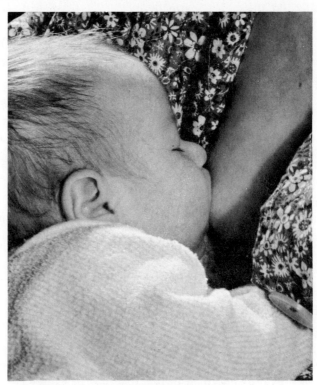

Fig. 23. Breast feeding.

are not evident when these infants are breast-fed. This, of course, does not include those infants who, because of some metabolic defect, cannot tolerate any form of milk.

Probably the majority of women can successfully breast-feed their infants if they understand and follow principles of hygiene and nutrition. Nurses themselves need to understand the principles underlying successful breast feeding. A normal infant is born with a "rooting" reflex, so that he seeks with his mouth the source of nourishment. Anything that touches his cheek is interpreted as a source of food, and if he is hungry, he immediately turns his head in that direction. Therefore, a nurse who puts her hand on a baby's cheek and tries to turn his head toward the breast, is defeating her purpose. A better policy is to let the breast lightly brush the infant's cheek, and he will then turn in that direction to seek the nipple. He may need some help in learning to grasp the nipple properly.

We have learned much about the behavior of young infants. The baby who is allowed to eat when he is hungry, to determine for himself

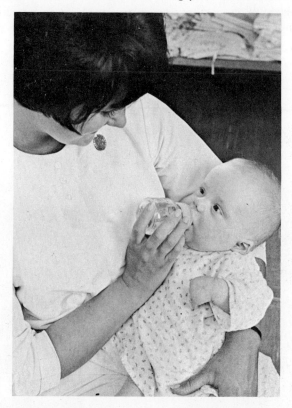

Fig. 24. Positioning of an infant for bottle feeding.

the amount of food that satisfies him, to sleep as long as he chooses without being disturbed, appears to have a much better chance to develop a sense of security as well as physical well-being.

Self-demand feeding is often considered impractical in the newborn nursery. Nurses are apt to react in a conservative manner to new ideas. Certainly there are practical difficulties, but it is actually poor nursing to reject an idea that is for the welfare of the patient without meaningful consideration. Almost always, the sole insurmountable obstacle to carrying out a new but desirable technique is a closed mind.

The healthy infant soon adjusts his appetite to his own rhythmic metabolic needs and sets up his own feeding schedule if allowed to do so. In the majority of vigorous, full-term infants, this schedule approximates a 4-hour interval. Smaller infants may need food every 3 hours, or, occasionally, at a 2-hour interval. The rate of stomach emptying also varies in individuals. It appears far better to satisfy an infant's normal desires than to force him to adopt a predetermined schedule. After a short period of adjustment, the household can learn to plan activities around the infant's schedule.

The nursing infant may be permitted to suck for the period of time

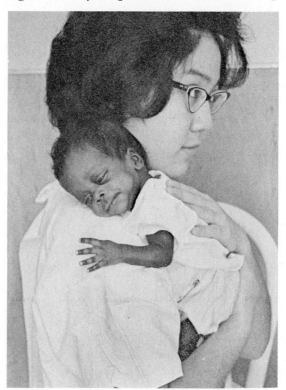

Fig. 25. Bubbling a baby against the shoulder.

it takes to satisfy him, provided of course that there is sufficient milk. Some babies seem to get right down to business and get all they want in 5 or 10 minutes. Others may be more leisurely and enjoy 15 or 20 minutes at the breast. An infant who is not satisfied in 20 to 30 minutes is signaling that things are not entirely right. Perhaps the mother has found it difficult to relax, or has not had enough rest or proper nourishment. This results in an interruption in the flow of milk, causing the baby to be irritable and unsatisfied. In turn, baby's unhappiness causes more worry and unrest for mother. Frequently, a third person—such as a nurse— understands the difficulty and helps to straighten things out.

Artificial Feeding

The mother who, for whatever reason, chooses to feed the baby a formula, can be assured that present day formulas approximate human milk and are entirely satisfactory.

Probably of greater importance to the average infant than the type of feeding is the feeling of acceptance and security he receives. The bottle fed baby needs to be held closely and lovingly in the same manner as the breast-fed baby. Bottle propping has no place in either the newborn nursery or in the home. It is dangerous for the infant and deprives him of needed physical contact. (Fig. 24)

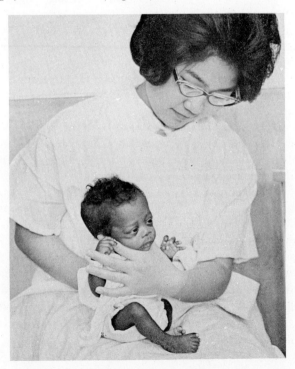

Fig. 26. Bubbling a baby sitting upright.

Babies are apt to swallow air when they nurse and need bubbling once or twice during feeding. This is true both of bottle fed and breast-fed infants. The baby may be held up over his mother's shoulder and his back gently rubbed, or he may be sat upright on her lap with his head supported. (Figs. 25 and 26)

The formula is usually warmed, although recent studies have shown no ill effects from cold milk, and it appears to be well accepted this way. Mothers should be made aware that healthy babies regurgitate small amounts of formula at times. They should know that there is a difference between regurgitation and vomiting.

Regurgitation means the simple spitting up of small amounts, actually an overflowing, perhaps from an air bubble, too rapid nursing, or just too much milk for the stomach to hold.

Vomiting is used to designate the expulsion of an appreciable amount of fluid. Although this also may be the result of rapid feeding or inadequate "burping," it may also indicate an abnormal condition, and requires careful watching.

Types of Formulas

Commercial formulas. Commercially prepared formulas come either completely ready for use, or may require dilution with sterile water. Some preparations are available to the consumer completely prepared in their own disposable containers, with nipple attached. These formulas have been prepared to approximate quite closely human milk and are easily digestible. They are a great help to mothers who have to consider the amount of time and work required in the preparation of formulas. They are, however, rather expensive, and the mother may prefer to do the preparation herself.

Evaporated milk is probably the most popular form of milk for home preparation. It is inexpensive, safe, and easy to use. It can be kept in the can until opened, is easily diluted and well tolerated by most infants. Most brands have been irradiated with vitamin D.

Whole milk is not so frequently used today for young infants. It requires careful handling, is easily contaminated, and must be fresh. Grade A pasteurized milk should be used, and it should be boiled before use, both to soften the curd and to destroy harmful bacteria. Whole milk may also have been irradiated with vitamin D.

Dried milk may be either whole milk or skim milk that has been processed into powdered form. When reconstituted, whole dried milk is similar to liquid milk, although vitamin A has been destroyed during the processing. It is useful while traveling or in areas where refrigeration is not available.

Any of these forms of milk must be kept refrigerated; whole fresh milk immediately following production, evaporated milk after the can is opened, and dried milk after being liquefied.

Special formulas are available for infants allergic to milk. These are usually made from soy beans or have a meat base. Formulas are also available for infants with certain metabolic defects, such as phenylketonuria.

Preparation of Formulas

The type of milk used needs dilution with sterile water and the addition of a carbohydrate in order to meet the infant's needs. The carbohydrate may be in the form of simple sugar, or a dextrin-maltose preparation. Formulas for full-term babies are calculated to provide 20 calories an ounce. The average infant takes 2 to 3 ounces at a feeding during the first weeks of life, with gradual increases in strength and amount.

There are two methods of preparing a formula at home. One, known as the *aseptic method*, requires that all utensils be sterilized before use, and that these utensils be used for no other purpose than formula preparation. This includes saucepan, mixing spoons, measuring cups and can opener. Bottles, bottle caps and nipples are boiled, the tops of cans washed with soap and water and rinsed in hot water. The person preparing the formula should scrub her hands and wear a clean apron or dress.

The method known as *terminal sterilization* is simpler and more commonly used. In this method, the formula is mixed in clean utensils and poured into clean bottles, nipples put in place and then covered with paper, metal or glass caps. The filled bottles are placed on a rack in a kettle, partially submerged in water, and covered and boiled for 25 minutes. They are then cooled at room temperature and placed in the refrigerator as soon as possible. Specially made utensils for sterilizing may be bought, but are not essential.

Additions to Feeding

Whether breast or bottle fed, the infant needs supplements of vitamins C and D. These can be fed directly with a dropper into the infant's mouth. Orange juice, of course, is an excellent source of vitamin C. If used, it should be diluted, and started in amounts of a teaspoonful. As some infants are allergic to orange juice, many prefer to start off with vitamin drops and switch to orange juice as the baby grows older.

Vitamin D may also be given in pediatric drops, or may not be necessary at all if the infant is getting enough irradiated milk to supply his requirements. This is seldom the case, however, and additional vitamin D must be supplied. An alternate source of vitamin D is cod liver oil. The chief objection to this is the possibility of the young infant aspirating the oily substance.

Milk is not a source of iron in the diet, but the normal, full-term infant has stored enough iron during the last month of fetal life to meet his needs for the first few months of his neonatal life, after which he needs iron-rich supplementary foods.

Fluorides. The role of fluoride in strengthening the calcification of dental tissues in formation has been documented in recent years. In areas where the fluoride content of drinking water is inadequate or absent, its administration in appropriate dosage to infants and children is recommended by the American Dental Association and by the majority of pediatricians.

Fluoride preparations come in tablet or liquid form. Drops may be started at approximately one month of age as prescribed by the pediatrician, the usual dosage at this age being approximately one drop daily, with dosage increases at intervals throughout childhood. Topical application of a fluoride preparation to erupted teeth is a recommended additive, rather than a substitute for the internal preparation.

BIBLIOGRAPHY

Aldrich, C. A., and Aldrich, M.: Babies are Human Beings. New York, MacMillan, 1955.
American Academy of Pediatrics:
Standards and Recommendations for Hospital Care of the Newborn. Evanston, Illinois, American Academy of Pediatrics, 1964.
————:
Resuscitation of the Newborn Infant. Evanston, Illinois, American Academy of Pediatrics, 1958.
Apgar, V.: Proposal for a new method of evaluation of the newborn infant. Current Res. Anesth. & Analg., *32:*260, 1953.
Barnes, G. *et al.:* Management of breast feeding. J.A.M.A., *151:*192, 1953.
Blake, F. G.: The Child, His Parents and the Nurse. Philadelphia, J. B. Lippincott, 1954.
Fonkalsrud, E., and Clatworthy, H. W.: Accidental perforation of colon and rectum in newborn infants. New Eng. J. Med., *272:*1097, 1965.
Nelson, W. E., (ed.): Textbook of Pediatrics. 8th ed., p. 346. Philadelphia, W. B. Saunders, 1964.
Spock, B.: Baby and Child Care. New York, Pocket Books, 1963.
Ziegel, E., and VanBlarcom, C. C.: Obstetrical Nursing. 5th ed. New York, Macmillan, 1964.

SUGGESTED READINGS FOR FURTHER STUDY

Blake, F. J., and Wright, F.: Essentials of Pediatric Nursing. 7th ed., pp. 140–204. Philadelphia, J. B. Lippincott, 1963.
Brazelton, T. B.: The early mother-infant adjustment. Pediat., *32:*931, 1963.
Birchfield, M. A.: A mother's views on breast feeding. Amer. J. Nurs., *63:*88, (Mar.) 1963.
Close, K.: Giving babies a healthy start in life. Children, *12:*179, 1965.
O'Keefe, M.: Advice from a nurse-mother. Amer. J. Nurs., *63:*61, (Dec.) 1963.
Ribble, M.: The Rights of Infants. 2nd ed. New York, Columbia University Press, 1965.

Ross Laboratories: The Phenomena of Early Development. Columbus, Ohio, Ross Laboratories, 1962.

Rubins, R.: Maternity Care in Our Society. Nurs. Outlook, *11:*519, (Jul.) 1963.

————: The family-child relationship and nursing care. Nurs. Outlook, *12:* 36, (Sep.) 1964.

Sarto, Sister Joseph: Breast feeding: preparation on, practice and professional help. Amer. J. Nurs., *63:*58, (Dec.) 1963.

Strang, R.: An Introduction to Child Study. 4th ed., pp. 33–48. New York, Macmillan, 1959.

8

Nursing Care of the Newborn
With Illness or Abnormality

NEONATAL HAZARDS

Neonatal mortality. In the previous chapter we considered the healthy newborn baby, and we feel quite contented and comfortable now that he has made his appearance safely, and has become an independent person. There are probably few experiences (indeed, if there are any) more awe inspiring than that of seeing a new life appear—and of speculation about the future for this tiny creature.

Unfortunately, there are still too many babies who do not live long enough to fulfill the promise of their birth. The young infant, even today, faces many dangers as he takes his place in the world. Although picking the right parents and assuring himself of good heredity help him considerably, it is true that the first year of life is the most hazardous. It is still true that during this first year, the first 24 hours have the highest mortality rate of the entire span of childhood.

Mortality rate in the United States. In the United States the mortality rate for infants (from one month to one year of age) has shown a steady decline since 1915. Infant and neonatal mortality rates are figured as the rates of death per 1000 live births. In 1915, the infant mortality rate was 99.9; in 1964 it was 25.2.

The first 28 days of life, the neonatal period, accounts for the greatest part of this figure. In 1961, out of a mortality rate of 25.3 for infants from birth to one year, 72.7 per cent of the deaths occurred during the neonatal period. Furthermore, a large percentage of these deaths occurred during the first 24 hours.

It is no cause for pride to discover that the United States has not kept pace with other nations of the world in lowering the rate of infant and neonatal mortality. Among the countries that keep reliable birth and death records, the United States stands in 10th place in proportion of infant deaths, and in 12th place for neonatal deaths.

Rate by states. The infant mortality rate by states for 1961 presents an interesting picture. The Children's Bureau reports that the difference between states reflects, at least to some extent, the per capita income

TABLE 8-1. DEATHS IN AGE GROUPS PER 1,000 LIVE BIRTHS (1959–1961)*.

COUNTRY	UNDER 1 YEAR	Rank	UNDER 28 DAYS (NEONATAL)	Rank
Sweden	16.3	1	13.2	2
Netherlands	17.7	2	13.2	3
Norway	18.5	3	12.1	1
Australia	20.4	4	14.6	4
Switzerland	21.4	5	16.3	9
Finland	21.8	6	15.1	6
Denmark	21.9	7	16.2	8
United Kingdom	22.6	8	16.0	7
New Zealand	23.1	9	14.6	5
United States	25.9	10	18.7	12
Canada	28.0	11	18.2	11
Ireland	30.6	12	20.7	14
Japan	31.0	13	17.4	10
Luxembourg	31.6	14	19.3	13
Federal Republic of Germany (West)	33.2	15	23.3	15

* Adapted from: Trends in Infant and Childhood Mortality, 1961. P. 63. Children's Bureau, Statistical Series No. 76, 1964.

position, with the state showing the lowest per capita income having the highest mortality rate.

Main causes of infant deaths in the United States (1961). The causes of infant deaths are here listed in order of frequency:

1. immaturity and other prenatal and natal causes
2. asphyxia and atelectasis with mention of prematurity
3. congenital malformations
4. birth injuries
5. influenza and pneumonia

Other important causes of infant deaths, though of lesser frequency, are digestive system conditions, accidents, blood dyscrasias and others.

With the picture above in mind, we now need to spend some time considering ways of preventing these conditions. Following this, we must turn our attention to care and treatment for the large number of neonates who suffer from these and from other handicaps to life and health, and finally, to consideration of the nurse's part.

The first condition to be considered is the condition that is the major cause of death among the newborn—prematurity.

THE PREMATURE INFANT

The greatest hazard that can face a newborn infant is that of being born too early. About two-thirds of all deaths among newborn infants occur in the relatively small per cent born prematurely. The causes of death among prematures are the same as those among term infants, anoxia, birth injuries, malformations, respiratory distress syndrome, and other infections.

Definition of Prematurity

The term prematurity (or immaturity) has been used by international agreement to designate any live-born infant weighing 2500 gm. (5 lb. 8 oz.) or under, at birth. This definition has not been entirely satisfactory in that a child may have a low birth weight and yet be a product of a full term pregnancy, whereas others weighing more than this figure may be true prematures who would have been large babies if carried to term. The birth weight itself is not as significant as the length of the period of gestation.

In 1961, the Expert Committee of the World Health Organization made the recommendation that the term *prematurity* be replaced by the term *low-birth-weight* for infants of 2500 gm. or less. The American Academy of Pediatrics has adopted this term in its manual, emphasizing that it in no way wishes to discourage the use of *premature* when the known gestational period is less than 37 weeks, or the use of *full-term* for an infant of 37 or more weeks of intra-uterine growth. At present, the majority of hospitals admit all infants of 5½ pounds or less to the premature nursery, recognizing the fact that some may be sturdier and require less specialized care than others.

Causes of Prematurity

Causes appear to be diverse, with many falling into the frequently used category of "unknown." Maternal toxemia is one cause, multiple pregnancy another. Malformed fetuses are frequently aborted or born early. We know that certain factors are often present in the mother when she gives birth early, such as poor nutrition, excessive fatigue, poor prenatal hygiene; but we cannot, with certainty, call these causes in themselves. Too often, we just do not know the reason.

Prevention of Prematurity

Obviously, prevention of prematurity is the best cure. Unfortunately, we have made very little progress despite our concern. Certainly better and earlier prenatal care is of great importance to both mother and child. When a woman places herself under medical care as soon as she suspects pregnancy, there is opportunity to offer her guidance. Infections or other abnormal conditions can be detected and treated, often prevented. Education about nutrition and prenatal hygiene should be offered. These measures in themselves are not necessarily going to prevent premature delivery, but they can contribute toward the mother's physical and mental health, and in that sense, improve chances of healthy childbirth.

Better prenatal care. This includes many things. Public education is one, financial assistance may be another. Prenatal clinics must be available in the areas where they are most needed; but even then are of little use if not patronized by those whom they are supposed to serve.

The impersonal manner with which patients are often treated in the clinic does not encourage its use. The young woman who must lose several hours of working time as she sits and waits is going to be hesitant about attending. The mother who must bring her children along into the crowded, noisy clinic—or else worry about what is happening at home as she sits for hours—may not think attendance worthwhile.

If the nurse can do little about changing general conditions, she can develop a friendly, helpful manner toward her patients. She can treat them as people, try to be helpful and sympathetic, and show a willingness to listen.

In some present-day clinics, the waiting time is put to good use. This is seen as an opportunity to develop discussion groups, involving patients and staff. Play space and recreation is provided for the children, and mothers come and go as they are called for examination. All of this seems to make good sense.

Appearance of the Premature Infant

The appearance of the premature infant is not beautiful. In fact, he falls far short of the idealized baby picture. His early birth prevented him from laying down the subcutaneous fat that makes the full-term baby appear pink and chubby. Consequently, the premature infant is wrinkled and red, appearing thin and scrawny.

Care of the Premature Infant

The premature infant needs highly skilled nursing care. Here is a situation for which the nurse should either acquire the necessary skills, understanding, and observational power, or decline a responsible position in the premature nursery. The infant's well-being, in fact his very survival, depends to a large extent on the nursing care he receives.

Immediate care. Immediately after birth, he must be placed in a warm, controlled-temperature environment, which can best be secured by the use of an incubator. The incubator can also provide humidified air, thus aiding respiration. It is equipped to provide oxygen as needed, and it provides the necessary isolation from infectious atmospheric agents.

No person except those involved in his care should have access to a premature infant. Scrupulous cleanliness must be observed, and those persons involved in his care must stay out of the nursery entirely if they suffer from any kind of infection.

Temperature. The premature infant requires help in raising his temperature to a physiologically normal level. Atmospheric temperature of 80°–90°F is usually necessary to maintain a body temperature of 96°–

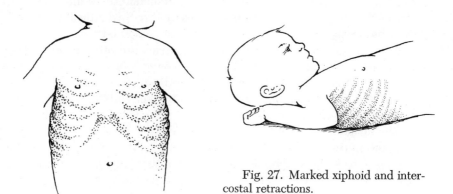

Fig. 27. Marked xiphoid and intercostal retractions.

98°F, although higher atmospheric temperature may be needed during the initial warming up period. Body temperature should be obtained by the axillary method unless the incubator is equipped with a skin-temperature detection unit.

Specific nursing care. The small newborn infant needs a minimum of handling and a maximum of observation. Not only must he be continually watched, but the nurse must have a good understanding of the characteristics she needs to observe. The infant must be observed for adequacy of breathing, for color, state of activity, vigor, type of cry, and for any sudden change in these patterns. Any one infant may develop a pattern that is generally adequate for him, and a change in this pattern may have serious meaning. This change may be in the character of the cry, in activity, in quality of respiration, or in feeding pattern. An alert nurse reports any change, even though it may appear to be insignificant.

Respiratory System Sufficiency

The premature infant has a respiratory system that is still immature, and poorly suited to meet the needs of extra-uterine living. Weakness of the thoracic cage and of respiratory muscles cause retraction during inspiration, which in turn inhibits adequate lung expansion. Incomplete development of the alveolar structure of the lungs themselves, together with feeble cough and gag reflexes, adds to the difficulties. Breathing is irregular and of the abdominal type, and some degree of cyanosis is frequently present. (Fig. 27, *left* and *right*)

Humidified air helps to keep secretions moist and movable. Oxygen is administered if necessary, but is no longer given routinely. If given, atmospheric oxygen concentration should be kept at the lowest level consistent with respiratory relief for the infant, and should be discontinued as soon as possible. However, oxygen can be a life saving measure and there should be no hesitancy about giving it in adequate amounts.

The nurse should note increased difficulty in breathing, or deeper retractions, as well as the appearance of cyanosis, or increase in the present degree of cyanosis.

Activity

The small premature infant is relatively inactive and has a feeble cry. His muscle tone is poor, so he lies limply, and does not assume the tensed leg and arm positions characteristic of the full-term infant.

Feeding Patterns

For the very small premature infant, a delay of 24 hours or longer before the first feeding is usual, as early feeding introduces extra hazards. Because of the small stomach capacity, feedings are given every two to three hours, depending on the size of the infant. The first feedings are usually of glucose water, followed by small amounts of formula or breast milk.

Method of feeding. The larger and more vigorous low-birth-weight infant may be able to suck on a small, large-holed nipple without undue fatigue. He should be supported in a semi-erect position within the incubator while being fed, and positioned on his side after he is finished. Feeding time should be limited to 20 minutes, to avoid over fatiguing the infant.

Gavage feeding is preferred for the small or weak infant. A sterile, soft rubber French catheter, size 8 to 10, is passed through the infant's mouth and down into the lower esophagus. This distance may be estimated by measuring from the tip of the infant's nose to the lower end of the sternum, and marked on the catheter. The position of the catheter is tested by placing its free end under water and watching for air bubbles. If bubbles appear as the infant breathes, withdraw the catheter and try again. If no air bubbles appear and the infant breathes easily, a glass syringe, without the plunger, is attached to the catheter's end, the formula poured in and allowed to enter the tube by gravity. The syringe should not be held more than 6 or 8 inches above the infant. As the last of the formula appears in the tip of the syringe, the catheter must be occluded by pinching or doubling over, and quickly withdrawn to prevent any dribbling of milk into the air passages.

Daily Care

The small infant tires easily with minimum effort and strain, therefore he should be handled as little as possible. He can lie in the incubator unclothed, cutting down on handling as well as affording the best opportunity for careful observation.

Bathing. At best, this should be a quick sponging off with soft, sterile cotton. Hexachlorophene in soap or solution may lower incidence of skin infection.

Weighing. This is possible without removing the infant from the incubator. Whether he is weighed daily or not depends on his size and condition, as well as the philosophy of the physician in charge.

Prevention of infection. The premature baby is especially susceptible to infection. All linen used in his care should be delivered to the nursery in sterile packs. He must have his own individal thermometer and equipment. Nursing personnel wear gowns that are put on when entering the nursery, changed daily, and not worn elsewhere. On entering the nursery, personnel wash their hands thoroughly with a hexachlorophene material for three minutes, paying particular attention to fingernails, spaces between the fingers, and arms and elbows if exposed. Masks have limited use and may be dangerous to the health of the infants if improperly used. They must be replaced every 20 to 30 minutes, and worn to cover the nose and the mouth. They must never be used to allow a person with an upper respiratory infection to enter the nurseries. Their use is usually limited to the occasional visit of the physician or of the laboratory technician.

Rings and watches are not worn in the nursery.

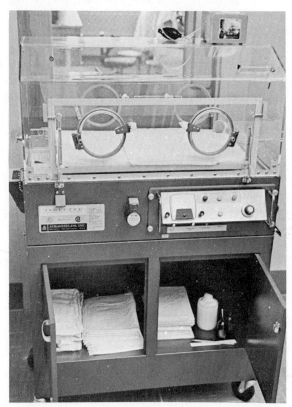

Fig. 28. Isolette with servo-control unit.

Incubator Care

The ideal way to provide the necessary warmth and humidity is with the use of an incubator. The incubator also provides the optimal aseptic environment and makes the administration of oxygen a simple procedure. Today, it is the accepted practice to care for the premature infant in well-equipped, specialized nurseries. Where incubators are not available, an attempt to maintain a satisfactory level of body temperature may be made by use of a large box or basket as a crib. A large, folded blanket may be used for a mattress, with hot water bottles placed under the blanket. Hot water bottles may be placed along the sides of the box if there is something to keep them from direct contact with the infant, such as a blanket lining the box, with the bottles between the box and the blanket. The temperature of the bottles should not be over 100°, and they will need frequent changing. The temperature of the room should be maintained at 85° to 90°.

One of the greatest factors in saving the lives of small premature infants has been use of the Isolette. This provides an entirely closed area, with air entering through a filtered inlet and circulated by a unique

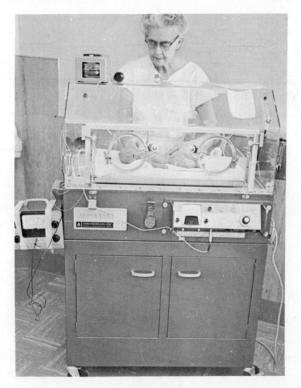

Fig. 29. Use of isolette for small premature
infant. Servo-control in use.

system throughout the incubator. Humidified air and oxygen are provided and easily regulated. The infant is entirely visible through a plexiglass hood, and receives all nursing care through the arm ports. (Fig. 28)

If a small baby is expected to be admitted, the incubator can be heated and made ready before the infant arrives. The thermostat is set to the desired temperature, and the humidity chamber filled with sterile, distilled water and set at the desired rate.

An additional feature of the Isolette now available is the Servo Control Unit. It provides a means of stabilizing the infant's temperature at a normal physiological level. A temperature sensing thermistor (called a Patient Probe) is attached to the skin of the infant's abdomen with a piece of tape. The Patient Probe detects changes in skin temperature as low as 0.2°, and regulates the heat of the incubator accordingly. A skin temperature of 97°F approximates a body temperature of 98° The Servo Control Unit, therefore, is pre-set at 97° but can be easily raised or lowered. A safety cut-off thermostat automatically turns off the heat at 98° to 100°, sounds an alarm, and illuminates a red warning light if the incubator should become overheated for any reason. (Fig. 29)

Other features of the Isolette include an incubator weighing scale, a tilting deck to permit the assumption of either a Fowler or a Trendelenburg position, as well as an oxygen concentration control that limits oxygen concentration inside the incubator to 40 per cent. This control can be set aside if necessary, to raise the concentration to 70 to 80 per cent.

As the infant progresses, he acquires, with increasing success, the ability to regulate his own body heat. He can graduate from incubator to heated crib, and be ready to tolerate the nursery atmosphere before he is discharged.

The Infant's Parents

The nurse should give some thought toward helping the parents of the premature infant. They have been anticipating this birth for a long time, and undoubtedly have made preparations for the baby's care at home. Now they will have to go home empty-handed, and it may be weeks, or even months before they can take their baby home. These babies are usually kept in the nursery until they weigh 5 or 5½ pounds and are progressing in a satisfactory manner. Not only do the parents go home empty-handed, they experience considerable anxiety over the frail baby left in the nursery.

During this waiting period, the parents need an opportunity to learn how to care for the baby when he comes home. Their experience tends to make them uncertain and wary of handling such a small, delicate child. Some nurseries are able to provide practice and teaching rooms where parents can attend classes and demonstrations of bathing and dressing small babies, preparing formulas and feeding techniques. The parents

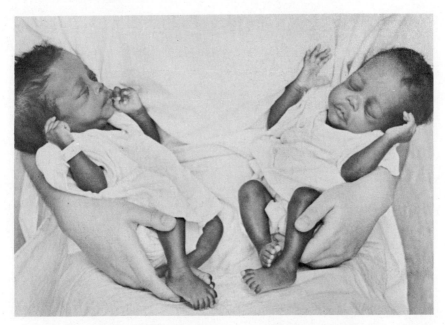

Fig. 30. Prematurely born twins ready for discharge.

practice these and other skills, and acquire confidence in their own ability. These occasions also provide an opportunity for parents to get together and to exchange ideas, discuss problems, and meet socially.

If this kind of help is unavailable, the mother (the father too, if possible) must have a chance to bathe, dress and feed the baby before taking him home, and receive instruction about formula preparation.

This preparation helps the parents in handling their child, and guards against the tendency to overprotect. There will be fewer panic calls to the nursery or pediatrician, and greater security in the home. (Fig. 30)

CARE OF THE NEWBORN INFANT WITH CONGENITAL ANOMALIES
The Infant With a Cleft Lip Anomaly

A young, prospective mother is naturally excited over the forthcoming birth and the prospect of bringing home her first baby. There have been charming new babies among her relatives and friends, and everyone is looking forward to the new arrival. There has usually been much preparation in anticipation of the homecoming.

Mary White was such a mother. She was told in the delivery room that she had a healthy son, but she became considerably puzzled when no one brought him to her for immediate inspection.

After she had rested, however, the nursery nurse appeared in her doorway, holding the newborn baby lovingly and tenderly in her arms. "Mrs. White," she said, "you have a husky son of whom you can be very proud. I am anxious for you to see him, but I must tell you first that he has a facial defect, a cleft in his upper lip. Fortunately, this defect can be repaired early. It is not pretty to look at now, but plastic surgery can give you a very good looking baby. He surely is a fine boy altogether."

Mary eagerly accepted her child, but could not help the feeling of shock that she experienced when she looked at his face. Perhaps one of the greatest dreads at the moment was the thought of the reaction of her family and friends when they saw her child's disfigurement.

Mary was not alone in her unhappiness, because this defect appears in about one out of 800 births. The cause is not entirely clear. There seems to be a genetic influence in some instances, for the incidence is higher in families in which there is a history of the defect, but it also occurs in isolated instances. It has been known to occur in infants whose mothers have had rubella during the first trimester of pregnancy, but, in this instance, this defect does not occur so frequently as do others.

The defect itself is the result of a failure of the maxillary and premaxillary processes to fuse during the fifth to eighth week of intra-uterine life. The cleft may be a simple notch in the vermilion line, or it may extend up into the floor of the nose. (Fig. 31)

Plastic surgeons differ as to the best time for repair. Some are in favor

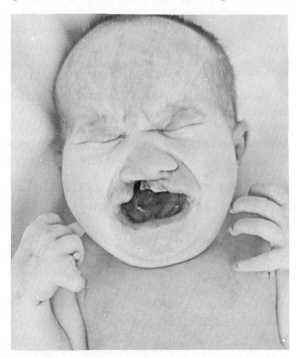

Fig. 31. Unilateral cleft lip extending into the floor of the nose.

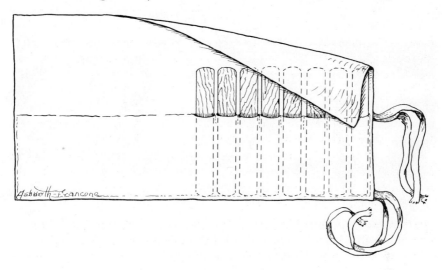

Fig. 32. An elbow restraint.

of early repair, before the infant goes home. Another group prefers to wait until the infant is two or three months old.

There are certain obvious advantages to early repair. The mother's emotional comfort in being able to take home a normal-looking infant needs to be considered. Another advantage concerns feeding: because of the divided upper lip, he cannot suck, and has to be fed by dropper, spoon or Asepto syringe. This presents difficulties for both mother and child.

If early surgery is contemplated, the baby should be healthy, of average or above average weight, and must be placed where he can be—and is—watched constantly. A newborn child has greater difficulty dealing with excess mucus than does an older infant. Good results are obtained when these infants are in the hands of competent plastic surgeons and experienced nurses.

The surgeons who decide to wait can also cite advantages. They have more tissue to work with in an older child, of particular advantage when dealing with a wide defect. They believe they are more certain of good results, and also believe that the parents can be realistic enough to face facts as they are.

Nursing Care

There is little preoperative preparation for the infant who has surgery during the first few days of life. For the older infant, it would be well to accustom him to elbow restraints, for he has to wear them for several days following surgery. It is also helpful if the nurse becomes accustomed to feeding the infant with an Asepto syringe. This requires a special technique that is difficult to acquire without practice.

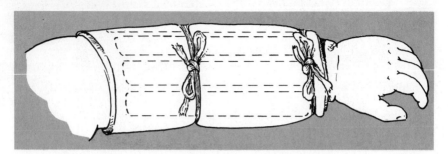

Fig. 33. Elbow restraint applied.

Immediate postoperative care. This demands continuous and intelligent observation. The swollen mouth tissues cause an excessive secretion of mucus that is poorly handled by a small infant. For the first few hours, he must never be left alone because he can quickly and easily aspirate the mucus.

A sore mouth calls for a comforting thumb, and this can quickly undo the difficult and costly repair. This is one occasion when the child's ultimate happiness and well-being must take precedence over his immediate satisfaction.

Elbow restraints. These must be properly applied and checked frequently. These are made with canvas and with tongue blades, which are tied firmly around the arm, and pinned to the infant's shirt or gown to prevent them sliding down below the elbow. (Figs. 32 and 33) The child can move his arm around, but cannot bend his elbow to reach his face. The restraints must be applied snugly, but not allowed to hinder circulation.

Restraints need to be removed frequently to provide physical relief. This is done by removing them from one arm at a time and controlling movements of the child's arm. A sufficient supply should be kept on hand in order to change soiled restraints.

The baby suffers emotional frustration because of the restraints, so satisfaction must be provided in other ways. He needs rocking and cuddling as any baby does, but probably in larger measure. Mother is the best person to supply this loving care, and no doubt the most willing. Nurses come next.

Care of suture line. The suture line is left uncovered after surgery and must be kept clean and dry to prevent infection with subsequent scarring. In many hospitals, a wire bow—called a Logan Bar—is applied across the upper lip and attached to the cheeks with adhesive tape. This prevents tension on the sutures. (Fig. 34)

The sutures are carefully cleaned as often as necessary to prevent the collection of dried serum. Frequent cleaning is quite essential for the first two or three days, as well as after every feeding as long as the sutures are in.

A *tray* containing the articles needed for suture care is kept at the bedside and changed daily. It should contain a covered jar of sterile cotton-tipped applicators, a sterile container of solution for cleansing and a paper bag for waste. The solutions used are commonly hydrogen peroxide or sterile saline.

With clean hands, dip an applicator into the solution and gently clean each suture with a rolling motion. The sutures inside the lip also need cleaning. Application of an ointment following the cleansing may be ordered.

Technique for feeding. Have ready a sterile Asepto syringe with the tip protected by a piece of sterile rubber tubing about one inch long. Plastic tubing is unsatisfactory as it may slide off and lodge in the infant's throat.

Place the syringe and warmed formula on the bedside stand within easy reach. Hold the infant in your arms in an upright position. Pour the formula into syringe and place the rubber covered tip in the child's mouth, away from the suture line. The formula usually drips quickly enough without squeezing the bulb. The nurse must learn to regulate the drops to the infant's breathing and swallowing, but both she and the baby soon learn. The baby swallows considerable amounts of air and needs burping frequently. About 30 minutes should be allowed for a feeding.

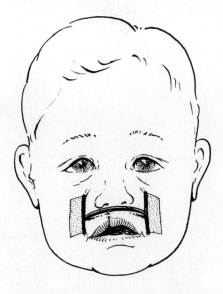

Fig. 34. Logan Bar for easing strain on sutures.

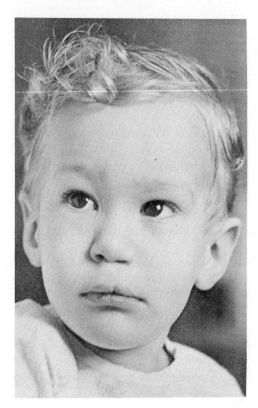

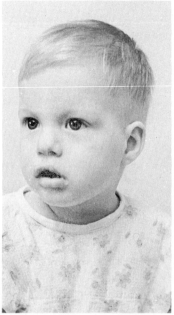

Fig. 35. (*above*) This child has returned for slight revision of cleft lip repair.

Fig. 36. (*left*) This child may need a revision of the vermilion line.

The baby is much safer when placed in his crib after his feeding if he is positioned on his side, in order to prevent aspiration if he vomits or regurgitates. If he cannot be satisfactorily restrained in this position but must instead be placed on his back, his head should be kept elevated and the child watched carefully.

The sutures are removed 7 'to 10 days after surgery. The infant will probably be allowed to suck on a soft nipple at this time. Following effective surgery and intelligent, careful nursing care, the appearance of baby's face should be very good.

Mother should be told that this baby can be fed and treated as any other. The scar fades as time goes on. She needs to know that he is probably going to need a slight adjustment of the vermilion line in later childhood. With today's surgery, she can expect that the child will not have the unsightly, thickened tissue seen in early days. (Figs. 35 and 36)

Some infants who have a cleft lip also have a cleft palate. In such instances, the lip is repaired as described, but the palate repair is delayed until sometime during the second year. The baby is able to suck after the lip repair and should progress normally until ready for palate surgery. Some milk may seep through the cleft palate and out through the nose, but most of these babies learn to handle this without too much difficulty.

Esophageal Atresia With Fistula

A much more serious anomaly is that of esophageal atresia, with or without fistula into the trachea. There are several types of atresia, but 90 per cent of them fall into one category. This most common type consists of the upper, or proximal end of the esophagus ending in a blind pouch, with the lower, or distal segment from the stomach connected to the trachea by a fistulous tract. (Fig. 37)

About 25 per cent of infants with esophageal atresia are born prematurely. Anomalies associated with this condition include congenital heart defects and anal atresia.

The child with congenital esophageal atresia can be expected to live only a very short time without corrective surgery. The premature or low-birth-weight infant may need special care for a period of time before he is able to tolerate the type of surgery demanded, but the average full-term infant can usually tolerate it shortly after birth.

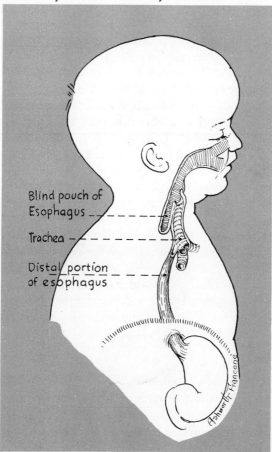

Fig. 37. The most common form of esophageal atresia.

Symptoms. It is obvious that mucus, or any fluid that a newborn baby with this condition swallows, goes into the blind pouch of the esophagus. This pouch soon fills and overflows, with the usual result of aspiration into the trachea.

Probably few other conditions are as dependent on the watchful observation of the nurse for early diagnosis, which in turn, greatly influences the child's chances for survival. This newborn infant has frothing and excessive drooling. He has periods of respiratory distress with choking and cyanosis. It is true that many newborns have difficulty with mucus, but the nurse should be alerted to the possibility of an anomaly, and report such difficulties to a responsible person. She may, and should, take the responsibility for delaying the first feeding until the infant has been checked.

If early signs are overlooked and the nurse tries to feed the child, she experiences a situation that she could very well do without. The baby chokes, coughs and regurgitates as the food enters the blind pouch. He becomes deeply cyanotic and appears to be in severe respiratory distress. During this process, he aspirates some of the formula with resultant pneumonitis. Naturally, this sequence does much to make surgery more of a hazard to the child. In a very real sense, the infant's life may depend upon the careful observation of the nurse.

Diagnosis. Diagnosis is not difficult to make if the possible presence of this condition is recognized. A rubber catheter passed through the infant's nose is blocked at the site of the atresia, and X-ray film shows the catheter coiled upon itself in the blind pouch. Frequently, the catheter alone is sufficient, but if contrast media is used, it should be a small amount of iodized oil. Barium is never used. The fistulous tract into the trachea may be demonstrated by the appearance of air in the gastrointestinal tract.

Surgery. Surgery consists of an anastomosis of the two esophageal segments when these are close enough for the purpose and of closure of the fistula. Occasionally, the gap is too wide for this, in which case, the upper segment is brought to the skin surface, and a gastrostomy performed for feeding purposes. Later, a colon transplant is done. In either type of surgery, many surgeons routinely perform a gastrostomy to permit early feeding.

Preoperative Care

The infant needs to be placed in an incubator where highly saturated air, constant temperature, and oxygen are available. He is usually placed in a semi-sitting position to prevent regurgitation.

The blind pouch is kept free of mucus by continuous suction, or by frequent pharyngeal aspiration. Either must be carefully performed to avoid injury to the blind pouch.

The child needs constant watching, with prompt attention to choking if it occurs. Naturally, he is given nothing by mouth. Intravenous fluids are started, generally by means of a cutdown. These children develop pulmonary edema easily, so the nurse must be unusually observant of the rate and flow of the fluid.

Surgery may be delayed until the infant's condition is improved, and, here again, the nurse must be constantly aware of his condition. She must watch for changes in color, temperature, pulse, and state of activity. She must keep in mind the ever present danger of pneumonia or pneumonitis. The child must be turned frequently.

Not the least of the nurse's duties is to give adequate attention to the infant's family. It must be remembered that this is a newborn infant who has never been home. Perhaps he is also premature, thus enhancing the family's anxiety. Frequently, the infant has been removed from the place of his birth and taken to a center where more skilled care is available. This means that the mother does not get to see her child, and must rely on reports from her husband or from other members of the family.

Perhaps she is fortunate at that. It is certainly frightening to see the child enclosed in the incubator with so many tubes attached to his body. Families are often afraid to ask too many questions, and so bring back only gloomy reports to the anxious mother.

It does nothing for the family for the nurse to say, "The baby is doing as well as can be expected." They certainly hope he is doing a little *better* than the picture allows them to expect. However, the nurse must guard against giving a false impression of well-being and optimism. A brush-off of "You will have to ask the doctor" is not well accepted either. If the nurse does not know what is going on, or is not interested, the child is indeed in a sorry plight!

Time must be taken to listen to the family, and to give honest answers. The nurse refers them to the doctor as necessary, but she can give much supporting care herself. She can explain the various types of equipment, thus removing the mystery from them. She can explain the defect and its repair in simple, nonmedical terms. She can show a warm, human interest in the mother's progress and well-being. Above all, she does not show a feeling of irritation or hurriedness, but by her manner, she convinces the family that these interviews are an important part of nursing.

Postoperative Care

While the infant is still in surgery, his nurse prepares for his return. The incubator must be clean, warm, and be functioning properly. Ample supplies must be readied so that she will have no difficulty obtaining them, because she must resume her careful, constant observation on the infant's return.

Following surgery, treatment is resumed much as before. The child

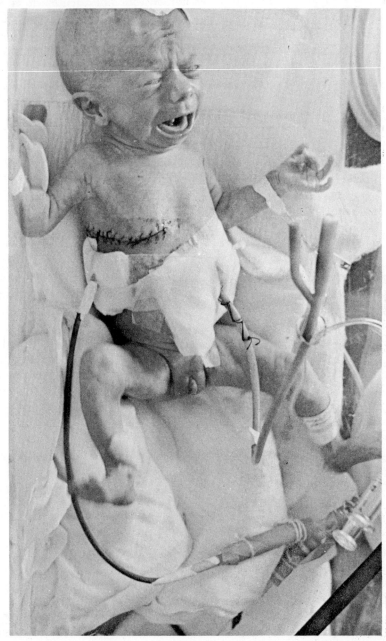

A

Fig. 38a. Repair of tracheal esophageal atresia and fistula showing chest incision and drainage tube. Gastrostomy tube also in place.

Fig. 38b. The infant is being given a gastrostomy feeding.

is given intravenous fluids, placed in a constant, humidified atmosphere, and kept free of excessive mucus.

Feeding. Feedings by gastrostomy tube are usually started on the second or third day. For this, the nurse needs the warmed formula, a sterile funnel or Asepto syringe (without the bulb), and a clamp. The syringe (or funnel) is attached to the gastrostomy tube and formula placed in the funnel or syringe before the tube is unclamped. The formula is allowed to run in slowly, and the tube is again clamped when the formula has reached the lower edge of the funnel, to avoid introducing air into the stomach. (Figs. 38a and 38b)

PSYCHOLOGICAL NEEDS. The infant has psychological needs, one of which is the need to suck. Following an anastomosis, he can be given a sterile nipple stuffed with cotton or a pacifier to suck when he receives his gastrostomy feedings. After the feeding, he needs to be held and cuddled.

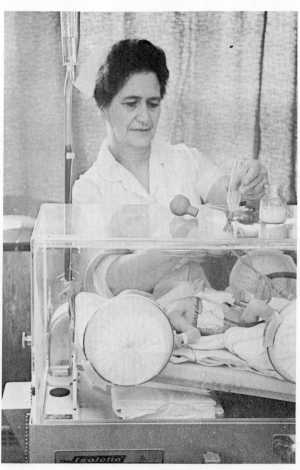

Fig. 38b.

The infant who has not yet had an anastomosis cannot be permitted to suck, thus he has an even greater need for physical contact and warm acceptance. These infants continue to need gastrostomy feedings until further surgery.

Most of these infants, however, have had an anastomosis, and are ready for oral feedings after 8 to 10 days. A small-holed nipple should be used, and feedings given very slowly. Stenosis at the site of the anastomosis is not uncommon, so the nurse must be particularly watchful for choking or difficult swallowing.

When the mother is able to, she should be encouraged to spend some time observing and helping with the care of her baby. Remember that this child has never been home before, so the mother needs practice in the routine care of her newborn infant as well as in special procedures. She needs to develop confidence in bathing and weighing as well as in dressing a small infant.

GASTROSTOMY FEEDING. The mother should also learn how to give gastrostomy feedings. Hopefully, she will not have to give them, but many babies develop strictures at the site of the anastomosis, requiring temporary use of the gastrostomy tube for feeding. The wound itself should be well healed at the time of baby's discharge and require no special care or any dressing, so that baby can be put in the tub for bathing.

The mother also needs to practice oral feeding, and to learn what symptoms indicate impending trouble, such as a stenosis at the site of anastomosis. She should be told to call her doctor or the hospital resident if baby chokes over feedings or regurgitates, and to stop feeding until baby has been checked. With all of this, she must not be made too apprehensive.

A fair proportion of these infants develop stenosis at the site of the anastomosis and require dilatation, which probably will be done at the hospital. Mother should also know of this possibility.

The gastrostomy tube may be left in place for several months until the surgeon is satisfied that all need for its use is past. Frequently, several dilatations of the esophagus are necessary during the months following surgery.

Prognosis is somewhat guarded, much depending on the infant's condition at time of surgery. Early diagnosis, especially before feedings are attempted, is an important factor in the infant's survival. For many infants, the condition is complicated by prematurity and by other congenital anomalies. However, through careful management, together with devoted nursing care, the mortality rate has been greatly reduced from the former prediction of "hopeless," and a normal life is now possible for many.

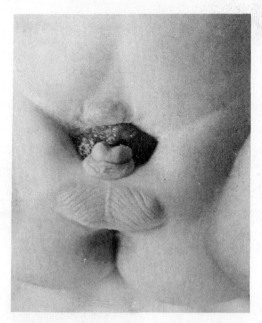

Fig. 39. Exstrophy of the bladder in male infant.

In this condition there is a failure of the union of the lower abdominal walls, leaving the entire bladder exposed. There is continuous urinary leakage. Surgery may consist of a ureteral transplantation into the colon, or a ureteroileostomy may be done.

CONGENITAL METABOLIC DEFECTS

Recent research has greatly extended our knowledge concerning congenital metabolic defects, commonly called inborn errors of metabolism. Each year, many reports are presented concerning newly described conditions. Many of these are still in the process of study, with sufficient information as yet unavailable. An article by Waisman* describes 26 such "new inborn errors," and provides interesting, informative reading. The majority of these disorders involve mental retardation or mental deterioration.

Some metabolic errors that have been studied in the past, and also involve mental retardation or deterioration are listed here.

phenylketonuria	Gaucher's disease
galactosemia	Tay-Sachs disease
maple syrup urine disease	Niemann-Pick disease
gargoylism	Wilson's disease

* Waisman, H.: Some newer inborn errors of metabolism. Pediat. Clin. N. Amer., 13:469, 1966.

A concise, well-written article by Garell* concerning these and other metabolic defects associated with mental retardation, provides information concerning the type of defect, manifestations, and treatment, if any has been found to date.

The conditions of phenylketonuria and galactosemia have been quite well described, and some time will be taken here to discuss them.

Phenylketonuria

Phenylketonuria is a recessive hereditary defect of metabolism that if untreated causes severe mental retardation. In this condition, there is a lack of the enzyme that normally changes the essential amino acid, phenylalanine, into tyrosine.

As soon as the newborn baby with this defect begins to take milk, either breast or cow's milk, he begins to absorb phenylalanine in the normal manner. However, because of his inability to metabolize this amino acid, phenylalanine builds up in his blood serum to as much as 20 times the normal level. This takes place at such a rapid pace that by-products of this high serum phenylalanine begin to appear in the urine somewhere between the first and sixth week of age.

Children with this condition develop severe and progressive mental deficiency, apparently because of the high serum phenylalanine level. The infant appears normal at birth, but commences to show signs of mental arrest within a few weeks. It is therefore imperative that these infants be discovered as early in life as possible and placed immediately on a low phenylalanine formula.

Diagnostic tests. Phenylpyruvic acid appears in the urine in this condition after the first or second week of life. The presence of this acid can be detected by a simple urine test. A few drops of 10 per cent ferric chloride when placed on a wet diaper causes a blue-green spot to appear immediately if phenylpyruvic acid is present. Variations of this test include the following.

TEST TUBE TEST. Two or three drops of 10 per cent ferric chloride added to about 5 cc. of urine turns the urine blue-green.

PHENISTIX TEST. A paper strip (Phenistix) that has been impregnated with ferric salt, is dipped in urine or pressed against a wet diaper. The color reaction of the Phenistix is the same as that for the ferric chloride test.

For any of these tests, the blue-green color starts to fade quickly, sometimes within 30 seconds. Color reactions from other chemicals giving a false-positive reaction are usually longer lasting.

FILTER PAPER TEST. A strip of ordinary white filter paper may be placed in the infant's diaper or dipped in urine. When dried, it is sent

---

* Garell, D.: Metabolic defects associated with mental retardation. Amer. J. Dis. Child., *104*:401, 1962.

to a testing laboratory. This is more useful for home testing, for filter paper urine gives results for several days following use.

One disadvantage of relying upon the urine test is that most newborn infants have left the hospital before the test can be useful. In statewide programs, envelopes containing filter paper and directions are given to mothers leaving the hospital or mailed to mothers whose babies were delivered at home. Unfortunately, the busy mother too often forgets, or fails to sense the importance of the testing, and damage occurs before the condition is diagnosed.

BLOOD TEST. A blood test devised in recent years gives good results as early as the third or fourth day after birth, but is of no value until the infant has received dietary protein, which is present in his milk feedings. This screening procedure, called the Guthrie inhibition assay test, utilizes blood from a simple heel prick. It is becoming standard procedure in many newborn nurseries, being performed just before the infant is discharged.

The advantage of this test lies in the ability to discover suspicious cases before serum phenylalanine levels have built up with the resultant risk of brain damage. A follow-up urine ferric chloride test is useful, particularly for those infants born into families in which there is a history of mental retardation or known phenylketonuria.

Early dietary treatment for infants with this condition offers the best preventive measure known against brain damage.

GALACTOSEMIA

Galactosemia is a recessive hereditary metabolic disorder in which the enzyme necessary for converting galactose into glucose is missing. The infants generally appear normal at birth, but experience difficulties after the ingestion of milk—whether breast milk, cow's or goat's milk—because one of the component monosaccharides of milk lactose is galactose.

Early feeding difficulties, with vomiting and diarrhea severe enough to produce dehydration and weight loss, and jaundice, are primary manifestations. Unless milk is withheld early, other difficulties include cataracts, liver and spleen damage, and mental retardation, with a high mortality rate early in life.

The earliest diagnostic finding is the presence of galactose in the urine, but if vomiting or refusal to eat have been present, the test may be negative. Galactose tolerance tests have been used, but may present definite hazards to the infant. Recently, a blood test using the Guthrie inhibition assay method, has proved a reliable diagnostic test. It can be performed in conjunction with a test for phenylketonuria.

Treatment consists of omitting galactose from the diet, which, in the young infant, means a substitution for milk. Nutramigen and soybean preparations such as Sobee or Mulsoy, are satisfactory substitutes.

Although withholding of galactose later in infancy may cause a regression of symptoms, the mental retardation is irreversible.

The nurse holds an important role as the person with the responsibility for noting feeding difficulties early in the postnatal period, and reporting these difficulties promptly and accurately.

CONGENITAL RUBELLA

Following a major rubella epidemic in Australia in 1941, the teratogenic effect of the virus on the developing fetus during the first trimester of pregnancy, as it passed the placental barrier, was noted and eventually well documented. A resulting combination of defects discovered in the newborn, consisting of congenital cataracts, heart disease, deafness and microcephaly, became known as the rubella syndrome.

In 1962, the rubella virus was successfully propagated in tissue culture. Techniques for isolation of the virus and detection of antibodies are now perfected, although time-consuming and expensive. Facilities for detection are not widely available at the present time.

The most extensive rubella epidemic in history occurred in the United States in 1964, resulting in a large number of babies with congenital malformations from maternal infection. It has been estimated that as many as 10,000 to 20,000 babies may have been so affected. One result of this epidemic with its unfortunate consequences has been an increase in our knowledge concerning congenital rubella.

Recent advances. It is now apparent that the rubella virus infection acquired by the fetus in utero generally persists throughout fetal life, is present at birth, and for an undetermined time after birth. Virus has been recovered from aborted fetuses and from infants throughout the first year of life. One preliminary study has given the figure of 63 per cent of infected infants remaining contagious at one month of age, with 7 per cent still contagious at 10 to 12 months of age. Persons coming into intimate contact with these babies may develop the disease, and such cases are on record.

Congenital defects. A large variety of defects have been reported in association with congenital rubella, in addition to those previously documented. Malformations constituting the rubella syndrome are now found to include the following.

cataracts and other eye defects, occasionally glaucoma
deafness
cardiac anomalies, especially patent ductus arteriosus and septal defects
intrauterine growth retardation
subnormal head circumference and retarded functional development

Less commonly found, but probably associated with rubella, are meningocele, purpura, enlarged liver and spleen, defects of long bones, and many others.

Care of Infants With Congenital Rubella

An infant may be suspected of harboring rubella virus if there is a history of maternal infection during the first trimester of pregnancy, and if the presence of one or more of the malformations described is observed. There does, however, appear to be evidence that some infants, infected in utero, excrete rubella virus even when no abnormalities are noted.

The infant suspected of having congenital rubella should be isolated while in the hospital. Airborne risk is probably insignificant, but personnel caring for the child should have a clear past history of rubella, and not presently pregnant. Duration of contagion is uncertain, but until viral studies become more easily available, it should be remembered that the condition may be contagious for perhaps a year, if not longer.

The infant needs the same kind of nursing care offered any small infant. In addition, he should be examined daily for skin petechiae and purpura, carefully checked for heart murmur, eyes examined, and abdomen examined for liver or spleen enlargement.

Follow-up evaluation should include audiometric testing. Surgery later in infancy or early childhood for cataracts brings good results. Other abnormalities are treated according to the specific defect. At present, there is no known therapy to eliminate the carrier state.

Prevention of Congenital Rubella

It seems quite clear that a pregnant woman may transmit rubella to the fetus even though she may have a subclinical case of which she is unaware. Protection of the fetus therefore appears more difficult than has been previously supposed, and reliance on gamma globulin for protection may be unsound. Many childhood rashes may be termed "German" measles, so that the pregnant woman who considers herself immune because of a supposed childhood rubella infection, may not, in fact, be immune at all.

A list of viral conditions that produce rashes similar to rubella follows.

1. Erythema infectiosum. (fifth disease.) A mild erythematous eruption occurring in epidemics among children.
2. Exanthem subitum (roseola infantum, sixth disease). An acute, mildly infectious illness with maculopapular rash, and high fever.
3. Rubeola (or regular measles.) Mild cases may be misleading. Koplik's spots are present in the mouth, but occurring before the rash appears, are frequently missed.
4. Scarlet fever. The rash of rubella may resemble either that of measles or scarlet fever. Scarlet fever has diminished in severity and extent in the United States, and may not be recognized.

5. Rashes produced by other viruses, such as the ECHO or the Coxsackie viruses.

Rubella, as it appears in a child or adult, is a mild, febrile disease characterized by mild catarrhal symptoms, low or absent fever, enlarged lymph nodes of the neck, and a macular rash. Koplik spots are not present.

Rubella produces few, if any, constitutional symptoms in a healthy child. Deliberate exposure of girls (well below the child-bearing age) to the disease is advocated by many, although this does not preclude the possibility that the girl's mother or other female relatives, unaware of beginning pregnancy, may not become infected. The difficulty of protecting pregnant women is obvious, because exposure of the mother of small children frequently occurs before the disease is diagnosed, and before the mother is aware of her pregnancy.

A rubella vaccine has not as yet been perfected, but laboratory studies indicate a promise of an effective vaccine, hopefully not far in the future.

BIBLIOGRAPHY

American Academy of Pediatrics: Standards and Recommendations for Hospital Care of Newborn Infants. Evanston, Illinois, American Academy of Pediatrics, 1964.

American Journal of Diseases of Childhood: Rubella syndrome. Amer. J. Dis. Child., *110:* (Oct.) 1965.

Cooper, L. Z., and Krugman, S.: Diagnosis and management: congenital rubella. Pediatrics, 37:335, 1966.

Crosse, V. M.: The Premature Baby. 5th ed. Boston, Little, Brown & Co., 1961.

Fishbein, M. (ed.): Birth Defects. pp. 235–240. Philadelphia, J. B. Lippincott, 1964.

Garell, D.: Metabolic defects associated with mental retardation. Amer. J. Dis. Child., *104:*401, 1962.

Geddes, A. K.: Premature Babies: Their Nursing Care and Management. Philadelphia, W. B. Saunders, 1960.

Holdsworth, W. G.: Cleft Lip and Cleft Palate. 3rd ed. New York, Grune & Stratton, 1963.

Nelson, W., (ed.): Textbook of Pediatrics. 8th ed. Philadelphia, W. B. Saunders, 1964.

United States Department of Health, Education and Welfare, Children's Bureau: Trends in Infant and Childhood Mortality, 1961. Washington, United States Government Printing Office, 1964.

Waisman, H.: Some Newer inborn errors of metabolism. Pediat. Clin. N. Amer., *13:*469, 1966.

World Health Organization: Technical Report Series, 1961, no. 217. *in* Standards and Recommendations for Hospital Care of Newborn Infants. American Academy of Pediatrics, 1964.

Ziegel, E., and Van Blarcom, C. C.: Obstetrical Nursing. 5th ed. New York, Macmillan, 1964.

SUGGESTED READINGS FOR FURTHER STUDY

Callon, H. F.: The premature infant's nurse. Amer. J. Nurs., *63*:103, (Feb.) 1963.

Campbell, M.: Clinical Pediatric Urology. Philadelphia, W. B. Saunders, 1951.

————: Principles of Urology. Philadelphia, W. B. Saunders, 1957.

Cornblath, M., *et al:* Research and nursing care in the premature nursery. Amer. J. Nurs., *62*:92, (Jul.) 1962.

Creevy, D.: Ileac diversion of the urine. Amer. J. Nurs., *59*:530, (Apr.) 1959.

Davens, E.: A view of health services for mothers and children. Children, *12*:47, 1965.

deVries, P., and Barrett, A. C.: Care of the infant with an esophageal anomaly. Amer. J. Nurs., *61*:51, (Jun.) 1961.

Goulding, E., and Koop, C. E.: The newborn: his response to surgery. Amer. J. Nurs., *65*:84, (Oct.) 1965.

Groves, K., and Schloesser, P.: A state program to control phenylketonuria. Amer. J. Nurs., *64*:74, (Aug.) 1964.

Guthrie, R.: Blood screening for phenylketonuria. J.A.M.A., *178*:863, 1961.

Heggie, A.: Current concepts in epidemiology and teratology. Pediat. Clin. N.A., *13*:251, 1966.

Hepner, R.: Care of the premature. Current Therapy, *6*:617, 1964.

Holinger, P., *et al:* Congenital anomalies of the tracheobronchial tree and of the esophagus. Pediat. Clin. N.A., *9*:1113, 1962.

Holt, L. E., *et al:* A study of premature infants fed cold formulas. J. Pediat., *61*:556, 1962.

Hsia, D., and O'Flynn, M.: Diet in relation to hereditary metabolic disorders. Pediat. Clin. N.A., *9*:945, 1962.

McLenahan, I.: Helping the mother who has no baby to take home. Amer. J. Nurs., *62*:70, (Apr.) 1962.

Owens, C.: Parents' Reactions to defective babies. Amer. J. Nurs., *64*:83, (Nov.) 1964.

Parmelee, A. H.: The doctor and the handicapped child. Children, *9*:189, 1962.

Ragsdale, N., and Koch, R.: Phenylketonuria, detection and therapy. Amer. J. Nurs., *64*:90, (Jan.) 1964.

Silverman, W., and Parke, P.: Keep him warm. Amer. J. Nurs., *65*:81, (Oct.) 1965.

Solnit, A., and Stark, M.: Mourning and the birth of a defective child. Psychonal. Study Child., *16*:523, 1961.

Thompson, L. R.: Nursery infections: apparent and inapparent. Amer. J. Nurs., *65*:80, (Nov.) 1965.

Tollefson, D. M.: Nursing care of the patient with an ileac diversion. Amer. J. Nurs., *59*:534, (Apr.) 1959.

Ross Laboratories: Your Premature Baby. Cleveland, Ross Laboratories, 1962.

UNIT 3

THE INFANT

9

Age Four Weeks to One Year

We do not expect to see healthy Johnny in the sick babies' nursery at this age, but how are we to understand his development and to care for his needs if he should appear, unless we know something about the road he has traveled since we saw him as a newborn infant? We need to know certain landmarks along that road.

The infant who has lived through the first month of life has a busy year ahead. This year he grows and develops at a faster rate than he is ever going to again. It seems incredible that this helpless, tiny bit of humanity, in the short space of one year, is going to become an individual with strong emotions of fear, jealousy, anger and love; that he will be able to rise from a supine to an upright position, and move about purposefully.

He is going to gain both weight and height extremely rapidly. During the first six months, his growth is going to be so rapid that he will double

TABLE 9-1. GROWTH DURING THE FIRST YEAR.

WEIGHT		HEIGHT	
First 5 to 6 Months			
birth weight (average) range	7½ lb. 5½ to 10 lb.	birth height (average) range	20 inches 18 to 22 inches
physiological weight loss during first week of life, due to loss of body fluid and inadequate intake.	Up to 10% (normal loss)	grows approximately	6 to 7 inches
Weekly gain	6 to 8 oz.		
5 to 6 months doubles birth weight		5 to 6 months has grown 6 to 7 inches	
Second Half of First Year			
Now he slows down slightly.		grows approximately 3 to 4 inches during this 6 to 12 month period.	
Weekly gain	4 to 6 oz.		
At 12 months, triples birth weight		Has grown 10 to 12 inches since birth.	

117

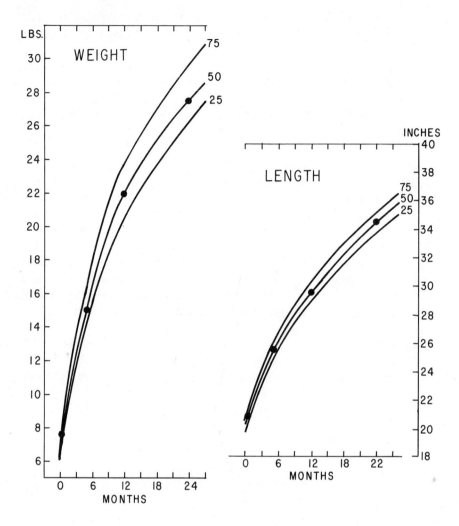

Fig. 40. Growth chart showing average growth in weight and height.

his birth weight at 5 to 6 months and add about 6 inches to his height.

The second six months will also be a period of rapid growth, but at a slightly slower rate. At one year of age, he should triple his birth weight and have added an additional 3 to 4 inches to his height.

A table of Johnny's growth during his first year is shown in Fig. 40.

Remember that the average child is no one particular child at all. To determine properly whether Johnny is reaching acceptable levels at the proper time, he must be measured in relation to his own birth weight and height. A baby weighing 6 pounds at birth cannot be expected, at five or six months, to weigh as much as a baby who weighed 9 pounds at birth, but each should have doubled his own birth weight. It is important to learn how to use a growth graph in assessing Johnny's progress. (Fig. 40)

Because of the normal infant's rapid growth, his appetite is excellent; in fact, he eats more in proportion to his weight than he does during his second year. Mothers become so accustomed to the intense hunger of their healthy infants that they tend to become alarmed when this appetite begins to slacken during the toddler and pre-school years.

MATURATION AND DEVELOPMENT

As the young baby develops, his nerve cells mature, his fine muscles learn to coordinate, and he follows the developmental schedule of his peers. Naturally, his mother is full of pride if he learns to sit or to stand before the baby up the street, but actually such precocity means very little. Each child follows his own rhythm of progress. That is why it is difficult to write a table and say in it "The infant smiles at one month, he sits at six months." Perhaps he does, or perhaps he does not, but in all probability, he is perfectly normal. If we need averages (and we do for purposes of evaluation) a useful table is as follows.

smiles	6 to 10 weeks
head control (no lag if pulled to sitting position)	3 to 4 months
rolls from back to abdomen	5 to 7 months
transfers toy from hand to hand	6 to 7 months
crawls, sits with slight support	6 to 7 months
creeps and pulls to standing position	9 to 10 months
walks with support (cruises)	10 to 15 months
walks alone	12 to 16 months

In order to illustrate the variations that fall within the normal range, some infants walk at a much earlier age, whereas some never toddle but wait instead until they can walk firmly before they make any serious attempt. Some do not seem to get the "hang" of creeping, and slide along in a sitting position, but they still manage to get to their destination. They do not seem in the least worried about not conforming, and they eventually reach their normal development along with all of the rest.

Why then use tables? If an infant lags too far behind in his progress toward maturity, whether it is in the motor, the intellectual, or in the social area, he is entitled to a careful and complete study of all the factors influencing his behavior. Is his environment so deprived that he has no incentive to learn? Does a physical examination reveal deficiencies? Is his nutrition adequate?

Perhaps he exhibits a strong tendency toward slowness in all areas, and this is significant. Perhaps he is so intent on learning one skill that he postpones learning another. It may mean a "wait and see" attitude, or it may indicate that help is needed. Certainly he is entitled to a careful evaluation. Therefore, some understanding of normal behavior for the various age groups is important.

Average Rate of Achievement During the First Year

The first three months. During the first three months of life, the normal baby makes amazingly rapid developmental progress. He soon commences to become a social being, learning to smile at another person at 8 or 10 weeks. He is undiscriminating in his social response, relating well to anyone who pays attention to him. He learns to make cooing and babbling sounds very early, and at three months, he is able to use these sounds with pleasure on socal occasions.

It is important to remember that the small baby is *responding* to overtures made toward him by the adults in his life, whether these are his parents, baby sitters or nurses. He cannot achieve emotional maturity consistent with his age level either at home or in the hospital if he has no one to stimulate him. The infant who does not respond with a social smile at three months needs to be studied.

At three months, the baby should be able to support his head if he is held upright, although his control is not perfect and his head wobbles about.

He learned to fix his gaze on an object within his immediate line of

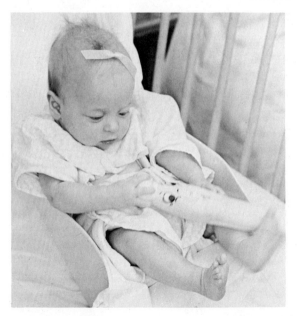

Fig. 41. Three to four months. Enjoys being propped. Focuses attention on toy.

vision during his first weeks of life, and by the age of one month, follows the object briefly with his eyes and his head. At three months, he has developed sufficient hand and eye coordination to attempt to make contact with an offered object, and even holds it briefly if it is put in his grasp.

Most infants at this age sleep throughout the night and have well-defined nap periods during the day, with intervals between for play and feeding.

Three to six months. By the fourth month, the tonic neck reflex is fading, and the child is coordinating the movements of his arms and legs. At this time he enjoys being supported in a sitting position, and holds his head quite steady without bobbing. If placed in a supine position, he raises his head and chest and turns his head from side to side. In another month he learns to roll over. Then let mother or nurse beware when turning her back on him while reaching for those safety pins. (Figs. 41 and 42)

Six to nine months. The six- to seven-month-old has begun to sit, although he still needs some support. He is readily able to grasp objects

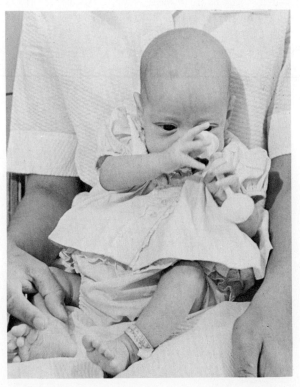

Fig. 42. Eye and hand coordination are good at four months.

which he examines in a purposeful manner. They are transferred from hand to hand, to mouth, looked at critically, then back to hand and then to mouth again. (Fig. 43)

His delight with his own growing abilities is such that he has little time to spare for others. He does enjoy having people around him, however. He experiments with vocal sounds, startling people with sudden loud squeals and crows. His babbling has definite vowel and consonant sounds that he delights in repeating to himself.

At this age it is an excellent practice for mother to babble back to him. He learns by imitation, and it has been observed that an infant learns best if there is social interaction in his environment. Later, he needs clear speech to imitate, but now he is preoccupied with sounds.

An infant at this age enjoys a playpen, as it gives him freedom to roll and to exercise.

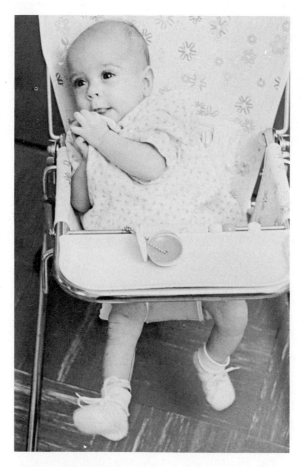

Fig. 43. Six months. Can sit with slight support.

Before the end of this nine-month period, he has probably learned to wave bye-bye and to play pat-a-cake. He has learned that when he says "Ma-ma" or "Da-da," his favorite people come running. He has now learned to distinguish his mother to the extent of complaining when she leaves the room. (Figs. 44 and 45)

At six to eight months, the first teeth may appear, usually the lower central incisors. Babies in good health and showing normal development may differ in timing of tooth eruption. Some families show a tendency toward very early or very late eruption, without other signs of early or late development. At nine to eleven months, the average baby has eight teeth. (Fig. 46)

Some babies appear to experience considerable discomfort as their teeth erupt, and manifest this by fretfulness, disturbed sleep and salivation. The gums may be sensitive and inflamed. Fever or other disturbance is probably due to other causes than normal tooth eruption. A clean, hard teething ring may be helpful.

Nine months to a year. This is an interesting period. The infant learns

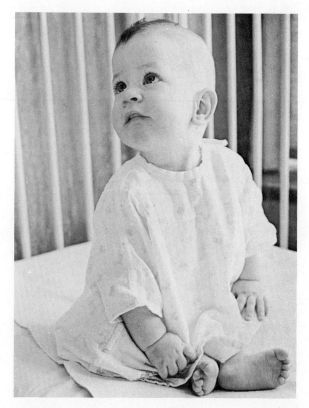

Fig. 44. Eight months. Sitting alone is no problem now.

to shift from a prone to a sitting position, and is soon able to pull himself up to his feet. He doesn't know how to sit down again, however, and cries for help. His mother has barely helped him down when he is up again, a performance repeated many times. This lasts for only a short time; he soon learns. He does refuse to lie supine when he is awake, and the simple task of changing a diaper may become quite a chore.

He learns to creep and gets around faster than his mother anticipates. He begins to resent bars on his playpen and commences a campaign for greater independence. He usually is able to stand alone at 10 or 11 months, and begins to cruise sideways by holding on to objects. (Fig. 47)

The end of the first year is not as much of a landmark, developmentally, as is the 10th or 15th month. Our one-year-old has developed socially to the point where he enjoys being the center of the family group, as he usually is. If his antics are laughed at, he repeats them. (Fig. 48)

He listens intently to words, and his parents have read meaning into two or three of the one-syllable words he uses. He can respond to simple

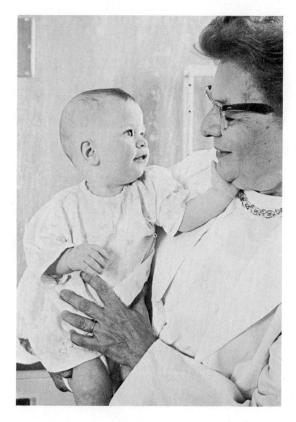

Fig. 45. Eight months. Interested and friendly with people she knows.

directions such as "Wave bye-bye" or "Give it to me." He may even understand "no–no"; whether he heeds is another matter.

At this age, his emotions are differentiated so that he is able to experience fear, anger, love and sympathy. He is beginning to recognize familiar friends and turns away from strangers.

The first year of life is of absorbing interest both to the child himself and to his parents. Changes occur rapidly as the infant reaches new levels of maturity. They occur so rapidly that many mothers are reluctant to be separated from their babies for any length of time for fear of missing a new and fascinating aspect of development. (Fig. 49)

INFANT NUTRITION

There is no rigid, set time for starting the baby on solid foods. There seems to be no advantage to starting solid foods during the first weeks of life, and the experience may be frustrating to a hungry baby. An energetic, fast growing baby, however, may demand more food at an earlier

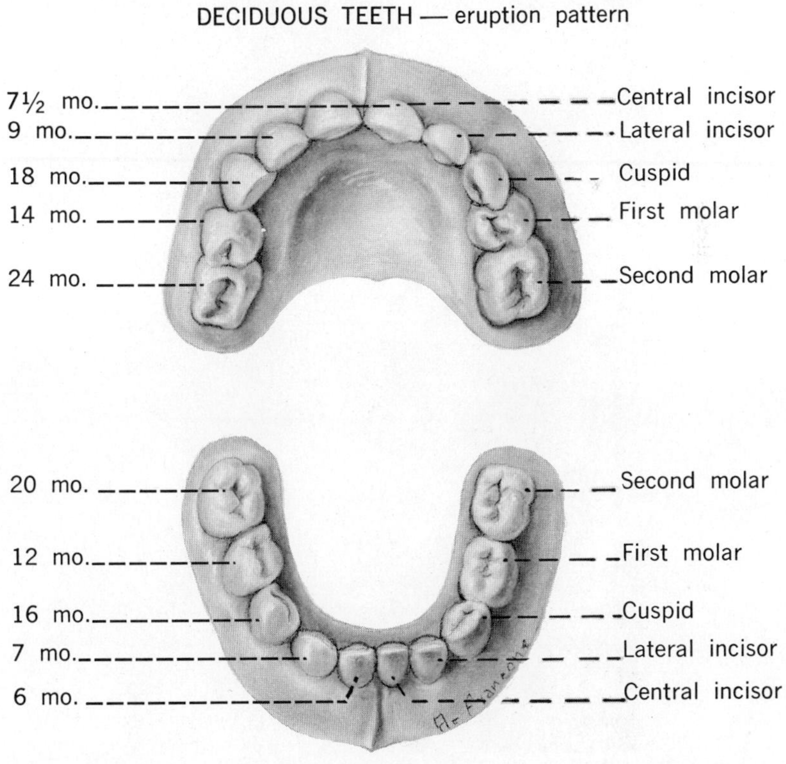

DECIDUOUS TEETH — eruption pattern

7½ mo.	Central incisor
9 mo.	Lateral incisor
18 mo.	Cuspid
14 mo.	First molar
24 mo.	Second molar

20 mo.	Second molar
12 mo.	First molar
16 mo.	Cuspid
7 mo.	Lateral incisor
6 mo.	Central incisor

Fig. 46. Graph showing approximate age for the eruption of deciduous teeth.

age than a more placid infant. If this is the case, a supplement of cereal may be the answer.

The immediate needs during the neonatal period are for the nutrients found in milk, and for vitamins C and D. These vitamins can be supplied in various ways. Vitamin C through orange juice or vitamin drops, vitamin D through fortified milk, cod liver oil or vitamin drops. Although the milk diet is also deficient in iron, the healthy full-term baby has stored enough iron before birth to last him from four to six months.

Somewhere between the ages of one and four months we introduce our baby to solid foods. This first food is usually cereal, for its taste is bland and it is of a smooth consistency, a condition that makes the food more acceptable to the baby who, until now, thought that all food came in liquid form.

This cereal may be a wheat, rice or barley cereal cooked at home, or it may be one of the commercially prepared baby cereals that require only mixing to the right consistency with a little formula.

Bland, strained fruit may be the first food offered, or it may be intro-

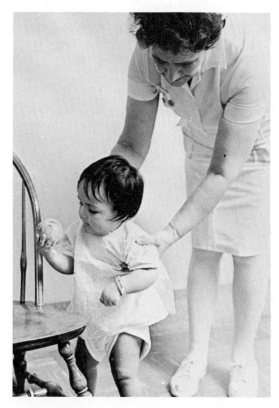

Fig. 47. One year old. Just a little support and she will soon be walking alone.

duced after he is accustomed to cereal. Mashed, ripe bananas are usually enjoyed, also pureéd prunes or peaches.

The baby knows only one way to take food, and that is to thrust his tongue forward as if to suck, which of course has the effect of pushing the food right out of his mouth. The process of transferring food from the front of the mouth to the throat for swallowing is a complicated skill that must be learned. The eager, hungry baby is quite puzzled over this new turn of events, and is apt to become frustrated and annoyed over this routine. "What is all this nonsense, anyhow? Where's my bottle?" he is likely to protest in loud and clear terms. In fact, it is best to let the very hungry baby take the edge off his appetite with part of his formula before proceeding with this new procedure. (Fig. 50)

Babies like their food smooth, thin, lukewarm and bland. If a mother understands that the queer look she gets from her baby is one of astonishment, and that the pushing out of food with the tongue does not mean rejection, she can be patient.

The baby's clothing (and his mother's too) needs protection when he is sitting in his mother's arms. A small spoon fits his mouth better than

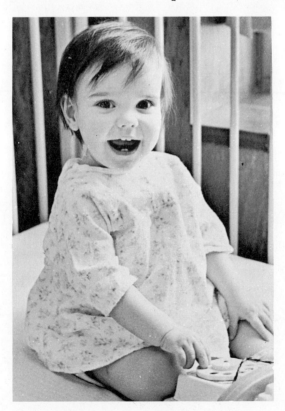

Fig. 48. It's fun to be nearly one.

a large one, and makes it easier to put food further back on the tongue, but not far enough to make the baby gag. The mother needs to catch the food if it is pushed out and offer it again, but her baby soon learns how to manipulate his tongue, and comes to enjoy this novel way of eating.

Foods are started in small amounts, one or two teaspoonsful daily. The choice of mealtime does not matter. It works best, at first, to offer one food for several days until the baby becomes accustomed to it before introducing another.

Strained vegetables are added next, the green and yellow vegetables being a moderately good source of iron. Egg yolk (also a good source of iron) may also be started sometime between three and six months of age. Whole eggs should not be given until much later, because many infants are allergic to egg albumen. The yolk is hard-boiled, finely mashed and started in amounts of about one-fourth of a teaspoonful.

It is difficult to make a formal schedule for infant feeding, because times and amounts vary for individual infants. A full-term, healthy baby may progress from 6 feedings in 24 hours to omission of the late evening formula sometime during the first half of the year.

At six months, most healthy babies are enjoying daily portions of strained vegetable and fruit, cereal twice a day, with egg yolk or strained

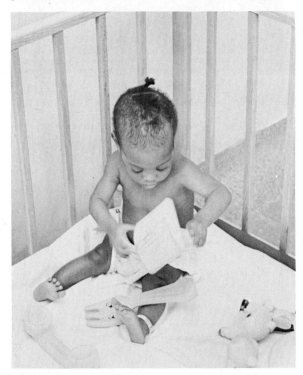

Fig. 49. What does the book say?

meat added to the noon meal. The formula may have become whole milk by now, and the baby is probably learning to drink from a cup, although he still derives much comfort from his bottle.

About this time, teeth are erupting, so a piece of zweiback or of crisp toast is appreciated.

Toward the end of the first year, a baby is usually ready for his three meals a day, with a snack of orange juice and zweiback at midmorning. Chopped foods can be handled now, and whole eggs if he has shown no allergy to egg albumin.

A great variety of pureéd baby foods, chopped junior foods and prepared milk formulas, are on the market, and they certainly relieve mother of much preparation time. It should be remembered, however, that prepared foods involve a considerable expense that many families can ill afford.

The nurse can be helpful and point out that there is no magic in prepared baby food, that vegetables and fruits can be cooked and strained at home, and are just as well accepted by the baby. Cereals can be

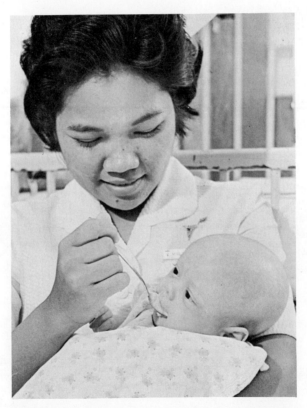

Fig. 50. First solids. A baby tends to push foods out with his tongue.

cooked, and formulas prepared at home as well. Some families prefer to spend more for the convenience and economize elsewhere, but no one should be made to feel that a baby's health or well-being depends on commercially prepared foods.

The well baby's appetite is the best index of the proper amount of food. Healthy babies enjoy eating and accept most foods, preferring those that are slightly sweet or slightly salty, but not strong-flavored or bitter. Realizing that a baby learns by imitation, we should be careful not to show our dislikes or prejudices against certain foods in his presence. If the baby does show a definite dislike for any particular food, there is no point in forcing it, because this is one of the best ways to make certain that he sees feeding time as an occasion for a battle of will power. However, a dislike for a certain food does not need to be permanent, and the rejected food may be offered again at a later date. The important point is to avoid making an issue of likes or dislikes. As has been aptly put, "A child will find it much easier to learn to like squash, for example, if he does not have a reputation as a squash hater to live up to."

MAINTENANCE OF HEALTH

Every infant is entitled to the best possible protection against disease, and because he cannot take the proper precautions himself, our duty is to do it for him. This care extends beyond his daily needs for food, sleep, cleanliness, love and security, to concern for his future health and well-being.

Within a very short span of time, medical science has discovered measures providing immunity against a number of serious or crippling diseases without the person having to provide his own immunity by contracting the disease itself. Because of the means at hand (which, at a very minimum of risk, assure protection against conditions such as diphtheria, smallpox, tetanus, and now polio and measles) we cannot afford to take chances with our children's health with inadequate immunization.

The chronically ill child may not need to forego this protection, depending on his condition and our present knowledge; but whether he is given immunization, or protected from contact from these diseases, is a matter to be discussed in connection with the condition itself. The immunization schedule here presented concerns the healthy child.

Immunization Schedule

The Academy of Pediatrics, through its committee on the control of infectious diseases,* has recommended a schedule of immunization for healthy children living under normal conditions. Children with certain chronic or acute conditions, or children who can be expected to be

---

* Report of the Committee on the Control of Infectious Diseases. 15th ed. Evanston, Illinois, American Academy of Pediatrics, 1966.

TABLE 9-2.

RECOMMENDED SCHEDULE FOR ACTIVE IMMUNIZATION
AND TUBERCULIN TESTING OF NORMAL INFANTS
AND CHILDREN.*

2 to 3 months	DPT	type 1 OPV or trivalent OPV[2]
3 to 4 months	DPT	type 3 OPV or trivalent OPV
4 to 5 months	DPT	type 2 OPV or trivalent OPV
9 to 11 months	tuberculin test	
12 months	measles vaccine	
15 to 18 months	DPT—trivalent OPV—smallpox vaccine[2]	
2 years	tuberculin test	
3 years	DPT—tuberculin test	
4 years	tuberculin test	
6 years	TD—smallpox vaccine—tuberculin test	
	trivalent OPV	
8 years	tuberculin test[4]	
10 years	tuberculin test[4]	
12 years	TD—smallpox vaccine—tuberculin test[3,4]	
14 years	tuberculin test	
16 years	tuberculin test	

Abbreviations—DPT (diphtheria and tetanus toxoids and pertussis vaccine combined); OPV (oral poliovaccine—if trivalent OPV used—interval should be 6 weeks or longer); TD tetanus and diphtheria toxoids, adult type).

[1] Immunization may be started at any age. The immune response is limited in a proportion of young infants, and the recommended booster doses are designed to insure or maintain immunity. Protection of infants against pertussis should start early. The best protection of newborn infants against pertussis is avoidance of household contacts by adequate immunization of older siblings. This schedule is intended as a flexible guide that may be modified, within certain limits, to fit individual situations.

[2] Initial smallpox vaccine may be given at any time between 12 and 24 months of age.

[3] Frequency of repeated tuberculin tests depend on risk of exposure of children under care, and the prevalence of tuberculosis in the population group.

[4] After age 12, follow procedures recommended for adults: i.e., smallpox vaccine every 5 years and tetanus toxoid booster every 10 years as TD.

exposed to certain infectious conditions such as typhoid, need a modification of schedule.

Present day recommendations include inoculation of all healthy children against diphtheria, pertussis, tetanus, measles, poliomyelitis, and smallpox.

The triple antigen, consisting of diphtheria and tetanus toxoids and pertussis vaccine (DPT) is given intramuscularly, preferably into the midlateral muscles of the thigh or the deltoid.†

Polio vaccine may be given intramuscularly as inactivated poliovaccine (IPV—Salk), or as oral poliovirus vaccine (OPV—Sabin). There are

* Report of the Committee on Control of Infectious Diseases. P. 5. Evanston, Illinois, American Academy of Pediatrics, 1966.

† ibid, p. 4.

no contraindications for oral poliovirus vaccine for children under the age of eighteen, it is accepted more readily by the child, and appears to have a superiority to IPV in its protective capacity and immunization effect.

If inactivated poliovaccine is used, a basic course of inoculation requires 4 doses, the first 3 at monthly intervals, and the fourth, 6 to 12 months later. Repeated biennial booster doses are necessary for maintenance of antibody levels.†

Smallpox vaccination is accomplished by the use of the multiple pressure method.

Contraindications to Inoculations.

1. Any acute respiratory disease or some other active infection. Prolonging intervals between injections, up to six months, does not interfere with final immunity.

2. Infants with eczema or other forms of dermatitis should not receive smallpox vaccination because of danger of eczema vaccinatum. The infant with dermatitis may receive cross infection from any freshly vaccinated person. Thus all exposure must be avoided. Infants with eczema vaccinatum are seriously ill, with a mortality range of 30 to 40 per cent.

3. Individual conditions, such as leukemia, may make inoculations inadvisable.

Research is proceeding rapidly in the field of preventive measures against infectious disease. Any table giving timing of immunization agents is subject to change as newer knowledge is acquired. The literature should be studied for recent advances.

DAILY LIVING

Emotional Development

The change from hospital to home living may be disrupting to the young infant as well as to his family. For a short time everyone needs to adjust to the situation while the baby and his family learn together. Many "problems" really turn out not to be problems at all, but only trial-and-error methods of learning new adjustments.

Being held, loved and cherished is the birthright of any child. It is important to understand very clearly the way a young infant behaves. Remember that he has had no background experience. He cannot reason with himself thus: "Although my stomach is contracting in painful spasms because it is empty, it is not yet time for my feeding, and my mother is busy at the moment. She will have to pick me up and change my diaper, but right now she is soothing my two-year-old brother who just fell and scraped his knee. Therefore, I must be patient because I know that she

† ibid, p. 51.

will attend to me as quickly as possible." No, he knows only that he hurts, and he knows only one way to react; that is to cry.

Neither can he reason "I know that my mother loves me, she has shown it before when she held me and attended to my needs." No, he can only feel that his pains are soothed when his mother satisfies his hunger. After repeated experiences of satisfaction, experience teaches him that mother is the source of his pleasure, and that the warm, blissful feeling of repletion and loving care comes when she holds him and attends to his physical needs.

Pleasure Principle versus Reality Principle

We say that the young infant operates on the pleasure principle, and this is true. It is impossible to learn in an atmosphere of *uncertainty* and *insecurity*. If you have ever been in a classroom and struggled with some problem about which you had not grasped the fundamental principle, you can understand this. The problem did not become clear, and you never did catch up until you learned the *fundamentals*. Why, then, do we expect the infant to learn to wait, to stand discomfort, when he has not yet learned the *fundamentals?* Would it not be better to pick him up when he cries, love and soothe him, feed him, make him comfortable, until he finally learns the meaning of *security* and *love?* Then, and only then, can he move on to greater maturity, toward the advanced *reality principle.* Then he can begin to learn the satisfaction that comes when immediate satisfaction waits on a more desirable future goal.

Certainly we need to use common sense. In the same way that a young baby exercises his muscles, he exercises his lungs by crying. He may also become too tired through excessive handling or stimulation, and respond the only way he knows, by crying. Perhaps mother or nurse has to learn by experience too; but it takes only a small amount of practice to learn when baby is uncomfortable, when he is crying just for exercise, or when he just wants to be left alone.

Do we "Spoil" the Baby?

The infant in the hospital seldom becomes over-stimulated from play or fondling. At this early age, he does not discern his mother as a particular individual, but rather as a being who provides satisfaction and security for him in generous quantities. Anyone who fits the picture will do. Later, during his first year of life, he becomes more perceptive, and attachment to his mother is extremely close, making separation intolerable to him. Of course the word "mother" when used in this connection, means the person who is with him and cares for him constantly. A "mother figure" is not necessarily his natural mother, but may perhaps be a grandmother or some other mother substitute whom a baby has learned to accept as a mother. She must, however, be a constant figure with warm, accepting qualities in order for the baby to learn the meaning of trust and security. He needs to develop maximum security before he can cope with frustration.

Of one thing we can be confident; the young infant needs no more frustration than the experience of birth gives him. Sometimes mothers, and nurses as well, worry that they will "spoil" the infant or young child by giving prompt, consistent attention to his distress signals. Miss Blake puts this very well when she says of frustration in early infancy

A 'spoiled' child is one who does not know what he wants. He was never satisfied in his infancy, and because it happened before he was able to understand he is in a perpetual state of fear lest his needs remain unsatisfied. Meeting an infant's needs does not 'spoil' a child—it is lack of confidence that gratification will come that makes an infant or child overwhelmingly demanding, perpetually dissatisfied, unhappy and fearful.

As the infant matures, he learns to differentiate between himself and others. If his previous experience has been satisfying, his sense of trust and security will become well established, and he will be able to take the next step in development; that of being able to postpone immediate satisfaction for a greater future fulfillment.

The Infant's Relationship to Mother

As we have seen, the young infant has awareness of only his own needs, and is unable to distinguish between himself and his environment. As he matures, however, he gradually learns that the gratification of his needs comes from a source outside himself. The person who attends to these needs, who supplies comfort and satisfaction, does of necessity become the one to whom he turns for gratification.

The mother who gave him birth is the person whom we expect to provide security for the young infant. However, it is probable that the infant himself is unaware of this particular relationship, and responds to the person who meets his needs despite the possibility that she is not responsible for his birth.

The young infant does not, apparently, need to have one person only to whom he makes his response, as he responds to the comfort and security provided rather than to visual identification. His need is for the stimulation and interaction provided in a warm, close relationship. Without this, he does not develop: deprived of a previously satisfactory relationship, he regresses, physically and emotionally.

As the infant's development continues, his world widens and he becomes more visually aware of those who care for him. Somewhere around the sixth month, most infants manifest this growing awareness by sobering at the sight of an unfamiliar face. He takes longer to respond to the overtures of strange persons, but he can be won over quite easily by kindness and understanding.

At about nine months, or perhaps a year, the infant is comfortable in the familiar, but now perceives the unfamiliar as potentially dangerous. This is the response that is to be foremost in his experience for some time to come. Even when he matures enough to enjoy the challenge of the unknown and adventurous, he needs some connection with the tried and familiar for his security.

The working mother. With the knowledge mentioned above, how do we satisfy the needs of those infants whose mothers work away from home during much of the day? A look at today's world confirms the fact that many mothers of young children are employed outside the home.

The Children's Bureau supplies some interesting statistics. Of the 22 million women in the United States who were employed outside their homes in 1958, 7.5 million had children under the age of 18. Of this number, 2.9 million had children under the age of 6.

Although these figures tell us that the largest proportion of these women were mothers of older children, the nearly 3 million mothers of children under the age of 6 make a large group.

It is true that many mothers who have planned to go back to work shortly after the birth of their babies find themselves unwilling to do so. They realize how much pleasure they are depriving themselves of and their infants by separation. However, for the mother who must resume employment while baby is small, what is the best course for her to take?

In view of the young infant's dependency and need for individual care, day nurseries and care centers are quite unsatisfactory. These children thrive best in individual day care homes. Care should be exercised in chosing a home that would be right for the child. The day care mother probably should not attempt to care for more than two babies, or only one if she already has one of her own.

The person caring for the infant should be genuinely fond of babies, and show the warmth that the young infant must have to develop normally. She must be physically and emotionally capable of giving the necessary care. A majority of states require that such day care homes be licensed, and that they meet certain standards of cleanliness, hygiene and wholesome environment.

A better solution to the problem of care for the young infant who must have a substitute mother, for at least part of the time, is the employment of a satisfactory person to come into the child's home instead of taking him away from his own environment. This is not always possible, and many babies do make good adjustment to a part time day-mother in her own home.

When the infant needs total care, however, he still thrives best in a good foster home rather than in a residential nursery, however good it may be. Such nurseries for young infants are gradually disappearing from today's scene. At most, the infant is likely to be kept in a nursery until a proper home for him can be found. At present, the infant who is physically or mentally handicapped is still the child who is probably going to be given care in a custodial nursery, but additional steps are being taken. Foster homes for all infants who cannot be cared for at home are being sought, and the public is being educated to the needs of these children.

The difficulty, of course, in any of these plans is in finding good foster homes for infants, whether this includes only day care or complete care. It is also true that most women who offer short-term care to small infants or children do so primarily for the financial reward, small though it is. This does not preclude loving care, but it does place a somewhat different emphasis on the care involved. The situation is difficult in any case, because the foster mother hesitates to become emotionally involved with a child who must leave her after a short time.

In homes in which the family is broken by sickness or absence of the mother, or in which the mother is incapable of giving the kind of support needed for the child's healthy development, homemaker service may be very helpful, especially if the family is reluctant to be separated. In any case, although it is generally agreed that baby is best served when he is in his own home with loving parents who have feelings of pride and fulfillment in him, he is not necessarily deprived unduly if circumstances make it necessary for a suitable person to share in his care.

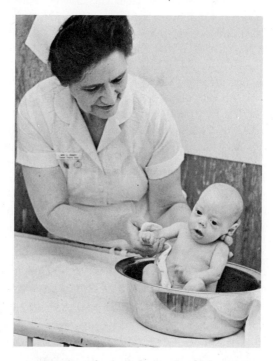

Fig. 51. The bath basin should be set in the crib for safety.

HOSPITAL CARE OF THE INFANT
Physical Care

A patient enters the hospital for one purpose only, to become physically well. We know that his physical welfare is greatly affected by his mental and emotional state. We have come to realize that a child cannot thrive physically if he is emotionally disturbed or if he is allowed to stagnate mentally. We must continually keep in mind that all of his needs must be met as nearly as possible in the highly artificial hospital setting.

In all of this, however, our basic goal remains the same: to restore the child to physical health and return him to his parents. Whether a hospital is the place for sick children is a question open to serious doubt, but we can not debate this at the moment. We are now speaking of the child who has already been admitted to the hospital. What type of care will we give him that can be instrumental in speeding him toward that day of discharge for which he so ardently longs?

The everyday routine care is important, and the nurse who has had little experience in handling infants in the hospital can profit by learning the practical application of basic principles of infant care and hygiene.

Bathing the Infant

A daily bath is desirable if the infant's condition allows this. The baby in the hospital should have his own bath basin, his own soap, and his individual bathing table. If the baby has no dressing or other contraindications, placing him in the bath rather than giving him a sponge bath can have a soothing and comforting effect.

Procedure for a Tub Bath for a Small Infant. Gather together all equipment before starting.

> large basin or small tub
> soap (hexachlorophene soap may be used)
> clean cotton balls
> soft wash cloth
> large soft towel or small cotton blanket

Water in the basin should be about 95° to 100°. A bath thermometer may be used, or the temperature may be tested by the time-honored elbow test. The water should feel comfortably warm to the elbow.

Small babies squirm and move about much more than an inexperienced person might expect. A basic rule in their care is never to turn one's back on an infant when the crib side is down. A very sensible precaution when bathing a baby is to put the bath basin right in the crib and thus do away with the need for turning from the baby. Crib mattresses are plastic covered and sheets can be changed, so splashed water is no problem. (Fig. 51)

Before undressing a baby, wash his face with clean water, using either the washcloth or cotton balls. This includes washing eyes and ears. Cotton balls are useful if any discharge is present, as a clean one can be used each time and then discarded.

If dried mucus is present in the anterior nares, a wisp of cotton may be twisted, dipped in clean water and used for cleaning the nose. This may cause baby to sneeze and bring down more mucus which can be wiped away.

Applicators have no place in the ordinary cleansing of a baby's eyes, ears or nose. Injury to the mucus membrane easily occurs as the baby squirms. Any material in the ears or nose that is too deep to remove without probing should be removed by the use of appropriate instruments in the hands of a trained person if it is important that it be removed.

The baby's scalp may next be soaped, then the baby picked up by sliding your hand and your arm under him, grasping his head firmly as you hold it over the basin to rinse the soap away. (Fig. 52)

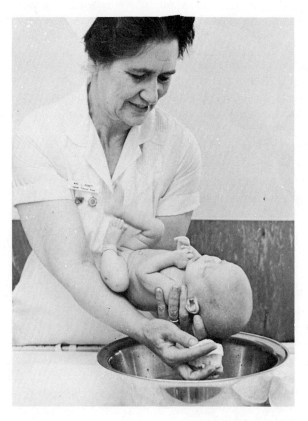

Fig. 52. Hold the baby securely while washing her head.

After drying his head, undress the baby and examine his body for rashes or excoriations. You may then soap his body all over and lift him into the basin, supporting his head and shoulders on your arm. Some nurses prefer to soap the infant with their free hand while he is still in the tub, because a soapy baby is slippery and difficult to pick up.

If the baby is enjoying this experience, make it a leisurely one, and let him stay in the water for a few minutes as you take this opportunity to talk and to play with him. After he is finished, lift him out, wrap him in a towel or a blanket and pat him dry, paying attention to creases. Perhaps it should be noted that if the baby's diaper was soiled when it was removed, the feces should be wiped from his buttocks before placing him in the bath.

After the bath, the labia in girl babies should be separated and cleansed with cotton and clean water if this is needed. Boy babies have usually been circumcised and need only be inspected for cleanliness. An uncircumcised boy needs to have the foreskin gently retracted and any accumulation of smegma or debris washed off. If the foreskin does not easily retract, do not force it, but report this to the pediatrician.

For the baby with healthy skin, powders, lotions and ointments are unnecessary. Powder tends to cake in the creases and cause irritation. A baby may have an allergy to the ingredients in baby lotion; in any case, a clean baby smells sweet enough without adding any trimmings.

An excessively dry skin may benefit from the application of mineral oil or a neutral lubricant. If powder is needed, corn starch is non-irritating. Various medicated ointments are available for excoriated skin areas.

A baby's fingernails need to be inspected and cut if they are long, because he can scratch his face with his aimless arm movements. The nails should be cut straight across, using care to hold the arm and the hand firmly while cutting.

Bathing the Older Infant. For the older infant, the procedure is essentially the same. When the baby is old enough to sit and move about freely, he may enjoy the regular bathtub, but usually this is frightening to him. Splashing about in a small tub may be more fun, especially with the addition of a floating toy. Try to schedule your time so that this can be a leisurely process, a time for nurse and baby to enjoy together.

Sponge Bathing. For the infant who cannot be placed in a tub, a sponge bath has to be sufficient. There are several points to remember.

1. The face and head must always be washed with clean water and a washcloth before handling the rest of the body. Never does the nurse go back to the face after changing the diaper or washing the perineum without first thoroughly washing her hands. Usually it is best to wash the face and head before undressing the child.

2. Use sufficient, *warm* water in the basin. The water can be warmer

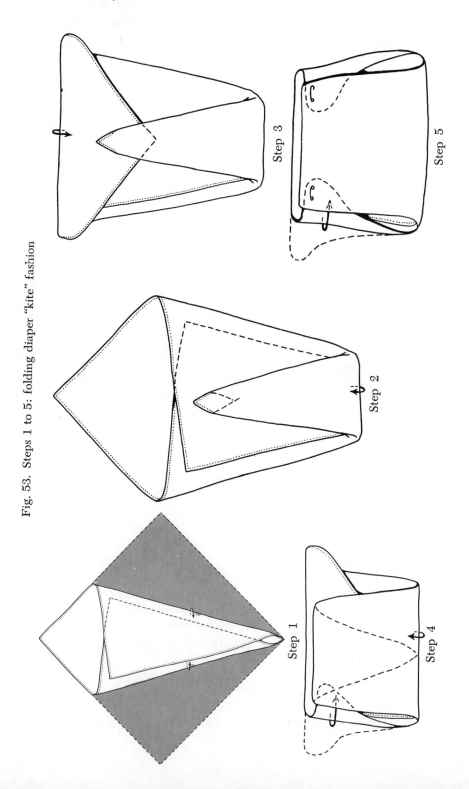

Fig. 53. Steps 1 to 5: folding diaper "kite" fashion

Step 1

Step 2

Step 3

Step 4

Step 5

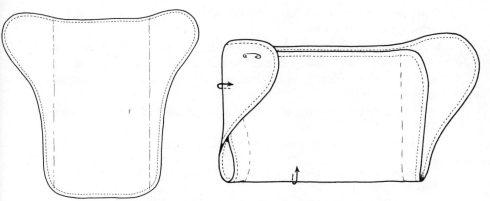

Fig. 54a. Diapers may be purchased ready shaped.

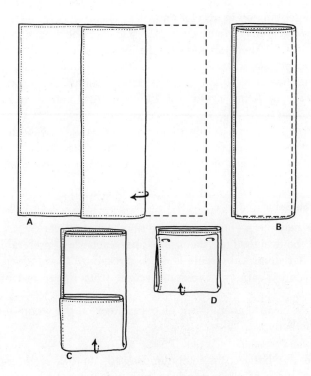

Fig. 54b. Steps to follow for folding a diaper in an oblong fashion.

for a sponge than for a tub bath. Make an effort to keep the baby from becoming chilled.

3. After washing the child's body, wash the perineum using downward strokes, moving from front to back. Do not use a washcloth to go over the area more than once; if more than one stroke is needed, use a clean cotton ball each time.

4. Turn the baby on his abdomen if possible, and wash the rectal area last.

Naturally all precautions outlined for tub bathing are necessary here as well.

Dressing the Baby

Babies in the hospital wear cotton shirts or gowns and diapers except in hot weather when a diaper alone is sufficient. The easiest way to dress a small baby is to grasp his hand and pull his arm through the sleeve. If gowns that tie in back are used, care must be taken to see that they fit properly, are not too tight around the neck, or too loose, thus allowing the baby to get tangled in his clothing.

Diapers come in various sizes and shapes. The important point to remember is that there should not be bunched material between the thighs. Two popular diaper styles are either the oblong strip pinned at the sides, or the square diaper folded "kite" fashion. The latter kind has the advantage of being useful for different ages and sizes. (Figs. 53 and 54)

The older infant needs his diaper pinned snugly at both hips and legs to prevent feces from running out at the open spaces. The nurse needs only to clean a soiled crib and smeared baby once or twice to remember this.

Weighing the Baby

A baby may be weighed daily, semi-weekly, or weekly, as ordered. He should be weighed at the same time each day, preferably before breakfast. A regular baby scale is used. Procedure is as follows:

1. Ascertain the baby's previous weight from the record of the last weighing.

2. Place a clean diaper, sheet, or paper liner on the scoop of the scale in which the baby is to lie.

3. Balance the scale.

4. Place the baby, completely undressed, on the scale and weigh. Use a small piece of clean paper to manipulate the scales if this is the practice in the nursery.

5. In case of a significant discrepancy from the previous recorded weight, check the scale balance and have your findings checked by a second person.

6. Remove the infant from the scale, discarding the scoop liner.

7. Enter weight in the appropriate space on the chart with weight recording countersigned by a second person if necessary. (Fig. 55)

Taking the Baby's Temperature

In most sick baby nurseries, rectal temperatures are routine, although some favor axillary temperature taking. Each baby should have his own thermometer which should be cleaned after each use. The thermometer should be kept in a special container in the bedside stand, or in a container attached to the wall of his cubicle.

Before taking the temperature, inspect the thermometer for breakage, especially at the bulb. If the thermometer has been kept in a solution, rinse it and shake it to below 98°.

If the baby has his temperature taken rectally, hold his ankles firmly as you raise his legs to expose the rectum, and insert the thermometer into the rectum just past the bulb of the thermometer. Both the thermometer and the baby should be held firmly, and the nurse should keep her mind on the business at hand, because thermometers have been broken by kicking and squirming babies. Three or four minutes is considered a sufficiently long insertion to get an accurate temperature.

After use, clean the thermometer with a soapy cotton ball, rinse it with water, and soak it in an antiseptic solution for the designated time, then dry it, and replace it in its container.

Feeding

Principles and techniques of feeding have been discussed in the section on infant nutrition. Every effort should be made to make eating an

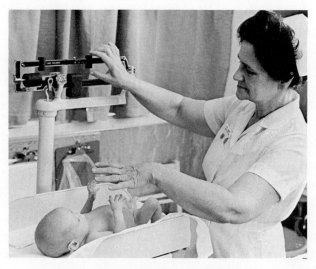

Fig. 55. Weighing a baby.

enjoyable experience for the infant. To this end, care should be taken to allow no disagreeable or painful procedures to interrupt feeding time. Only a little consideration and forethought is necessary to accomplish this.

Medications and Treatments

Oral Medications. A small baby is not too partcular about the taste of his food if he is hungry. Almost anything liquid can be sucked through a nipple, including liquid medicines, unless they are quite bitter. Medications that come in syrup or fruit-flavored suspensions are easily administered this way. Another method of administering oral medications is to drop them into the baby's mouth with plastic medicine droppers. If a small medicine cup is used, remember that an infant only swallows a few drops at a time. Too much poured into his mouth may cause him to choke and perhaps to aspirate, or he may simply let the medication run out of his mouth.

When giving medicine to an infant, raise his head and shoulders from the bed, or hold him in a semi-upright position. Be certain to make a positive identification of the child. He is entirely dependent on you, and he cannot tell you if you have the wrong patient.

After giving him the medication, open his mouth to see if he has swallowed all of it. Leave him lying on his side, or with his head elevated, as a precaution against aspiration should he vomit.

Elixirs contain alcohol and are apt to make him choke unless they are diluted. Syrups and suspensions do not need dilution in themselves, but are thick, and they may need dilution to insure that the baby gets the full dose.

The nurse, of course, should be aware of the purpose of the medication she is giving as well as its composition and side effects. She should

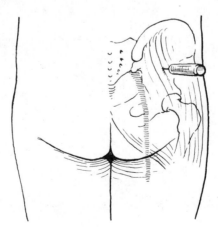

Fig. 56. An intramuscular injection
into the gluteal muscle.

double-check the dosage and make certain that her computations are correct. She should watch for any untoward effects from the drug and report them promptly.

Errors in medications. Nurses are human and can make errors. To admit an error, is often difficult, especially if there has been carelessness or laxity concerning the rules. A person may be strongly tempted to adopt a "wait and see" attitude. This, of course, is the gravest error of all. It is much easier for a nurse to accept the censure of the doctor or the head nurse, whether deserved or undeserved, than to endure anxiety and guilt she feels while she waits to see if there are to be any ill effects. She certainly should want to avoid, at all costs, the terrible guilt that comes if the child suffers any serious consequences from her error, and which might have been avoided had the mistake been disclosed promptly.

Intramuscular injections. Certain precautions must be taken when intramuscular medications are used, especially if they are for infants. Many of the antibiotics irritate subcutaneous tissue and cause sloughing or form abscesses if they are not injected deep into the muscle. An inexperienced nurse may be fearful of plunging the needle deeply enough into muscular tissue, especially if she is treating a small baby. A 21 or 22 gauge needle, one inch in length, is preferable for intramuscular use with infants.

Intramuscular injections for the adult are routinely given into the gluteal muscle. The nurse, using reasonable caution and applying her

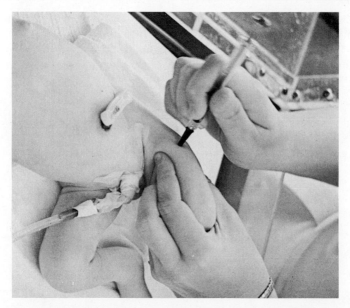

Fig. 57. An intramuscular injection into the anterior-lateral aspect of the thigh.

knowledge of anatomy, has little difficulty in selecting the correct site. She knows that she must inject into the upper outer-quadrant of the buttock in order to avoid striking the sciatic nerve. She divides the buttock into quarters and selects the correct area. (Fig. 56)

With an infant, the selection of the proper site is much more difficult. The area is very small, the crest of the iliac, which forms the upper boundary, is higher than she expects. Because serious injury has been done to the sciatic nerve by improperly administered injections, many pediatricians prefer that the injection be given in the lateral or anterior midthigh, where the quadriceps muscle offers a wider area. Care must be taken to avoid the femoral cutaneous nerve by choosing the lateral or anterior portion of the thigh, midway between the knee and the hip. (Figs. 57 and 58)

Following any injection or painful treatment, the baby must be soothed and comforted.

Assisting with intravenous therapy. Intravenous therapy is quite commonly used for sick infants, either to correct electrolyte imbalance, as a medium for medication, or as a method of feeding.

The small veins of infants are difficult to enter and tend to collapse easily. It is most disheartening to find intravenous fluid infiltrating into the subcutaneous tissues after a doctor has spent a long time starting the infusion. It is difficult to tell who is more frustrated, the baby or the doctor. It follows then, that intravenous infusions must be watched very carefully.

A scalp vein is frequently chosen for the site, because in small infants, it is relatively easy to enter and easier to manage. Special scalp-vein needles attached to small tubing are obtainable. The area on the scalp to be used needs to be shaved and to be cleansed with antiseptic. (Fig. 59)

The baby should be mummied (see Fig. 60) for the insertion, and his

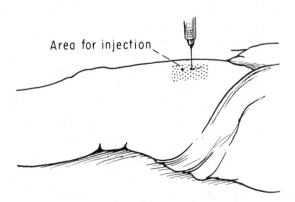

Area for injection

Fig. 58. An intramuscular injection into the midposition of the thigh.

head held firmly against the treatment table. After insertion, the needle should be firmly taped in place, and the plastic tubing taped to the side of the infant's head or cheek.

Sandbags are used to immobilize the head, and clove hitch restraints are useful to prevent the infant from reaching the needle or catching his arm in the tubing.

Other sites are on the back of the hand, the flexor surfaces of the wrist and the medial side of the ankle. The antecubital space is seldom used in small children because it is extremely difficult to restrain the child so that he cannot bend his arm.

Intravenous drip must be slow for the small child, in order to avoid overloading the circulation and inducing cardiac failure. It is extremely difficult to slow a regular intravenous drip to 4 or 6 drops per minute and still have it function properly. Various adapting devices are available which decrease the size of the drop to a "mini" or "micro" drop of 1/50 or 1/60 ml., thus delivering 50 to 60 mini- or micro- drops per cubic centimeter rather than the 15 drops of a regular set. Many intravenous sets also contain a control chamber that is designed to deliver controlled volumes of fluid, avoiding the inadvertent entrance of too great a volume of fluid into the child's system. (Fig. 61)

None of these safeguards obviate the necessity of frequent inspection of the therapy. The drops are counted frequently and the site of injection examined. The child's movements frequently cause the infusion to slow up or to speed up, or may cause the needle to slip out of the vein. Routine recording of the rate and the amount of fluid is necessary.

The intravenous infusion therapy is uncomfortable, and the necessary restraints increase the child's frustration. If the nurse is reasonably careful, and if the needle is securely taped, the infant can frequently be held for comforting and relaxation.

When long-term intravenous therapy is contemplated, an intravenous cut-down is usually performed. This is accomplished by cutting down to

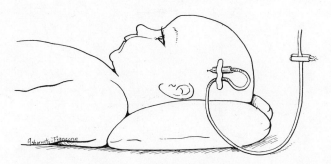

Fig. 59. A scalp vein infusion.

the vein and threading in plastic tubing, with two or three silk sutures required to close the wound. This requires a sterile dressing and subsequent removal of the sutures.

A more recent technique that modifies this surgical procedure is the use of an especially constructed needle through which tubing can be threaded into the vein and the needle then withdrawn, thus doing away with the dissection of a cut-down.

The infant needs careful restraint to avoid difficulties at the start of an intravenous infusion as well as to prevent him from dislodging the needle later. The mummy restraint is useful when attempting the scalp vein technique, or a modified mummy leaving an arm or a foot free if another site is used. A clove-hitch restraint for arms or legs gives the infant some freedom, and at the same time prevents interference with continuing therapy, or elbow restraints may be useful. Sandbags are necessary to immobilize the head if a scalp vein is used. (Fig. 62)

Types of intravenous fluids. Intravenous fluids are manufactured to meet many needs—for correcting electrolyte imbalance, for supplying additional protein or carbohydrate, and as vehicles for medications. Many of these, however, still need modification if they are to meet individual infant requirements.

Mixing intravenous solutions requires considerable technical skill, the use of aseptic technique, and correct calculations. It should be attempted only under supervision until the nurse has become proficient. The addi-

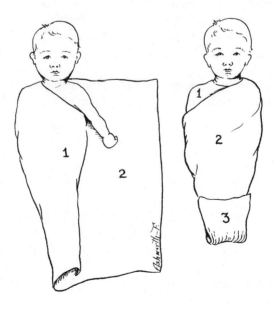

Fig. 60. Mummy restraint.

tion of medication to intravenous fluid also calls for conscientious and experienced personnel.

Obtaining Urine Specimens

Routine urine specimens are obtained from all infants and children on admission to the hospital. Many of these children need subsequent specimens for specific tests. In order to obtain a urine specimen from an infant, it is usually necessary to attach some kind of a collector to his perineum.

The simplest way to obtain a specimen is by the use of a plastic urine

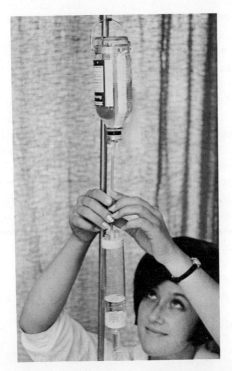

Fig. 61. Regulating intravenous flow.

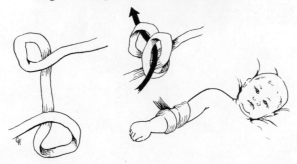

Fig. 62. The clove hitch restraint.

collector, popularly called a P.U.C.* This collector is made of a flexible plastic material secured to a sponge ring that surrounds a round opening made to fit over the infant's genitals and secured by pressure-sensitive adhesive. It is easily removed after the infant voids, and the adhesive surfaces can be pressed together to form a leakproof bag. (Fig. 63)

Other kinds of containers include glass bird-seed cups for girls and glass or plastic test tubes for boys, secured in place by a cotton belt or by adhesive. These containers should have their edges covered with adhesive and those with chipped edges discarded. Any type of collector should be inspected frequently when in place and removed as soon as the specimen is obtained.

Catheterizations are rarely performed on infants, a clean specimen being satisfactory in most instances. To obtain a clean specimen from a female infant, have a bowl of soap and water with cotton balls ready; separate the labia and clean with downward strokes moving outward to the perineum, and using a clean cotton ball for each stroke. For a male, the penis and perineum are cleaned in the same manner. An antiseptic solution, such as benzalkonium chloride (Zephiran) may be used in place of, or in addition to, the soap solution. The P.U.C. or sterilized container is then applied. Although a midstream specimen is desirable, it is unrealistic to try to get such a specimen from an infant.

Continuous urine collection. Continuous urine collections for a period of 12 or 24 hours are often necessary to help establish diagnoses. Various methods have been devised, with varying degrees of success. Usually, an incomplete specimen is unsatisfactory for diagnostic purposes; therefore it is important that no urine be lost during the collection period.

One method for males utilizes a rubber finger cot fitted over the penis with a small hole made in the closed end, fitted on to a rubber or plastic

---

* Pediatric Urine Collector. Sterilon Company, Buffalo, New York.

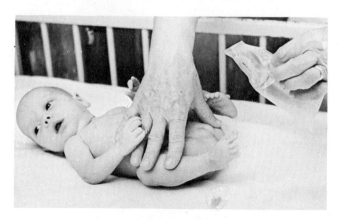

Fig. 63. Applying a plastic urine collector.

tubing that drains into a large container. The finger cot needs frequent inspection because it may become twisted and cut off the flow. A plastic or pyrex funnel may be used in the same manner for either sex, or an ileostomy bag placed over the genital area and tubing inserted through a small hole made in the closed end.

An ingenious device for continuous urine collection has been perfected and is useful for small infants. This consists of a nylon mesh screen stretched over a frame on which the baby lies. This frame fits into a bassinet, or may be used in a small crib. Urine filters through the screen and is funneled into a container between frame and mattress.

Emotional Care

The infant in the hospital finds his development retarded to the degree that his normal pattern of living is hampered. Probably a short-term illness is not going to present him with any grave psychological problems if he is given the affection and loving care that his nature demands, and if he is promptly restored to his family. A long-term hospitalization presents

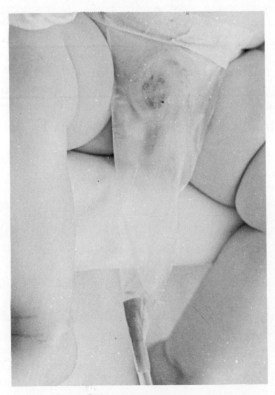

Fig. 64. Plastic urine collectors for continuous collection are now available.

different problems, even if the infant is receiving considerable attention during his stay.

What happens to the baby who lies in the hospital for long periods of time, with little manifestation of love that he can understand and little tactile stimulation? Illness in itself is frustrating, causing pain and discomfort, and forcing limitation of normal activity. None of this is understood by the infant. Add to all of this a cold, sterile atmosphere, little cuddling or rocking, and you find that cleanliness and treatment of illness is not enough. Not once or twice, but often, a pediatrician has sent home a baby who has not been responding to treatment in the hospital, to find that the baby commenced to thrive in a home that may lack cleanliness and proper hygiene, but is rich in warmth and love.

The pediatric nurse must thoroughly understand and accept the principle that rocking and cuddling a child, playing with him, or perhaps just the watchful observation of a sick infant, are all essential elements of nursing care. She may find that this principle is not always well understood by all personnel. If the nurse feels harassed or criticized for "standing around when there is much work to be done," she may need to clarify her objectives and examine her motives. Does she have the child's emotional welfare in mind? If so, has she made any effort to explain to others what she is trying to accomplish?

She may perhaps need to think things out rather like this: "To me, this form of support seems essential, but I can understand how it may look to a charge nurse who is under pressure from doctors, mothers, supervisors, and from the children themselves. Perhaps this is not the right time for this particular form of nursing care. It may be that there are other more important duties at this moment, and I can pick this up again later. In the meantime, what can I substitute for the personal attention I cannot give immediately?"

Seldom does one person have all the right answers, but team conferences or group discussions can be used to good advantage in exploring problems of emotional support.

Hospitalization for an infant may have other adverse effects. The small infant's maturation moves along largely as a result of his physical development. The infant hindered by his environment from reaching out and meeting the challenge presented to him by his developing senses becomes apathetic and ceases to learn. Therefore, it is natural that illness and confinement may cause regression.

We understand this well enough, but we do not always take into account the effect of the physical restraints that we put on the child. These may be mechanical restraints to his arms or legs, a restraint aimed at keeping him physically quiet, or a restraint to keep him away from other children.

Physical restraints are frequently necessary to keep the child from harming himself or undoing necessary procedures. This restraint must be compensated for by the nurse showing considerable evidence of affection, by alternate diversion in any way possible and by physical measures to relieve his discomfort.

The infant placed in an isolation unit for his own protection, or for the protection of others, suffers considerably from loneliness as well as from the discomfort occasioned by his disease. All too often, the only diversion we offer him is contemplation of the bare walls. Practical consideration of this problem is long overdue.

Parent-Nurse Relationship

The nurse's relationship with the parents of her patients is most important. A mother should be allowed, and encouraged, to feed her baby, change his diaper, hold him, and to do whatever she feels capable of doing. Many parents are timid or frightened, and think that they are not allowed to do this. The nurse should ask the parent if she (or he) would like to hold or to feed the child, using tact in order not to make the parents feel guilty if they do not feel adequate in the situation.

Sometimes mothers wish to care for other infants on the ward. A mother spending considerable time on the ward, perhaps because her own infant is very ill, often feels quite useless and asks if she can fill some obvious need of some other child. Perhaps you have not been able to get to Johnny's feeding promptly, and he is letting the world know in no uncertain terms what he thinks of this kind of service. Perhaps he is in obvious need of a change, or is holding up his arms beseechingly to be picked up.

No blanket statement can be made about this. The nurse must first find out the rules. Some departments have strict rules against any visitor handling another child, and tact will have to be used. However, if there is no reason why the visitor should not give the little attention to others that she wants to give, and she appears capable of handling the problem, this may be quite a morale booster to her. Care must be taken, however, not to ask the visitor to help "because I am busy" or to take for granted that because she once offered to feed Johnny that she will continue to do so. Abuse of this situation has sometimes been the cause behind the strict rules against allowing visitors to help.

BIBLIOGRAPHY

Aldrich, C. A., and Aldrich, M. M.: Babies are Human Beings. New York, Macmillan, 1953.

American Academy of Pediatrics: Report of the Committee on the Control of Infectious Diseases. 14th ed. Evanston, Illinois, American Academy of Pediatrics, 1966.

American Dental Association: Your Child's Teeth. Chicago, American Dental Association, 1962.

Blake, F.: The Child, His Parents and the Nurse. Philadelphia, J. B. Lippincott, 1954.

Blake, F., and Wright, F. H.: Essentials of Pediatric Nursing. 7th ed. Philadelphia, J. B. Lippincott, 1963.

Combes, M. A., et al: Sciatic nerve injury in infants. J.A.M.A. *173*:1336, 1960.

Gesell, A., and Ilg, F. L.: Infant and Child in the Culture of Today. New York, Harper & Brothers, 1943.

Gilles, F. H., and French, J. H.: Post-injection sciatic nerve palsies in infants and children. J. Pediat., *58*:195, 1961.

Silver, H. K., Kempe, C. H., and Bruyn, H. B.: Handbook of Pediatrics. 6th ed. Los Altos, California, Lange Medical Publications, 1965.

Spock, B.: Baby and Child Care. New York, Pocket Books, 1963.

Spock, B., and Lowenberg, M.: Feeding Your Baby and Child. New York, Pocket Books, 1956.

United States Department of Health, Education and Welfare, Children's Bureau: Children of Working Mothers. Washington, U. S. Government Printing Office, 1963.

————: Infant Care. Washington, U. S. Government Printing Office, 1965.

————: Nutrition and Healthy Growth. Washington, U. S. Government Printing Office, 1965.

SUGGESTED READINGS FOR FURTHER STUDY

American Dental Association: The Care of Children's Teeth: Some Questions and Answers. Chicago, American Dental Association, 1956.

Breckenridge, M. E., and Vincent, E. L.: Child Development. 5th ed., pp. 365–367. Philadelphia, W. B. Saunders, 1965.

Cooper, L. F.: Nutrition in Health and Disease. 14th ed. Philadelphia, J. B. Lippincott, 1963.

Gerber Products Company: Foods for Baby and Mealtime Psychology. Fremont, Michigan, Gerber Products, 1963.

Hanson, D. J.: Intramuscular injection injuries and complications. G.P., *27*:109, (Jan.) 1963.

Hurlock, E. B.: Child Development. 4th ed. New York, McGraw-Hill, 1964.

Illingworth, R. S.: The Development of the Infant and Young Child. 2nd ed. Baltimore, Williams & Wilkins, 1963.

Pitel, M., and Wemett, M.: The intramuscular injection. Amer. J. Nurs., *64*:104, (Apr.) 1964.

Spock, B., and Reinhart, J.: A Baby's First Year. New York, Pocket Books, 1956.

Strang, R.: An Introduction to Child Study. 4th ed., pp. 51–132. New York, Macmillan, 1959.

United States Department of Health, Education and Welfare, Children's Bureau: A Healthy Personality for Your Child. Washington, U. S. Government Printing Office, 1962.

Watson, E. H., and Lowrey, G. H.: Growth and Development of Children. 4th ed., pp. 128–132. Chicago, Year Book Publishers, 1962.

Winnicott, D. W.: The Child, the Family, and the Outside World. London, Penguin, 1964.

10

Nursing in Specific Conditions of Infancy

CONGENITAL ANOMALIES

Certain congenital anomalies are incompatible with life, causing death during the perinatal period. Other anomalies may be amenable to correction if treated very soon after birth. A sizable portion of the hospital infant population, however, is composed of infants who have survived the first months of life, and are now being evaluated for possible correction of anomalies that threaten their future development.

A few anomalies that bring infants into the hospital will be discussed here.

Hydrocephalus

Hydrocephalus is a condition characterized by an excess of cerebrospinal fluid within the ventricular and subarachnoid spaces of the cranial cavity. Normally, a balance is achieved between the rate of secretion of cerebrospinal fluid and its reabsorption; but in this condition, the balance has been disturbed.

The nurse needs to understand the process involved in the circulation of cerebrospinal fluid. The nurse should augment with her own reading the simple explanation that is to follow. (Ransohoff and Shulman give an interesting picture of the process as it is understood at the present time.*)

Briefly, cerebrospinal fluid is formed in the choroid plexus which lies in the ventricles of the brain. The fluid passes through the ventricular system, through the subarachnoid spaces, and is diffused down around the spinal cord and up over the outer convexity of the brain. It is probably reabsorbed into the venous system of the dural sinuses through the arachnoid villi. As far as is known, its only function appears to be protection, serving as a water jacket to guard the brain and spinal cord against injury.

* Fishbein, M., (ed.): Birth Defects. Chapter 25, pp. 253–259, Philadelphia, J. B. Lippincott, 1963.

Pathology

Hydrocephalus may occur as the result of an overproduction of cerebrospinal fluid in the rare instance of a tumor of the choroid plexus; as a result of defective absorption of cerebrospinal fluid; and, most commonly, as a result of an obstruction of the cerebrospinal fluid pathways.

Hydrocephalus is commonly designated as communicating hydrocephalus or noncommunicating hydrocephalus. The designation *communicating* implies free communication between the ventricles and the spinal theca; *noncommunicating* implies the presence of an obstruction to such free flow of fluid.

Major defects causing obstruction include:

1. The Arnold-Chiari malformation. A tongue-like projection of the cerebellum extends into the cervical canal, and the cerebellar tonsils are drawn into the foramen magnum. A myelomeningocele is frequently present in these cases.

2. Atresia of the aqueduct of Sylvius. This is a congenital narrowing of the upper portion of the channel in the posterior fossa.

3. Atresia of the foramina of Luschka and Magendie, causing obstruction at the fourth ventricle.

Hydrocephalus may be recognized at birth, or it may not be evident until after a few weeks or even months of life. Occasionally, the condition may not be congenital, but may instead occur during later infancy or during childhood as the result of a head injury, or an infection such as meningitis.

When hydrocephalus occurs early in life before the skull sutures close, the soft pliable bones separate to allow head expansion. This is manifested by a rapid growth in head circumference. The fact that the soft bones are capable of yielding to pressure in this manner may partially explain why many of these infants fail to show the usual symptoms of brain pressure, and may exhibit little or no damage to mental function until later in life. Other infants show severe brain damage, often occurring before birth.

Clinical Manifestations

A rapidly enlarging head may be the first manifestation of this condition. An apparently large head in itself is not necessarily significant. Normally, every infant's head is measured at birth, and the rate of growth is checked at subsequent examinations. Any infant's head that appears to be abnormally large at birth, or appears to be enlarging, should be measured frequently.

As the head enlarges, the suture lines separate, and the spaces can be felt through the scalp. The anterior fontanelle becomes tense and bulging; the skull enlarges in all diameters; the scalp becomes shiny, and its veins dilate. The eyes appear to be pushed downward slightly, with the sclera visible above the iris, giving the so-called "setting sun" sign. (Fig. 65)

As the condition progresses, the head becomes increasingly heavy, the neck muscles fail to develop sufficiently, and the infant has difficulty raising or turning his head. Unless the hydrocephalus is arrested, the infant becomes increasingly helpless, and symptoms of brain pressure eventually develop. These may include irritability, vomiting, failure to thrive, and arrested development.

Diagnosis

Diagnosis is made through pneumoencephalograms and ventriculograms.

Prognosis

Prognosis is guarded in all cases. A small proportion of cases are self-limiting, some becoming arrested before a significant amount of brain damage has occurred. Many affected infants exhibit severe damage at birth or shortly after. Although nerve tissue cannot be restored, surgical intervention to inhibit head enlargement may be resorted to in these infants in order to facilitate nursing care.

Surgical Treatment

Surgical procedures that have been curative, have been devised for certain rare types of hydrocephalus. For the majority of cases however, the only available procedure is a shunting device that bypasses the point

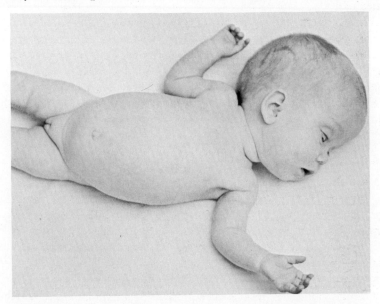

Fig. 65. A child with hydrocephalus. Note the pull on the eyes giving the "setting sun" appearance. Note also the site of incision for a ventriculo-auricular shunt.

of obstruction, draining the excess cerebrospinal fluid into a body cavity. This procedure produces arrest in head growth, and prevents further brain damage. Installation of a shunting device is considered to be indicated for any hydrocephalic infant whose condition permits, most surgeons being unwilling to wait for a possible spontaneous arrest.

Shunting Procedures. A number of types of surgery have been devised over the years for this condition, with varying success. The most successful kind of surgery has consisted of a shunting procedure, using a rubber or polyethylene tubing to bypass the point of obstruction and to drain the excess cerebrospinal fluid into a body cavity. The pleural and peritoneal cavities have been used, but these procedures have short-term effectiveness. Use of a ureter has been more successful, and many children today lead normal lives after a ventriculoureterostomy. This, however, necessitates the removal of one kidney, and also requires the addi-

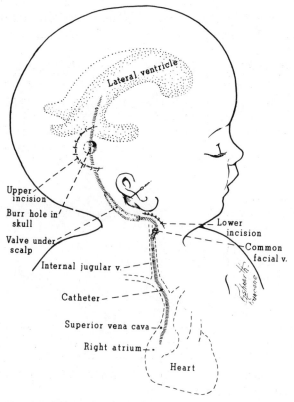

Fig. 66. An operative procedure for hydrocephalus, in which a catheter drains the ventricular system into the right atrium.

tion of measured amounts of salt to the diet, to be continued indefinitely. The amount of salt drained out of the body from the loss of cerebrospinal fluid seriously upsets the electrolyte balance unless it is replaced.

The procedure of choice, at present, is a bypass that uses the venous system, routing the excess cerebrospinal fluid into the right atrium of the heart, or into the superior vena cava. This procedure, called a ventriculo-auriculostomy, utilizes the internal jugular vein. A burr hole is made into the skull just above and behind the ear, through which the tip of a poly-ethylene or silicone rubber catheter is introduced into the ventricle of the brain. The catheter is then threaded into the jugular vein, with the distal end draining into the right auricle of the heart. A one-way valve built into the tube prevents reflux. Valves commonly used are the Spitz-Holter and the Pudenz-Heyer. (Fig. 66)

Difficulties also occur with this shunting procedure. Infection has frequently occurred at the site of the valve, for reasons not entirely understood. Ventriculitis and septicemia occur in many instances. These infections can seldom be cleared up without removal of the shunting device, together with vigorous antibiotic therapy. Following the clearing of the infection, the apparatus may be replaced, although reinfections do occasionally occur.

The valve can be easily felt under the skin. If it appears to be non-functioning, pumping of the valve may be ordered by the surgeon. This is done by applying rhythmic pressure with the fingers over the site of the valve. The soft tubing encasing the valve can be felt as it fills and empties. Pumping, if ordered, is usually carried out for fifty to one hundred or more times at designated intervals. This procedure is quite uncomfortable for the infant.

Postoperative Care

Following a ventriculoatrial shunting, the infant is kept with his head turned away from the operative site until the incision is well healed. If the child is able to turn his head, sandbags may be needed to keep it turned to one side. Vital signs are taken routinely as they would be after any surgical procedure. He should be watched carefully for change of color, excessive irritability or lethargy, and for abnormal vital signs. The fontanelle is frequently depressed after shunting; this is to be expected. A suction machine for removal of excessive mucus from the nose and the mouth should be readily available.

The side of the head on which the baby lies should be examined for pressure sores, particularly if the head is large and heavy. Sponge rubber under his head may be useful.

The child may receive intravenous fluids immediately following surgery, with oral feedings started when he is able to tolerate them.

Physical Care and Emotional Support of the Infant with Hydrocephalus

Every infant has the need, and the right, to be picked up, loved and held in a loving, comforting manner. When any child has suffered a painful or uncomfortable experience, his need for emotional support becomes much greater.

The chief way in which an infant can perceive such support is through physical contact, made in a soothing, loving manner. When a nurse has to be responsible for causing discomfort to a child, such as pumping a shunt or giving an intramuscular injection, she must realize that an integral part of the treatment is the immediate following of emotional support. Preferably, this support is given by the person who has caused the pain.

The nurse should *never* feel that she does not have time for this part of the treatment, any more than she would feel that she did not have time to wash her hands or put on sterile gloves when indicated. Occasionally, of course, it is not possible for physical reasons to pick up a child out of his crib. The nurse must convey her concern by her touch, her voice, her soothing manner. Convey it, however, she must.

Physical care is of course important. When the head is heavy and difficult for the child to turn, it must be turned for him to prevent skin breakdown. Tincture of benzoin applied to irritated places may prevent such breakdown. Any broken area should be reported at once.

Bathing. Sponge baths may be necessary if the infant has poor head control. Special care to the areas behind the ears and in the creases of the neck is important. As in everything done for these children, special attention can be a means of alleviating some of the inherent frustrations. There are many little comfort-promoting devices that nurses do not always consider important.

Comfortably warm bath water is soothing. Too often, one finds only a few inches of cool or lukewarm water in the bath basin, especially when the nurse has prepared the water before she has collected all of her equipment.

If back rubs are soothing for adults, might not a few minutes spent in giving a gentle rub be appreciated by an infant who must lie in his crib for long intervals? If a soft, gentle voice is pleasing to hear, this infant too may be soothed and pleased, perhaps even stimulated, if the nurse talks to him during the bathing process.

Feeding. Feeding technique also assumes importance for this child. These babies have a need to be held when they are fed even more than the healthy babies, but, in practice, this need is frequently not met. The nurse may need to select a chair with an arm on which to rest her elbow while supporting the heavy head. When these children have difficulty holding their heads erect, bubbling them becomes somewhat more difficult. Bottle feeding needs to be given carefully and slowly, with special attention to absence of air in the nipple.

When, for some reason, the baby cannot be held for feeding, there may be a temptation to prop the bottle; especially if the baby cannot move his head, and thus lose the nipple as easily as another child. There is no place for bottle propping in his care, however, or in the care of any hospitalized infant.

Head Measurement. The baby's head circumference should be measured daily, or at intervals ordered by the doctor. The tape measure is passed around the largest portion of the child's head, over the forehead and around the occipital region. In the interest of accuracy, it is better if the same person does the measurement each time, using the same tape measure.

Social Interaction. The infant in his crib needs social interaction. He needs to be talked to, played with, and provided with activity according to his ability. Toys commensurate with his physical and mental capacity must be provided for him.

If the child has difficulty moving about his crib, toys must be within his reach and within his ability to manipulate. A cradle gym tied close enough for him to reach may be good. If he cannot raise his head, or cannot turn in pursuit of an elusive toy, he receives additional frustration which he can well do without.

It is most important that the infant be allowed to become a part of the social environment, but this he cannot achieve if he is turned with his face toward a blank wall. Unless his nervous system is so impaired that all activity increases his irritability, he needs stimulation as much as any child. If turning an infant from side to side means turning him away from the sight of activity, turn the crib around so that he is not facing the wall or ward divider.

The effect of attention and stimulation on the average infant is amazing. One infant may lie in his crib day after day, receiving all necessary physical care, but no emotional stimulation. He is never played with, talked to, or picked up. Because of his limitations, he cannot provide self-stimulation. This child does not fit into our definition of a normal child, is not treated as one, and therefore does not act as one.

A second infant with the same handicap is given all the contact and support that any infant requires. His personality develops, growing by what it feeds on. His nurse uses the time she has for his physical care as a time for social interaction. She talks and laughs with him, plays with him, and visits him at times between the necessary occasions for giving physical care.

A person seeing the two infants might well remark about the personality development and mental alertness of the second child, finding the first child dull and apathetic. Yet both may have had the same capacity for development, but are products of differing environments. Once again, we become impressed with the concept that nursing is much more than the meeting of physical needs.

Help to Parents

A nurse does not find it difficult to understand the anxiety and apprehension parents feel if this condition is present in their child, but she may feel quite helpless in trying to give them support. Her own acceptance of the child with her tender care and concern for his welfare helps convey her warmth of feeling. Her matter-of-fact acceptance of his handicap, as well as her treatment of him as a baby with normal needs, helps put the situation on a more realistic basis.

Arrangements should be made to give much of the normal, daily care at times when parents are able to be present. They need to learn how to hold and handle the baby in as normal a manner as possible. Undoubtedly, they need much encouragement. Can they do him any harm by the

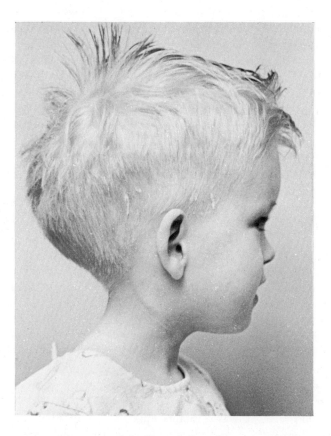

Fig. 67. Arrested hydrocephalus after a ventriculo-auricular shunt.

way they care for him? Should he not be kept quietly by himself to prevent too much stimulation? Many other questions may be asked of the nurse, and many misapprehensions may be cleared away.

A mother should be encouraged to help with her child's care when there are others present to give her support. She can be encouraged to feel the valve in the ventriculo-auricular shunting device, and to develop an understanding of its function. Both parents need to understand the importance of careful observation for any abnormal developments, and, at the same time, attempt to create as normal a life as possible for their child. (Fig. 67)

Spina Bifida

Another congenital anomaly of the central nervous system is a spinal malformation called *spina bifida.* In this condition there is a defect in the neural arch, generally in the lumbosacral region; the posterior laminae of the vertebrae fail to close, presenting an opening through which the spinal meninges and spinal cord may protrude.

The bony defect occurring alone, without involvement of the tissues, is called spina bifida occulta. In most cases, it is asymptomatic and presents no problems. A dimple in the skin or a tuft of hair over the site may cause one to suspect its presence, or it may be entirely overlooked.

Clinical Features

When a portion of the spinal meninges protrudes through the bony defect and forms a cystic sac, the condition is termed spina bifida with meningocele. No nerve roots are involved; therefore, no paralysis or sensory loss below the lesion appears. The sac may, however, rupture or perforate, thus introducing infection into the spinal fluid and causing meningitis. For this reason, as well as for cosmetic purposes, surgical removal of the sac, with closure of the skin, is indicated.

Spina bifida with myelomeningocele signifies a protrusion of the spinal cord and the meninges, with nerve roots embedded in the wall of the cyst. The effects of this defect vary in severity from sensory loss or partial paralysis below the lesion, to complete flaccid paralysis of all muscles below the lesion. The complete paralysis involves the lower trunk and the legs as well as bowel and bladder sphincters. It is not always possible however to make a clear-cut differentiation in diagnosis between a meningocele and a myelomeningocele on the basis of symptoms alone.

The condition myelomeningocele may also be termed meningomyelocele. The associated spina bifida is always implied, but not necessarily named. *Spina bifida cystica* is the term used to designate either of these protrusions.

Associated conditions. Hydrocephalus of the obstructive type is frequently associated with these two defects. Bypass procedures may arrest the hydrocephaly, but cannot affect or restore the neural function involved in a myelomeningocele. It was formerly thought that surgical repair of the spinal defect would frequently cause hydrocephaly not previously present, and parents were so advised. This has not been proved, however. The concept accepted by many neurosurgeons today is that hydrocephaly is already present, the surgical repair of the sac accelerating its development. Other defects are frequently present, the most common being talipes equinovarus. Hip displasia may also be present. (Fig. 68)

Surgical Treatment

Surgical repair of a myelomeningocele cannot be expected to decrease the neurological disability, although many surgeons believe that future function is improved to some extent in those carefully repaired. It has been observed that some newborn infants show a limited motor ability that rapidly decreases after birth. For this reason, many neurosurgeons advocate very early repair of myelomeningoceles, in an effort to prevent further deterioration of neural tissue.

A leaking sac calls for immediate repair to prevent meningitis. Some infants with a thin membrane over the sac, through which spinal fluid is leaking, show signs of meningitis at birth.

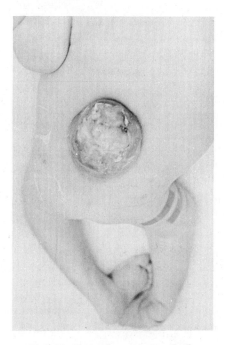

Fig. 68. A myelomeningocele showing an additional defect of club feet.

The primary objective of surgical repair is closure of the defect, with replacement of neural elements within the vertebral canal whenever possible. Nerve roots that can be freed are replaced in the canal, the sac amputated at its base or turned inward, and plastic surgery employed for covering the site of the defect.

Nursing Care of the Infant with Spina Bifida Cystica

Preoperative care. The infant needs the same kind of care outlined for the care of the child with hydrocephalus; in fact, he quite possibly has hydrocephalus. This infant's care, however, is complicated by the presence of the spinal lesion.

The infant with such a spinal lesion cannot be allowed to lie on his back, but must be positioned on his side or abdomen. His position must be frequently changed.

It is most important that the sac be kept clean and dry, with all pressure avoided. Any leakage of spinal fluid must be reported immediately. Avoidance of contamination from urine or fecal material is of particular importance. A sheet of plastic may be taped between the defect and the anus, and folded back on itself to form a barrier, and taped into place. If the sac covering is thin, a dressing may be ordered to be placed over it. This may be a dry, sterile dressing, or may be medicated. Adaptic, Vaseline gauze or Varidase may be used.

Perhaps the greatest nursing challenge is in keeping the perineum clean and in preventing excoriation when paralysis of the sphincter muscles is present, because the lack of sphincter control results in constant dribbling of urine and feces. Because the infant cannot be placed on his back, fecal material runs down over the perineum. The constant dribbling of urine and feces causes severe skin irritation. To help prevent excoriation, scrupulous cleanliness must be maintained. The perineum should be cleansed frequently with an unmedicated oil and left exposed to the air at all times.

In some hospitals the baby is placed on a Bradford frame to facilitate handling. The canvas frame must be covered with soft sheets to prevent skin irritation, and the edges of the open section below the perineal region protected with sheets of plastic that drape down into the receptacle placed on the bed below the frame.

The child is positioned on his abdomen with flannel restraints to hold him in place. A rolled towel under his ankles or a rolled blanket under his legs is needed to prevent pressure on his toes. It is possible to position a small infant on his side while on a Bradford frame, with the use of a rolled blanket against his back above the lesion, and restraints to hold him in place.

Nurses and parents are encouraged to hold the child at intervals, particularly for feedings. Of course he must be held in such a manner as to avoid pressure on the sac, but the child can be fitted comfortably into the nurse's arm. Parents may be frightened and need encouragement as well as help in correctly positioning the child.

Postoperative care. Following repair of a meningocele or myelomeningocele, the infant is placed in a prone or knee-chest position and not moved unnecessarily until the operative site is completely healed. This means that all procedures must be carried out with the infant in this position, including feeding and bathing.

Usual postoperative observations are followed. Perineal care must be continued, and special precautions for keeping the operative site clean and dry strictly observed. When feedings are begun, the nurse turns the baby's head to one side and holds the bottle, at the same time keeping baby in the prone position. The surgeon decides when he can be moved or turned.

Continuing Care

It is difficult to predict the future for these infants. Many of those with hydrocephalus and myelomeningocele appear to have a hopeless prognosis at birth. Many who do survive in spite of severe handicaps, succumb to infection during early life. Some, however, live through the hazardous early years. These children, with skillful help and favorable circumstances, may be able to achieve useful, satisfactory lives.

The majority of neurosurgeons and orthopedists prefer to give the child every possible assistance, even if the prospect does not appear particularly favorable. Shunting devices and repair of spinal defects are made early in life. If satisfactory results have been attained, orthopedic procedures should be carried out in anticipation of the possibility of future ambulation. These may include casting for talipes equinovarus and hip dysplasia, as well as intensive physical therapy to prevent progression of deformities.

As the child grows older, he can progress from a stroller to a wheelchair, with the prospect for many of learning to walk with the help of braces and crutches. Increasingly, as medical knowledge advances, more such handicapped children are helped to a relatively normal way of life.

Urinary control. The most difficult problem is that of urinary incontinence. If voluntary sphincter control is absent, the infant cannot be toilet trained. Dribbling of urine does not keep the bladder emptied, and reflux resulting in hydroureter and hydronephrosis is common, with resultant severe kidney damage.

The bladder can be emptied by mechanical expression, using the Credè method. Firm hand pressure is applied over the bladder region, with the hand moved slowly down below the symphysis pubis. This is done periodically to prevent the accumulation of urine in the bladder.

The parents should be taught this procedure before they take the child home.

A number of methods have been devised to achieve urinary continence for the child, none of which have proved to be entirely satisfactory. A very few children have achieved successful control after long-term, rigorous training. Control of fluid intake, with strict regularity of mechanical bladder emptying by the Credè method, combined with unlimited patience, has produced good results. Few parents or children are able to carry out these long-term programs. Even if control is achieved in this manner, the bladder may not be completely emptied.

Indwelling catheters may be useful for short periods, especially when an infection is being treated. Transplant of the ureters into the sigmoid is a procedure that has been widely used, but the ascending infection that usually results has been discouraging.

The most encouraging procedure employed at present is an ileal loop, or cutaneous ileoureterostomy. A small segment of the ileum is isolated, its distal end closed, and the proximal end brought to the skin surface of the abdomen. The remaining bowel is anastomosed for continuity of function. The ends of the ureters are inserted into the sides of the ileal segment, which then acts as a conduit for the urine to the surface of the body. An ileostomy bag fitted over the stoma receives the urine. The parents and child need careful instruction and practice in learning to apply the bag correctly to prevent leakage.

Bowel control is not so difficult to achieve. A slightly constipating

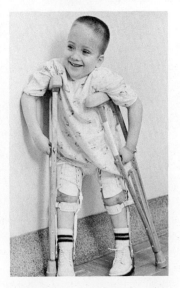

Fig. 69. Learning to walk again.

diet may be necessary at first. The parent places the child on the toilet at the time he usually has a bowel movement, perhaps using a suppository until habit is established. Accidents may happen at first, but intelligent regulation is usually effective.

The courage and persistence demanded from the parents of these children, as well as from the children themselves, is nearly more than the unaffected person can grasp. They deserve a great deal of emotional support and encouragement. Considerable physical and financial help is necessary for most families.

The child who does achieve ambulation through use of braces and crutches, and is able to take his place as a well adjusted member of society, rewards all those who gave so much time, effort and unending patience. The child in Fig. 69 is such an example. A myelomeningocele was successfully repaired in infancy. He learned to walk with crutches and braces; at the age of five he re-entered the hospital for new braces, an Achilles tenotomy, and urinary tract evaluation. He was a friendly, outgoing child with a sunny disposition, a lively imagination and quick mental ability. The picture shows him ready to leave the hospital with his new braces. Giving such a child hope for a relatively normal life seems well worth the effort put forth by so many—not the least of whom was the child himself.

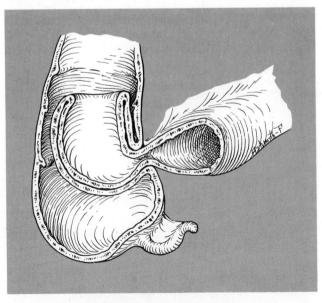

Fig. 70. Intussusception. Note the telescoping of a portion of the bowel into the distal portion.

CONDITIONS OF THE GASTROINTESTINAL SYSTEM

Intussusception

A healthy thriving baby, generally a boy, may some time after the first month of life suddenly develop extremely severe paroxysms of abdominal pain with no apparent predisposing cause. His mother may ascribe this to gas, especially when her baby resumes play after the colicky episode. Another spasm soon appears, however, and the mother realizes that something is seriously wrong.

Intussusception is the invagination or telescoping of one portion of the bowel into a distal portion. It occurs most frequently at the juncture of the ileum and the colon, although it can appear elsewhere in the intestinal tract. The invagination is from above downward; the upper portion, the intussusceptum, slipping into the lower, the intussuscipiens, pulling the mesentery along with it. (Fig. 70)

Incidence

The condition occurs more often in boys than in girls, and is the most frequent cause of intestinal obstruction in childhood. The greatest incidence, about 78 per cent, occurs in infants between the ages of six months to one year.

Etiology

The condition usually appears in healthy babies without any demonstrable cause. Its production is supposed to be favored by the hyperperistalsis and the unusual mobility of the cecum and ileum normally present in early life. Occasionally, a lesion such as a Meckel's diverticulum or a polyp may be present.

Clinical Manifestations

The infant who has previously appeared healthy and happy suddenly becomes pale, cries out sharply, and draws up his legs in a severe colicky spasm of pain. This spasm may last for several minutes, after which the infant relaxes and appears well until the next episode, which may be 5, 10, or 20 minutes later.

Most of these infants start vomiting early, a vomiting that becomes progressively more severe and eventually is bile stained. The infant strains with each paroxysm, emptying his bowels of fecal contents, after which the stools consist of blood and mucus, earning the name of "currant jelly" stools.

Symptoms of shock appear quickly. Rapid pulse, paleness, and marked sweating are characteristic. Shock, vomiting and currant jelly stools are the cardinal symptoms of this condition. Fortunately, these symptoms, coupled with the paroxysmal pain, are severe enough to bring the child into the hospital early.

The nurse does not, of course, make a diagnosis; however, because she is often consulted by neighbors, friends and relatives if things go wrong, she needs to be informed and alert. Therefore, a word of caution is needed. On rare occasions a more chronic form appears, particularly during an episode of severe diarrheal disturbance. The onset is more gradual and may not show all of the classic symptoms, but the danger of a sudden, complete strangulation is present. Presumably, such an infant is already under a doctor's care.

Diagnosis

Diagnosis can usually be made by the physician from the clinical symptoms, rectal examination, and palpation of the abdomen during the calm interval when it is soft. A baby is often not willing to tolerate this palpation, and sedation may be ordered. In about half of these cases, a sausage-shaped mass along the colon can be felt through the abdominal wall.

A barium enema is not only diagnostic, but may also reduce the intussusception.

Treatment

Unlike pyloric stenosis, this condition is a true emergency in the sense that prolonged delay is dangerous. The telescoped bowel rapidly becomes gangrenous, thus markedly reducing the possibility of a simple reduction. Adequate treatment during the first 12 to 24 hours should have a good outcome, with complete recovery. The outcome becomes more uncertain as the bowel deteriorates, making resection necessary.

Early Care of Infant After Admission

The baby is of course given nothing by mouth, and intravenous fluids are started. A cut-down or catheter into the vein will probably be used.

The young baby needs very careful watching because his condition can deteriorate rapidly. Vital signs need to be checked frequently, warmth applied if symptoms of shock are present, and general condition noted. Aspiration of vomited material is a very real danger, especially as the child becomes weaker. The baby will probably not tolerate being held to any extent. Although early reduction is imperative, the baby may be in the hospital for a few hours before surgery if symptoms are not entirely clear or if he is greatly dehydrated.

Surgical technique. Surgery consists of a gentle milking of the intussusceptum back into place. This is a simple procedure, requiring a small incision, and affords an opportunity for visual assurance of complete reduction as well as identification of any possible lesion that might be present. Should the bowel be found to be gangrenous or the intussusception irreducible, resection will be necessary.

Traditionally, surgery has been preceded by a diagnostic barium enema, and it has been observed in some cases that the reduction has been accomplished by the hydrostatic pressure itself. Most surgeons prefer to follow the enema with surgery to assure themselves of complete reduction and absence of other lesions. Some surgeons, however, are relying on the reduction by hydrostatic pressure under fluoroscopic observation when the diagnosis is made early and prostration is minimal. In every case the technique is carried out by the surgeon himself, with the operating room ready for immediate surgery if reduction is not accomplished.

Technique for reduction by hydrostatic pressure should be understood by the nurse for her own satisfaction, and to enable her to explain correctly to the child's parents. The child is taken to X-ray with intravenous fluids running. A Foley bag catheter is placed in the rectum, inflated, and barium solution allowed to flow by gravity into the colon. The reduction is shown by free filling of the small intestine, disappearance of the mass, and observable improvement in the infant's condition.* If any doubt exists, surgery is performed at once.

Prognosis

Early successful reduction gives complete relief with only rare recurrent attacks. Spontaneous reduction has been known to occur, but the condition is considered too dangerous to adopt a "wait and see" attitude. The mortality rate rises sharply with delay, and untreated cases are nearly always fatal.

Nursing Care

As in any abnormal condition affecting children or infants, a large portion of the nursing care is concerned with support of the parents.

Every parent is entitled to as complete and accurate an explanation as she or he can understand. The parents need to understand the condition, and its severity. Medical and nursing procedures are frequently complicated and extremely frightening to the uninformed person.

Many procedures that seem routine to the nurse do present an ominous aspect to a person who is unfamiliar with them, a fact that we too often overlook.

Jimmy, lying in his crib, has a tubing extending from his nose and connected to a continuous suction apparatus. Another tube extends from a bottle of fluid into a vein in his scalp. He may have still another tubing coming from his bladder into a drainage bottle. None of these may have

* Ravitch, M. M.: Intussusception in Infants and Children. Springfield, Charles C Thomas, 1959.

great significance, but even the most informed nurse might have a few qualms if this child was her own.

The untrained public has certainly become more informed about medical techniques through the popular magazines, television and other media. It is still difficult to be entirely objective, however, if the affected child is your own, and thus misunderstandings are still quite common.

In situations such as this, the doctor is quite busy and concerned about the patient, and looks to the nurse to give support to the family. An explanation of the whys and wherefores can clear up some of the mystery. Perhaps a nurse's greatest asset is the ability to listen. If she is really attentive, she can show her sympathy and understanding, help correct misunderstandings, and give assurance that the child's welfare is of the greatest concern to all.

The nurse should try to make the parents comfortable, and make them feel that they are part of the group and not hindrances or unavoidable nuisances. She gives them assurance that the child will be carefully watched when they take a much needed moment of relaxation in the coffee shop or restroom, and she has someone show them where to go. She does not insist that they go, however, against their wishes.

Occasionally, a nurse falls into the trap of giving false hope or of being unrealistically optimistic. She must remember that this is a sick child, and no one can predict a recovery with certainty.

Postoperative care. Following a simple reduction of the intussusception, treatment is symptomatic. Intravenous feeding is necessary until normal bowel sounds are present, at which time feedings are cautiously resumed.

The surgical area must be kept clean and dry, and care must be taken so that it is not contaminated by urine or fecal material.

If resection has been necessary, this assumes the gravity of any major abdominal surgery. Constant gastric suction is necessary to keep the stomach and upper intestinal tract empty. Drainage must be measured, and may be analyzed for electrolyte losses that must be replaced in the intravenous fluids.

One must not forget to turn these patients frequently. The small infant cannot learn to cough or breathe deeply to keep his lungs clear. A nasal suction machine must be on hand to keep the airways clear of mucus, and activity should be stimulated by frequent turning and, if necessary, by making the infant cry. Of course this must be explained to the parents, who will probably resent measures that make the child temporarily uncomfortable. When they understand the importance of deep breathing, which in a small child, can be stimulated only by crying, and the need for changes of position to facilitate the exchange of gasses in the lungs, they can willingly cooperate.

CONGENITAL HYPERTROPHIC PYLORIC STENOSIS

Pyloric stenosis is rarely symptomatic during the first days of life. It has on occasion been recognized shortly after birth, but the average affected infant does not show symptoms until about the third week of life. Symptoms rarely appear after the second month.

This condition is characterized by hypertrophy of the circular muscle fibers of the pylorus that causes a ring like constriction of the pylorus at the distal end of the stomach. When the peristaltic waves push the stomach contents toward the pylorus, this obstruction forces the material back, and causes forceful vomiting.

Incidence

The condition seems to be more common in male infants and is said to be more likely found in the first-born. Babies do not always abide by the rules, however, and the first infant you see with this condition could quite possibly be the third or fourth-born, and a girl.

Symptoms

The first weeks of such an infant's life are usually uneventful; he probably eats well and gains weight. Then he starts vomiting occasionally after meals. Within a few days the vomiting episodes increase in frequency and force, becoming projectile in character. The vomited material may contain mucus, but never bile, because it has not progressed beyond the stomach.

Because the obstruction is a mechanical one, the baby does not feel ill, is ravenously hungry, and is eager to try again and again. Unfortunately, the food invariably comes back.

As the condition progresses the baby becomes irritable, loses weight rapidly and becomes dehydrated. A condition of alkalosis develops from the loss of potassium and hydrochloric acid, and he becomes ill indeed.

Constipation becomes progressive because little food gets into the intestines, and the urine is scanty. Gastric peristaltic waves passing from left to right across the abdomen can usually be seen during or after feedings.

Diagnosis

Diagnosis usually can be made on the clinical evidence. The nature, type and times of vomiting, observation of gastric peristaltic waves, and a history of weight loss with hunger and irritability point in this direction. The olive-size pyloric tumor can often be felt through deep palpation by an experienced physician. Roentgen examination with barium swallow shows an abnormal retention of barium in the stomach and increased peristaltic waves.

Treatment

The condition is well-known and is suspected if a previously well infant commences to vomit his feedings. When under a pediatrician's care, either in a private office or in a clinic, these infants are carefully watched to prevent the critical degree of dehydration that was formerly so frequent. However, it still happens all too frequently that infants do not come into the hospital until dehydration and malnutrition are obvious, thus presenting an infant in very poor condition for surgical correction.

Treatment to correct pyloric stenosis is routinely surgical in the United States. The procedure commonly used is the Fredet-Remstedt operation. This procedure simply splits the hypertrophic pyloric muscle down to the submucosa, allowing the pylorus to expand so that food may pass. If performed by a competent surgeon on an infant in good condition, the operation is simple, and it gives excellent results.

In the United States, the older method of medical treatment is rarely used. This treatment consists of feedings of cereal-thickened formula, antispasmodic drugs and sedation. This treatment must of necessity be of long duration, is frequently unsatisfactory, and serves to increase the hazards to the child who is already malnourished and in poor condition. It may on occasion be used for a short time while a diagnosis is being established, but not for the child with pyloric stenosis who has lost much weight or who is already in alkalosis.

Nursing Care

Preoperative care. The infant who comes into the hospital after unsuccessful attempts at home treatment such as changes of formula and feeding techniques, is not, as a rule, in a condition for immediate surgery. He needs laboratory tests to determine his metabolic deficits and state of chemical imbalance.

Intravenous fluids are given to restore proper hydration and to correct the alkalosis. These are carefully calculated to restore lost electrolytes and bring the infant back into proper fluid balance.

The nurse should follow directions exactly as to the amount and type of fluid to be given. Mixing fluids, if this is required to meet the child's needs, is a very exact procedure, and should be done only by a nurse familiar with this procedure.

When the baby is in the hospital awaiting surgery, it would be very helpful if the mother could participate in his care. Both the mother and the baby are going to be happier if we can recognize their mutual needs. The nurse also needs a better opportunity to explain the purpose of waiting for surgery and the function of the intravenous fluids.

FEEDINGS. If the baby does need a period of hospitalization before surgery, a smooth-muscle relaxant such as atropine may be ordered prior to oral feedings. Feedings may be thickened by mixing cooked cereal with the formula, and the child fed through a large-holed nipple, in the hope that some nutrients may be retained.

RECORDING. The nurse needs to record accurately the amount of feeding given, and the approximate amount retained, as well as the frequency and type of emesis. Urinary output is estimated or measured; the skin turgor is noted as well as the general physical appearance, state of irritability, lethargy, or any change in response to external stimulation.

Immediate preoperative preparation includes bathing the baby, omitting oral feedings for a specified time, and giving the preoperative medication if any is ordered. When the baby is in surgery, the mother is given a comfortable place in which to wait, and some attention is paid to her needs. She may be invited to accompany the staff on their coffee break or lunch period. If she waits in the general waiting room, some member of the staff can seek her out for an occasional friendly word. Be sure that she understands the use of the recovery room, because many parents become alarmed at a wait of several hours after the doctor has assured them that surgery is simple and of short duration.

Postoperative care. Postoperatively, the child should be positioned on his side and watched carefully to prevent aspiration of mucus or emesis, particularly during the anesthesia recovery period. When fully reacted, but restless, he may relax if his mother holds him. If so, be sure to give her a gown to protect her clothing.

The first feeding is usually given about six hours postoperatively, and generally is glucose water. If well tolerated, this feeding can be alternated with small amounts of dilute formula at frequent intervals, gradually increasing in amount and in frequency. The baby may vomit a time or two, but should progress quite rapidly toward complete recovery. Intravenous feedings may be needed until the child can tolerate sufficient oral feedings.

With early diagnosis, and surgery before dehydration and malnutrition have become severe, the child has an excellent chance for returning to a satisfactory condition in a short period of weeks, and of progressing steadily on to complete recovery. Operative fatality rate under these conditions has become less than 1 per cent.

Malnutrition

Severe malnutrition from a protein-poor diet is not the acute problem among young children in the United States that it is in many countries. Malnutrition does exist, however, from a variety of causes. There are large numbers of families living on marginal incomes who find real difficulty providing proper nourishment for their small children. Some of this difficulty, it is true, is because of a lack of an understanding of the nutritional needs of infants and small children, and some is the result of ignorance of an inexpensive way of supplying those needs. Some mothers may be too preoccupied with their own problems or self-interest to be especially concerned.

As nurses, is it important that we know how to help a mother who cannot, or will not, buy the expensive prepared formula, baby foods and vitamin drops? If this is part of our responsibility, we must try to understand and accept the situation and work with the parents to find ways of helping the child to health.

Public health nurses report that large numbers of migrant worker's families with babies and small children have no refrigeration for keeping the baby's milk or food protected, and few facilities for sanitary preparation. Among them, diarrheal disorders are common. The breast-fed baby certainly fares better in these circumstances, yet relatively few are breast fed.

Perhaps before becoming too sharp with our criticism, we should consider the difficulties involved in breast feeding when a mother goes at day break to the fields, leaving her baby with whoever stays behind in camp.

It is difficult enough for the best informed and economically minded nutritionist to fit a well-rounded diet into a welfare family's budget. Thus it is not only the migrant worker's family, or the members of poor American Indian tribes who have problems providing proper nourishment for their children.

Causes of Malnutrition

Some infants, it is true, are severely malnourished through neglect, and are brought into the hospital for dietary treatment. Yet the mother who had six young children to feed, clothe and care for, could not be too severely judged when her six month old baby was brought to the hospital in an acute stage of malnutrition. A fretful, fussy baby, who vomited when someone took the time to feed him, somehow got overlooked in the general confusion at home. There didn't seem much point in working to get food down when it only came back again; she really must take the time to consider what to do about it, but right now, the two-year-old had just got into the kitchen cupboard and the four-year-old was playing out in the street.

Vitamin D deficiency. Malnutrition frequently accompanies chronic disease; the child has little energy and less appetite. Metabolic disorders such as celiac or fibrocystic disease cause severe malnourishment and may be complicated by rickets due to failure to absorb vitamin D or calcium.

RICKETS. Rickets is a deficiency disease caused by a lack of vitamin D. Children who live in the sunshine and wear little clothing may absorb sufficient vitamin D from the sun's ultraviolet rays, but the infant or small child in a temperate or an arctic climate rarely has opportunity to receive his antirachitic vitamin in this manner. Children of dark-skinned races also are particularly prone to rickets.

Vitamin D is not found in appreciable quantities in natural foods. Breast milk and cow's milk are poor sources; therefore, the infant needs additional vitamin D, which can be supplied through the use of fish liver oils or in water-miscible vehicles.

Rickets is a disease affecting the growth and calcification of bones. The absorption of calcium and phosphorus is diminished due to the lack of vitamin D, whose function it is to regulate the utilization of these minerals. Early manifestations include craniotabes (a softening of the occipital bones) and delayed closure of the fontanelles. There is delayed dentition, with defects of tooth enamel and a tendency to develop caries. As the disease advances, thoracic deformities, softening of the shafts of long bones and spinal and pelvic bone deformities develop. The muscles are poorly developed and lacking in tone, thus delaying standing and walking.

These deformities occur during the periods of rapid growth, and although rickets in itself is not a fatal disease, complications such as tetany, pneumonia and enteritis are more likely to cause death in rachitic children than in healthy children.

Infants and children require an estimated 400 units of vitamin D daily for the prevention of rickets. Because of the uncertainty of a small child receiving sufficient exposure to ultraviolet light in temperate climates, it is administered orally in the form of fish liver oil or synthetic vitamin. Whole milk and evaporated milk, fortified with 400 units of vitamin D per quart are available throughout the United States, but it does not seem reasonable to rely on this source alone.

Certain pathological conditions such as vitamin D-resistant rickets and renal rickets are not caused by vitamin D deficiency.

Vitamin C deficiency. scurvy. *Scurvy* is a deficiency disease caused by inadequate vitamin C in the diet. Early inclusion of vitamin C (ascorbic acid) in the form of orange or tomato juice, or a vitamin preparation, is insurance against the development of this disease. Febrile diseases seem to increase the need for vitamin C. A variety of fresh vegetables and fruits supply vitamin C for the older infant and child, although a considerable proportion of vitamin C content is destroyed by boiling, or by exposure to air for long periods of time.

Early clinical manifestations of scurvy are irritability, loss of appetite and digestive disturbances. A general tenderness in the legs, severe enough to cause a "pseudoparalysis" develops. The infant is apprehensive about being handled, and assumes a "frog" position, with hips and knees semi-flexed and the feet rotated outward. The gums become red and swollen, and hemorrhages occur in various tissues. Characteristic hemorrhages in the long bones are subperiosteal, especially at the ends of the femur and tibia.

Recovery is rapid with adequate treatment, but death may occur from malnutrition or exhaustion in untreated cases. Treatment consists in therapeutic daily doses of ascorbic acid.

Vitamin A deficiency. This occurs only if the diet is severely restricted or if absorption is impaired. Children on average diets receive sufficient vitamin A to prevent deficiency manifestations, and daily supplementary doses assure ample coverage. Children on low fat diets, or those with absorptive difficulties, need large daily doses of water-miscible preparations of vitamin A.

Other Causes of Malnutrition

Allergic reactions to foods may limit the child's diet to the point at which he is not getting the proper nutrients, and parents usually need a dietician's help in working out substitutes for the foods he cannot tolerate. Allergy to cow's milk has been recognized as a problem for a number of infants and children under the age of two years. Symptoms include vomiting and diarrhea, abdominal pain, asthma and rhinitis.

If milk is not withdrawn from the diet, an anaphylactic reaction with severe shock symptoms may result, and death may be the outcome. The infant with a milk allergy does well on a soybean formula such as Sobee or Mulsoy, or the newer formula, ProSobee.*

Diarrheal conditions, from whatever cause, or persistent vomiting, bring about a state of malnutrition requiring careful, skillful nursing.

Another condition, extremely difficult to remedy in many instances, is the marasmic state brought about in an emotionally deprived child. Diet may be satisfactory, and physical care meticulously given, but the infant who has a cold, unresponsive mother may suffer irreversible damage. A failure to thrive, when organic disease is ruled out and physical neglect is not a factor, may be the result of a lack of emotional warmth from the adult caring for the infant. This happens to the infant who is kept in his crib; whose bottle is propped; whose physical contact with other human beings is confined entirely to routine care with no interchange of mutual trust and understanding. The damage is much more than physical, of course, but the malnutritional effects can be startling, and may be fatal.

The infant who is being cared for by a tender, affectionate mother is much more likely to be a relaxed, comfortable being who eats well and sleeps well. On the other hand, when the mother is tense and irritable, the baby may be fitful, cry excessively, and eat and sleep poorly.*

* Mead Johnson.

* Chapman, A. H.: Management of Emotional Problems of Children and Adolescents. P. 40. Philadelphia, J. B. Lippincott, 1965.

Hospital Care of the Malnourished Infant

The malnourished infant admitted to the hospital presents problems that are not easily resolved. The underlying cause must be found and eliminated or treated. If the difficulty lies in the parent's inability to give proper care, whether because of ignorance, financial difficulty, or indifference, this needs consideration, with perhaps several services involved.

The nurse responsible for the daily care of the infant has her own particular problems when attempting to meet his needs.

One such problem may be in persuading the infant to take more nourishment than he wants. Inexperienced nurses find it very difficult to persuade an uninterested infant to take his formula, and it can become a most frustrating experience. Infants appear to be sensitive to the handling of an inexperienced, uncertain person. Perhaps the nurse's insecurity and uncertainty communicate themselves to the child in the way she handles him. It frequently happens that an experienced nurse is successful in feeding an infant three or four ounces in a short time, while, at the same time, the inexperienced nurse who seems to be going through the same motions, persuades the infant to take only an ounce or less. The nurse need not be too discouraged, because as she and the infant become accustomed to each other, they both relax, and the feeding ought to become easier.

In addition to a lack of interest in the feeding, the infant is weak and debilitated, with little strength to suck. Intravenous or gavage feeding may be employed, but in addition it may be most important for the infant to develop an interest in food and in the process of sucking. A hard, or small-holed nipple may completely discourage him. Whereas a strong, healthy infant delights in the process of sucking itself, this infant lacks incentive and strength. The nipple should be soft, with holes large enough to allow the formula to drip without pressure. However, a nipple may be so soft that it offers no resistance and collapses when it is sucked on, or the holes may be so large that milk pours out and causes him to choke. These experiences easily frustrate a weak infant, who soon gives up any attempt to nurse.

The baby who is held snugly in the nurse's arms, wrapped rather closely and rocked gently, will find it easier to relax and take a little more. An impatient, hurried nurse nearly always communicates her tension to the child. If the nurse is tense because of other feedings she must also attend to, she should ask for help. Never does she prop the bottle in the crib. This is a dangerous practice, and it has no place in a hospital nursery.

Some of the babies may be on a two- or a three-hour feeding schedule, because most weak babies are able to handle frequent small feedings better than the four-hour ones. In this case, it is more important than ever that the feedings be given on time. Also, as sucking takes consider-

TABLE 10-1. SOURCES OF NECESSARY NUTRIENTS, VITAMINS AND MINERALS AVAILABLE FOR INFANTS.

MILK	Main source of calcium and riboflavin. Supplies protein, vitamin A (not sufficient for needs) and thiamine. No vitamin D unless irradiated; insufficient in iron.
MEATS	Main source of protein. Vitamin B. Iron.
POULTRY	Protein, minerals.
EGG YOLK	High in vitamin A. Minerals and vitamin B.
LIVER	Iron. Protein.
VEGETABLES	Green leafy vegetables, cooked properly; an important source of iron, vitamins A and B. Yellow vegetables, high in vitamin A. Peas, soybeans, lentils, peanuts. Protein, iron, vitamin B. Tomato juice, vitamins C and A.
FRUITS	General: Iron, vitamin B. Citrus and strawberries: vitamin C. Yellow fleshed: vitamin A, iron. Dried: iron (mainly dried prunes).
WHOLE GRAIN PRODUCTS	Main source of vitamin B. Significant amounts of protein, vitamin B complex.
SUGAR	Carbohydrate. Concentrated energy food.
FATS	Best source butter or margarine, high in vitamin A and energy. Also egg yolk and peanut butter.

able energy, the weak infant tires easily. It is not good practice to take more than 20 or 30 minutes for feeding such an infant. If the baby does not take at least two-thirds of his formula, this should be reported. Accurate intake recording is essential, because these babies may need help in the form of small transfusions or parenteral fluids to furnish them with enough energy to take more oral nourishment.

Self-demand feedings, about which we hear so much, if used at all with these infants, must be used cautiously. A normal, healthy baby promptly makes his needs known if he is hungry, and will quickly fall into a routine, following the rhythmic filling and emptying of his stomach. If such a child sleeps through his feeding time only to waken an hour later in a near-famished state, he usually is the best gauge of his own needs. But the malnourished baby probably has lost the power to regulate his own supply and demand schedule.

CONDITIONS OF THE RESPIRATORY TRACT

The infant entering the hospital with an acute respiratory difficulty presents certain symptoms regardless of the causative factor. His respirations are shallow and rapid because of his body's effort to oxygenate the red blood cells. His nasal passages occlude easily, making sucking diffi-

TABLE 10-2. RECOMMENDED DAILY ALLOWANCES OF
NUTRIENTS, MINERALS AND VITAMINS DURING
FIRST YEAR OF LIFE.*

CALORIES	100–120/kg. of body weight.†
PROTEIN	2–4 gms./kg. of body weight.
FAT	No specific quantity set.
CARBOHYDRATES	No specific quantity set.
IRON	5–7 mg.
VITAMIN A	1500 I.U.
THIAMINE	0.4–0.5 mg.
RIBOFLAVIN	0.5–0.8 mg.
NIACIN	6–7 milliequivalents
VITAMIN C (ascorbic acid)	30 mg.
VITAMIN D	400 I.U.

* Table compiled from various sources.
† One kg. equals 2.2 lb.

cult or impossible. He undoubtedly has sternal retractions and some degree of cyanosis. In addition, he is likely to be very irritable.

The nurse must have an adequate knowledge of the normal respiratory system in order to provide satisfactory care. She should anticipate the child's need for a moisture saturated atmosphere in order to keep secretions liquefied and render his breathing easier. She understands the importance of a frequent change of position, at the same time recognizing the child's great need for rest to avoid complete physical exhaustion.

Case of Baby Jane

Baby Jane, four months old, was to be admitted to the sick babies' nursery with a diagnosis of Acute Bronchiolitis. Ruth Smith, student nurse, was assigned to get the room ready, as well as to care for Baby Jane on her arrival. The nurse was told to set up a Croupette and to prepare to maintain heavy moisture. If we follow her actions throughout the day, we may get a better picture of infant care under such conditions.

Before Baby Jane arrived, Miss Smith set up a Croupette in the crib, checking for good working order and following clearly marked directions on the Croupette itself. After this had been done, she put plenty of diapers, flannel gowns, pads and small blankets in the room, knowing that the infant would need frequent changes to prevent chilling in the moisture laden atmosphere.

Mrs. Brown and Baby Jane arrived on the ward just as Miss Smith finished setting up the unit. The mother looked apprehensive, and the nurse thought she had good reason to be. Baby Jane certainly looked sick. She had a pinched, anxious look, with a bluish pallor around her mouth. She was extremely fretful, twisting about and crying irritably, and breathing in a shallow, rapid manner.

"I just don't know what to do with her," said her mother. "She won't stop crying, she won't eat, but she still acts hungry. She looks awfully sick."

Miss Smith thought so too, but she sensed that the mother was looking to her for reassurance. "I think she will feel more comfortable if we get her in this Croupette as soon as possible. I will turn it on full while we undress her, so that she can get plenty of moisture. That should make her breathe easier. Shall I undress her for you?"

Mrs. Brown seemed relieved to have a competent nurse take over. Baby Jane was quickly put into a hospital gown and diaper, and lightly wrapped in a blanket. Her nurse cleaned the secretions from the anterior nares, using a cotton pledget moistened with water. Then she tucked the baby into the Croupette, carefully turning her on her side, with her head slightly elevated.

Baby Jane was too young and to exhausted to show any fear of the Croupette. As the moist air penetrated her nasal passages, she relaxed, breathed easier, and shortly fell asleep. Her mother also relaxed, and was happy to accept the suggestion that she go to the cafeteria for a cup of coffee.

Baby Jane required very careful nursing. In addition to maintaining moisturized air, Miss Smith kept close supervision of the sick child. As she became damp from the heavy moisture, Baby Jane required frequent change of clothing to prevent chilling. She had a great need for adequate fluid, inasmuch as a small infant can dehydrate very rapidly, and here the nurse experienced difficulty.

The baby appeared thirsty and made repeated attempts to suck her thumb, but would always pull it away angrily and cry. Miss Smith filled a nursing bottle with glucose water which she offered to Baby Jane through the tent opening. The baby sucked eagerly once or twice, and then fretfully drew away. This was repeated several times. When the doctor was informed of this he explained Baby Jane's puzzling behavior.

"Of course she is thirsty, but it is difficult for her to suck and to breathe at the same time because her nose is nearly occluded. Offer her glucose water at intervals, but do not persist if she has any difficulty. We will give her intravenous feedings to care for her liquid and nutritional needs, and this will also help to relieve her thirst."

To give a happy ending to the story, Baby Jane, who was essentially healthy and robust, recovered quite rapidly under the meticulous care she received, and went home to be once again the pride of her family. Thereafter, however, when any of the other children had a cold, they stayed completely away from Baby Jane.

Acute Bronchiolitis (Acute Interstitial Pneumonitis)

Acute bronchiolitis occurs with the greatest frequency during the first six months of life, and is rarely seen after the age of one year. The majority of cases occur in infants who have been in contact with older children or adults suffering from upper respiratory viral infections.

Etiology. The condition is assumed to be of viral origin in most cases, because a significant number of cases are associated with respiratory viral infection. Laboratory proof has not been available as yet, but present data does seem to support this contention.

Pathology. The bronchi and bronchioles become plugged with a thick, viscid mucus, causing air to be trapped in the lungs. The infant can breathe air in, but has difficulty expelling it. This hinders the exchange of gasses, and cyanosis appears.

Manifestations. Onset of dyspnea is abrupt, sometimes preceded by a cough or a nasal discharge. There is a dry, persistent cough, extremely shallow respiration and cyanosis, which is frequently marked. Suprasternal and subcostal retractions are present. The chest becomes barrel-shaped from the trapped air.

Body temperature elevation is not great, seldom rising above 101° to 102°F. Dehydration may become a serious factor if competent care is not given. The infant appears apprehensive, irritable and restless.

Nursing Care

Nursing care includes placing the infant in a highly humidified atmosphere. At present, cold humidification is preferred to steam. Various means for providing this kind of humidity are in use, and these will be discussed later in this section.

Elevation of the child's head and chest aids his breathing. Placing the child on his abdomen provides pressure on the chest to relieve the distension, but should not be done unless the nurse can observe the infant continuously, because he is undoubtedly too weak to protect his breathing if obstruction occurs. He should be turned at least every hour, and needs frequent changes of clothing because of the moist atmosphere.

If he is to be fed, clean his nares as much as possible before offering a bottle. Use a relatively small-holed nipple so that he does not choke, but do not make him work hard enough to tire him. If he can be removed from his Croupette, he no doubt will fare better when he is held for feeding. If he needs to stay in his humidified atmosphere continually, be certain that his head is elevated, and hold his bottle, watching for choking or signs of exhaustion.

The nurse must remember that the baby is working hard in an effort to breathe, and can become exhausted very easily. Handling should be at a minimum consistent with intelligent nursing care.

Medication is usually minimal because antihistamines, expectorants and sedatives do not appear to be useful. Antibiotics may be given to control secondary bacterial infections. Tracheostomy is not indicated in this condition.

With careful nursing care and intelligent treatment, the condition can be expected to improve within a few days. Mortality rate is low if adequate supportive care is given; it is considered to be under 5 per cent, even in severe cases. Complications, however, can include cardiac failure, respiratory failure from exhaustion, severe dehydration from loss of fluid because of hyperventilation, and bacterial bronchopneumonia.

Acute Bronchitis

Acute bronchitis in infancy is usually secondary to a previous infection, such as acute nasopharyngitis or one of the communicable diseases of childhood. Predisposing causes may be malnutrition, or some chronic infection of the upper respiratory tract.

Manifestations include a moderate fever with a dry cough which becomes looser as the disease progresses. The infant is not able to expectorate the loosened secretions and swallows or aspirates into the trachea and the bronchi.

Nursing Care

Nursing care is the same as in bronchiolitis, including moist air, change of position, and attention to nutritional needs.

The condition is rarely fatal with good nursing care and medical management. Serious complications are uncommon, although diffuse pneumonitis may occur. This is not the problem it once was, however, ever since the advent of antibacterial medicines. Chronic bronchitis is uncommon in small children.

Pneumonia in Infancy

Bacterial pneumonia in infancy is usually a bronchopneumonia rather than the lobar variety. Infecting agents include the pneumococcus, streptococcus, staphylococcus and *H. influenzae.* Pneumonia in infancy is often preceded by symptoms of an upper respiratory infection.

Manifestations. The infant with pneumonia is very sick. Temperatures reach 103 to 104°F early in the disease. Respirations are shallow and rapid, reaching as high as 80 a minute, and pulse rate of 140 to 180 is common in infants. Convulsions may occur at the onset, and vomiting is common.

Treatment. Treatment is concerned with the use of antibiotics, which generally give prompt and favorable response, and the use of oxygen and humidified air.

Prognosis. With early treatment, use of effective drugs, and conscientious nursing care, the mortality rate has dropped to below 3 to 5 per cent in all but staphylococcal infections.

Nursing Care

Nursing Care must be of a high order. Rest, removal of secretions by tracheal suction when necessary, dry clothing and frequent position changes are essential. Accurate observation and recording of vital signs, as well as of symptoms, is essential.

Staphylococcal pneumonia. Staphylococcal pneumonia, which threatened to reach serious proportions, especially in the newborn nursery, has not become as widespread as had once been feared. This condition is complicated by lung abscesses, empyema and pneumothorax. Case fatality can be high, although it now has been reduced by early recognition and prompt antibacterial treatment. Prophylactic measures are considered to be the principles of treatment in newborn nurseries. In view of the serious nature of the disease, and of the urgent need for early antibacterial drug therapy, the possibility of staphylococcal pneumonia should be considered in every pneumonia of infancy until laboratory reports prove otherwise.

Specific Nursing Procedures in Caring for Infants with Respiratory Disorders

Maintenance of High Humidity Atmospheres

A number of devices have been used to provide moisturized air for infants and children suffering from respiratory distress. In the past, steam kettles and "croup tents" were popular, but present-day methods favor the use of cold vapor.

The most commonly used apparatus for the administration of cold vapor is the Croupette. The Croupette is a "cool-mist croup tent,"* which is set up in a matter of minutes. The metal frame rests on the crib, and is covered with a plastic canopy. A jar of water outside the tent, out of the baby's reach, is attached to an atomizer assembly, delivering a fine

* Air–Shields, Inc., Hatboro, Pa.

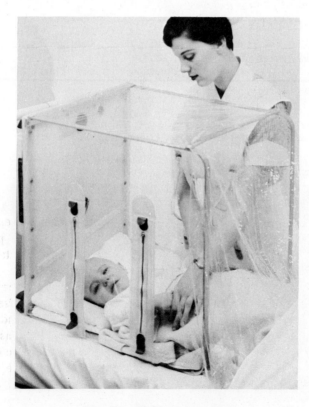

Fig. 71. Child in Croupette.

mist that fills the tent. Tubing from the atomizer may be connected to an oxygen tank or to a wall inlet if the use of oxygen is desired. If oxygen is not indicated, compressed air is used. An ice chamber situated at the back of the frame is useful for keeping the tent at a comfortable temperature, but need not be used if the baby's temperature is low. Directions for operating the Croupette are on the machine itself, and are easy to follow. (Fig. 71)

A baby is visible at all times through the plastic canopy, and complete care can be given through the zippered openings.

Another type of humidifier is the Mistifier.* (Fig. 72) This humidifier can be placed on the bedside stand with the outlet directed toward the patient. A plastic canopy draped over the crib with an opening to allow the vapor to enter is useful for direct inhalation. The Mistifier operates continually for about 10 hours before refilling is required, and has only to be plugged into any electrical outlet.

BIBLIOGRAPHY

Chapman, A. H.: Management of Emotional Problems of Children and Adolescents. Philadelphia, J. B. Lippincott, 1965.

Fishbein, M., (ed.): Birth Defects. Chapter 25. Philadelphia, J. B. Lippincott, 1963.

Gerber Products Company: Foods for Baby and Mealtime Psychology. Fremont, Michigan, Gerber Products, 1963.

Nelson, W., (ed.): Textbook of Pediatrics. 8th ed. Philadelphia, W. B. Saunders, 1964.

Ravitch, M. M.: Intussusception in Infants and Children. Springfield, Illinois, Charles C Thomas, 1959.

Wilson, C. B., and Raeburn, C. L.: The surgical management of meningocele and myelomeningocele. J. Pediat., *61*:595, 1962.

* Air–Shields, Inc., Hatboro, Pa.

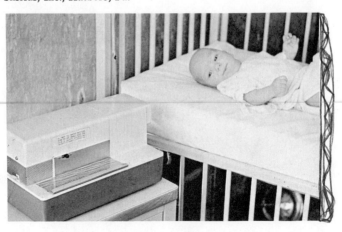

Fig. 72. Mistifier, ready for use.

SUGGESTED READINGS FOR FURTHER STUDY

Carrington, K. W.: Ventriculo-venous shunt: use of the Holter valve as a treatment of hydrocephalus. J. Mich. Med. Soc., 58:373, 1959.

Cooper, L. F., *et al.*: Nutrition in Health and Disease. 14th ed. Philadelphia, J. B. Lippincott, 1963.

Gucher, T.: The role of orthopedic surgery in long-term management of the child with spina bifida. Arch. Phys. Med., 45:82, 1964.

Merrill, R., *et al.*: Myelomeningocele and hydrocephalus. J.A.M.A., *191*:21, 1965.

Norton, P. L., and Foley, J. J.: Paraplegia in children. J. Bone Joint Surg., *41–A*:1291, 1959.

Potts, W.: The Surgeon and the Child. Philadelphia, W. B. Saunders, 1959.

Robins, M. M., and Plenk, H. P.: Intussusception in Childhood. Pediatrics, 25:592, 1960.

Willson, M. A.: Multidisciplinary problems of myelomeningocele and hydrocephalus. Phys. Ther., *45*:1139, 1965.

11

Orthopedic Conditions of Infancy

Infants with congenital orthopedic defects usually receive primary treatment on the general pediatric ward, and thus the nurse should be aware of the nature and treatment of these abnormalities. The two most common and important are clubfoot and dislocation of the hip.

CONGENITAL TALIPES EQUINOVARUS (CONGENITAL CLUBFOOT)

This is a deformity in which the entire foot is inverted, the heel is drawn up, and the forefoot is adducted. The Latin *talus,* meaning ankle, and *pes,* meaning foot, make up our word *talipes,* and is used in connection with many foot deformities. Equinus, or plantar flexion, and varus, or inversion, denote the kind of foot deformity present in this condition. The equinovarus foot has a club-like appearance, hence the term "clubfoot." (Fig. 73)

Congenital talipes equinovarus is the most common congenital foot deformity, appearing as a single anomaly, or in connection with other defects, such as myelomeningocele. It may be bilateral or unilateral. Etiology is not clear; an hereditary factor is occasionally observed. A theory that receives some acceptance postulates an arrested growth of the germ plasm of the foot during the first trimester of pregnancy.

Detection during the neonatal period. Talipes equinovarus is easily detected in a newborn infant, but must be differentiated from a persisting fetal "position of comfort" assumed in utero.

The positional deformity can be easily corrected by the use of passive exercise, but the true clubfoot deformity is fixed. The positional deformity should be explained to the parents at once, to prevent anxiety.

Nonsurgical Correction

If treatment is begun during the neonatal period, correction can usually be accomplished by nonsurgical methods. While the foot is held in as near normal a position as possible, without the use of force, a cast is applied over the foot and ankle (and usually to mid thigh) to hold the knee in right angle flexion. (Fig. 74) Casts are changed every few days to provide gradual, nontraumatic correction. Treatment is continued until complete correction is confirmed by X-ray and clinical observation, usually a matter of months.

An alternative method involves the use of a Denis Browne splint. The splint is composed of a flexible, horizontal metal bar attached to two foot plates. The child's foot is attached to the foot plate with adhesive tape, and the attachment of the horizontal bar permits changing the relationship of the bar to the plate as necessary. This splint must be used for a period of time, as long as seven or eight months, until a wide overcorrection is attained. (Fig. 75)

Following correction from a cast or a splint, a Denis Browne splint with shoes attached is used to maintain correction for another six months or so. After overcorrection has been attained, a special clubfoot shoe

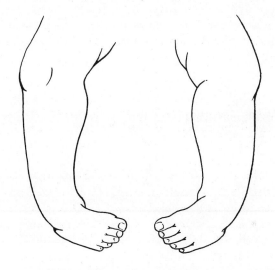

Fig. 73. Bilateral congenital talipes equinovarus.

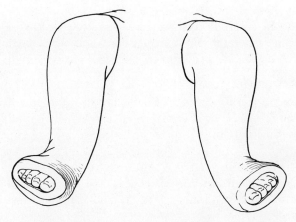

Fig. 74. Casting for correction of talipes equinovarus.

should be worn—a laced shoe with a turning out of the shoe and the outer wedge of the sole. The Denis Browne splint may still be worn at night, and passive exercises of the foot should be carried out by the child's mother.

Surgical Correction

Children who do not respond to nonsurgical measures, especially older children, need surgical correction. This involves several procedures dependent both upon the age of the child and upon the degree of deformity. It may involve lengthening of the Achilles tendon, capsulotomy of the ankle joint, release of medial structures, and, for the child over ten years of age, an operation on the bony structure.[*]

Prolonged observation, after correction by either means, should be carried out at least until adolescence, and any recurrence treated promptly.

Nursing Care in the Hospital

The infant or small child in a cast cannot explain to his nurses that his cast is too tight, impairing circulation, or is irritating his skin. Nursing observation should include the following:

Check the color and the temperature of the toes at frequent intervals. Check excessive irritability—indicating acute discomfort—with the attending physician.

Prevent the child from banging and denting his cast before it is dry. A clove-hitch restraint may be necessary.

Petal edges of the cast, when dry, with adhesive to prevent skin irritation.

Hold and comfort the child when possible. Better still, if his mother or father are present they can do this.

[*] Shands, A., Raney, R., and Brasher, H.: Handbook of Orthopedic Surgery. 6th ed., pp. 39–47. St. Louis, C. V. Mosby, 1963. (This is a good source for quick reference.)

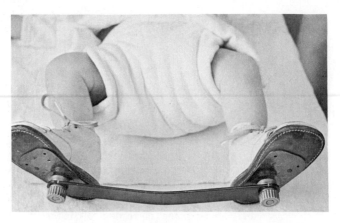

Fig. 75. Denis Browne splint with shoes attached.

If a Denis Browne splint is used instead of a cast, check the foot for irritation from adhesive tape, for swelling, or for any other indication of circulation impairment from the tight strapping.

Check frequently the position of the foot on the foot plate. These splints are uncomfortable until the infant becomes accustomed to them. He cannot kick the way he is accustomed to; in fact, there is less freedom of movement than when casts are used. These babies are in special need for comforting and being held.

Nursing Care Following Surgery

Check vital signs until they are stable.
Observe the cast for signs of bleeding.
Elevate the affected leg.
Observe circulation and temperature of the toes.
Be alert for any signs of infection.

Home Care

If the mother has helped with the hospital care, her baby is going to be much better served when he goes home. His mother must continue to watch for skin irritation and for signs of pressure from a cast that has become too tight. She must be prompt for any appointments, and understand the importance of notifying the physician or the clinic whenever the cast needs attention, or if the splint appears to have slipped.

The family must also be prepared to give additional emotional support to their baby until he becomes accustomed to his splint or his cast.

CONGENITAL DISLOCATION OF THE HIP

A defective development of the acetabulum, with or without dislocation, may be present in the newborn infant. The malformed acetabulum permits dislocation, the head of the femur becoming displaced upward and backward. The condition is difficult to recognize during early infancy. A family history is present in some instances, calling for increased observation of the young infant. The condition is approximately seven times more common in girls than in boys; and may be bilateral, but it is more commonly unilateral.

Diagnosis

Early recognition and treatment, before an infant starts to stand or walk, is of extreme importance for successful correction. Early signs include the following.

Asymmetry of the gluteal skin folds (they are higher on the affected side).
Limitation of abduction of affected hip. This is tested by placing infant on his back with his knees flexed, and then abducting both knees—passively—until they reach the examination table without resistance. If dislocation is present, the affected side cannot be abducted beyond 45°. Sometimes a clicking sound may be elicited as the head of the femur slips over the rim of the acetabulum.

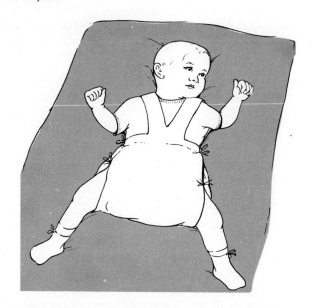

Fig. 76a. Frejka splint for the correction of a congenital dislocation of the hip.

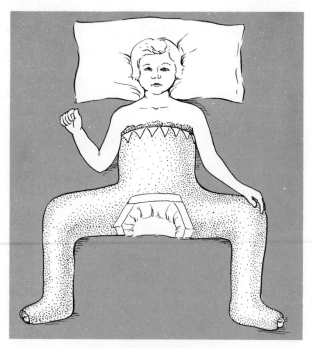

Fig. 76b. Frog leg cast.

Later signs, after the child has started walking, include: lordosis, sway-back, protruding abdomen, shortened extremity, duck-waddle gait, positive Trendelenburg sign. To elicit this sign, the child stands on his affected leg and raises his normal leg. The pelvis tilts downward rather than upward toward the unaffected side.

Roentgen studies are usually made to confirm the diagnosis. Uncorrected dislocation causes limping, easy fatigue, hip and low back discomfort, and postural deformities.

Treatment

Treatment begun before the first birthday, before displacement has taken place, is directed toward the formation of a normal joint by maintaining the head of the femur within the acetabulum. Good results are usually attained from the use of a Frejka pillow splint. The Frejka splint is a simple jumper-like device, with a pillow thickness between the thighs holding the hips in an abducted position. Plastic pants to protect the pillow should be worn over the diaper. The splint may be removed for diaper changing and for bathing. (Figs. 76a and 76b)

Treatment begun after the child has begun to walk includes traction on the affected leg for about a week or ten days in order to pull the head of the femur down to a point opposite the acetabulum, followed by casting in a frog-leg position for five to nine months. The frog-leg position is maintained whether the dislocation is unilateral or bilateral. After removal of the cast, physical therapy is needed, with use of a pool or a tank.

The child over the age of three years seldom responds to closed reduction, and surgical reduction becomes necessary. Traction may be applied prior to surgery, with a hip spica cast applied following surgery, to be worn for at least six months. Prognosis for replacement of the femoral head is poor after the age of six, and surgery is then performed to increase the stability of the hip and to improve its function.

Nursing Care

The infant in a Frejka pillow splint does not usually remain in the hospital. The child's mother is shown how to adjust the romper-like device, and the purpose is carefully explained to her. She is assured that she may hold him, or sit him in a chair or in a baby tender as she could any infant his age.

The child in a cast needs careful observation of circulation, attention to his skin, and comfortable positioning. A hard mattress is needed, with pillows for positioning while the cast is drying. Complaints of pain should be heeded and reported. The cast, which extends from the upper abdomen to the toes, should be petaled with adhesive around the waist and the toes, with a plastic sheet tucked under the cut-out pubic area and taped over the cast for protection from soiling and wetting.

If open reduction has been performed, the child should be watched for signs of shock and bleeding; fluids and diet are resumed as indicated.

The skin around and under the edges of the cast should be watched for irritation, particularly for crumbs of plaster, or food that may fall under the cast, or the child may stuff a small toy, or some food that he is supposed to have eaten, into the cast. The cast around the perineal area should be inspected daily for dampness or soiling, and the waterproof material washed, dried and reapplied.

The child may be held after the cast is dry; with a frog-leg cast he may be positioned in a sitting position on the nurse's lap, particularly for his meals. In bed, he must be turned frequently, and should be taken to the playroom or perhaps on rides about the hospital on a stretcher for diversion.

Parents need to learn the proper home care—learning most easily acquired through participation in the child's care before discharge.

BIBLIOGRAPHY

Fishbein, M., (ed.): Birth Defects. pp. 247–252. Philadelphia, J. B. Lippincott, 1963.

Furlong, M. B., and Lawn, G. W.: Evaluation of foot deformities in the newborn. G.P., *31*:89, (May) 1965.

Larson, C., and Gould, M.: Calderwood's Orthopedic Nursing. 6th ed. St. Louis, C. V. Mosby, 1965.

Ross Laboratories: Congenital Orthopedic Anomalies. Ross Laboratories, 1965.

Shands, A., Raney, R., and Brasher, H.: Handbook of Orthopedic Surgery. 6th ed., pp. 39–47. St. Louis, C. V. Mosby, 1963.

SUGGESTED READINGS FOR FURTHER STUDY

Coleman, S.: Treatment of congenital dislocation of the hip in the infant. J. Bone Joint Surg., 47–A:590, 1965.

UNIT 4

NURSING THE TODDLER

12

Normal Growth and Development from 1 to 3

Our infant, Johnny, has lived through one exciting year. What is in store for him during the period of transition from babyhood to childhood? We assume that he is normally healthy, and is living in a home in which he feels the love and security that is his birthright. His parents are just ordinary, everyday parents who make mistakes once in a while, who get cross, or occasionally tired and unreasonable, but who are willing to learn, are ready to use common sense, and, most important of all, have a large quantity of love and respect for their children.

PHYSICAL DEVELOPMENT

We can expect Johnny to have tripled his birth weight at one year, and to weigh four times his birth weight at two years. He grew about 10 to 12 inches during his first year; during his second year, he is going to add 3 or 4 more inches to his height. The growth chart in chapter 9 (Fig. 40) shows his normal progress up to two years of age.

Notice that his growth has slowed a little after the first year. Now he can concentrate on learning new skills and on perfecting those already attained. His voracious appetite gradually slows down as his world widens to include many things of more importance to him than food.

Deciduous Teeth

The toddler's teeth continue to erupt, but family patterns differ markedly. The chart in chapter 9 (Fig. 46) gives the sequence of tooth eruption and an indication of average time sequence. Marked delay in tooth eruption may occur in various growth and nutritional disturbances, but some families show early or late dentition without any other signs of deviation from normal.

Toothbrushing should be started early to establish good habits of tooth care. Plain water can be used until he acquires the ability to spit out the tooth paste. The American Dental Association recommends a general method of toothbrushing.* Brush down on the upper teeth, up

* American Dental Association: The Care of Children's Teeth. Chicago, American Dental Association.

on the lower teeth, and use a scrubbing motion on the grinding surface of the molars.

Fluoridation. If the toddler has been receiving fluoride drops since the neonatal period, his initial dose will be doubled when he has reached the age of 18 or 24 months, with increases in dosage during the second and third years of life. Fluoride preparations, in liquid or tablet form, are recommended for continuance into the ninth year, or until the crowns of the permanent teeth are calcified.

The fluoride ion taken internally strengthens the tooth formation, but is not effective in the preservation of teeth that have already erupted. Topical application of fluoride preparation is recommended as an additive, beginning at the age when the toddler accepts manipulative work in his mouth. This generally can be done at 30 or 36 months, but is of little value if much resistance is met, because the flow of saliva would be increased.

Topical application should be repeated at intervals of five to seven months, following tooth cleaning, and continued through college age. Topical application is advocated for those who drink fluoridated water, as well as for those receiving the pharmaceutical preparation.

The toddler should become acquainted with his dentist as early as possible. Between the ages of two and three is not too young for that first visit. He can become familiar with the office and equipment before dental care is necessary, thus never learning the fear that plagues so many children and adults.

Body Development

The *anterior fontanelle* normally closes by the age of 18 months, closing as early as 12 months in some children.

Big *muscles* are now well developed, and the toddler has a compulsion to use them. Coordination of the finer muscles is being perfected, allowing the toddler to manipulate eating utensils with increasing skill.

MILESTONES IN NORMAL GROWTH AND DEVELOPMENT DURING THE TODDLER YEARS

Twelve to Eighteen Months

At 18 months, the toddler is definitely an upright person, walking, and running with a somewhat stiff gait, and still using a wide stance. He is improving his motor skill and his muscular control. He enjoys pulling a wheeled toy while he walks, and he can climb stairs with help.

He can seat himself in a small chair, and he has learned to climb. He is becoming more adept at manual skills. He can place one block on another, and attempt a tower of three, although it may take some practice. He can hold a cup, using both hands, and drink, and he can hand the cup to his mother. He can throw a ball or hold a pencil, and can scribble vigorously.

His discriminating perceptions are mature in comparison with a one-year-old. He can point, on command, to pictures or objects familiar to him.

At 18 months, he is still self-absorbed, but now observes a newcomer with concentrated interest. He is aware of strangers, and probably shows fear of gestures of friendship from anyone he does not know. Although his urge to explore leads him into everything within his reach, he still takes refuge in the familiar, relying heavily on a blanket, favorite toy, or the ever-present thumb.

His linguistic abilities may have developed to the point at which he may have as many as ten words that now have definite meanings. He is beginning to imitate those occurrences that are familiar to him, such as pretending to read the paper. He is making the first gestures toward becoming a person in his own right. (Fig. 77)

Two Years Old

The two-year-old now runs quite easily and walks up stairs alone, a step at a time. He can not only throw a ball, but he can kick it too. Now he can build a tower of five or six blocks, which he appears to enjoy more than placing them in a horizontal line. He may be able to hold a cup with one hand, keeping the free hand close by. He is quite adept at handling a spoon, even though he may at times prefer to use his fingers.

He may have as many as 300 words in his vocabulary and is starting

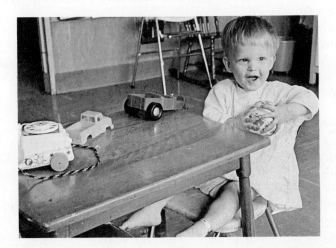

Fig. 77. Eighteen months of age—even a hospital can be fun.

to use short sentences. He is beginning to see himself as a person although his use of "you" and "I" may still be confusing, and he is more apt to use such expressions as "Johnny fall down," or, "Mommy come." He can, however, use the word "mine" with both purpose and determination. He is still self-engrossed, not yet entirely aware of himself and of others as individuals. Play is still largely parallel, although he enjoys having others around him.

Three Years Old

At three, most children have matured in a remarkable manner. Because of his ignorance of the world outside his home, the three-year-old's seeming maturity may lead older persons to expect more of him than he is able to give.

If his sense of security has been well supported, he should be ready for nursery school. He usually enjoys this form of independence. He is actually a "preschooler," and so we shall consider him.

Norms of Development

We have seen that the infant operates on the pleasure principle. He must develop security and trust before he can stand frustration. He has only begun to find himself as a person, and learned to differentiate himself from his mother.

Now, as a toddler, he has discovered his independence, and he must make the most of it. His development demands that he assert himself as a person. Much of his defiant behavior, his aggressiveness, comes from his "trying-on for size" of his newly developed personality. It is comforting to know that he is soon going to discard some particularly trying trait for a new one, equally unacceptable perhaps, but different. He can discard these much faster if he does not have his attention fixed on them by disapproving adults.

It is necessary to understand this important period in a toddler's development in order to give him the intelligent and satisfying care to which he is entitled.

Toilet Training

Johnny has matured in other ways since his previous admission to the infants' division. Now at two, he has, among other things, achieved at least a measure of bowel and bladder control. A brief look into his past year gives us some of the background of this development.

Toward the end of his first year, Johnny's muscles became sufficiently strengthened to support his weight, and he experienced the thrill of being able to stand and to walk. This was a wonderful experience, and Johnny became very proud of increasing ability to control his own movements.

He also became aware of pressure if his rectum was full, and had a dim comprehension of his own part in expelling feces.

Johnny's mother took advantage of these signs of maturation, and placed him on the potty-chair at the indicated times. Her approval when he performed properly filled him with gratification, because he was now old enough to value mother's approval more than his own immediate pleasure. He was pleased also to be able to offer her something of his own making.

Johnny felt no disgust over his products of elimination. The color and texture were rather pleasing to him, as well as the odor. In fact, he probably found this a convenient material at hand to satisfy his urge toward smearing.

If his mother was wise, she understood his feelings and did not shame him. When he had accidents, she quietly cleaned up the mess without comment. If he had used the feces as finger paint, she cleaned him up without showing disgust and provided more suitable play materials for him.

Sometime before the end of his second year, he was able to indicate his need to defecate, and was able to reach the proper place most of the time.

Johnny found control of his bladder sphincter rather more difficult. The start of his readiness to learn became apparent when he was able to connect the puddle on the floor with himself.

Mother had let Johnny watch other members of the family use the toilet. He was already familiar with the potty-chair, and was successful, most of the time, in using it for defecation. Now he perceived that mother would be pleased if he used it for that puddle as well.

Soon he was able to run to mother and indicate his need—usually after the fact! Not until he had sufficient control of his bladder sphincter to permit him to stay dry for two hours was there much benefit to be gained from serious training. With this degree of physiological control, together with his pride of accomplishment, it became not too difficult to stay dry, barring an occasional accident, during the daytime. For an average child, this control is usually achieved sometime during the latter half of the second year. Night control is not completely acquired by most children before the age of three; in fact, many normal children may be four or five before they achieve complete night control.

If a mother is sensible, she does not worry unduly if Johnny is slower in learning control than are her neighbor's children. It may be (and probably is) embarrassing for her when she takes him visiting, to hear relatives say, "Haven't you got that child toilet-trained yet?" She can take comfort knowing that Johnny must follow his own pattern of development and that few indeed are the healthy, well-adjusted persons who do not conform eventually.

PERSONALITY DEVELOPMENT

Developmental phases of this period are all concerned with the toddler's new awareness of the outside world and with his dim but growing understanding of his own power over his environment, and with his ability to manipulate it for his own ends. In general, we may speak of the normal developmental behavior of the toddler period as fitting into certain categories. Each child may, of course, exhibit these traits in a greater or lesser degree, or perhaps certain characteristics are not apparent at all. The average child, however, goes through most of the following stages.

1. Dependence/Independence
2. Negativism
3. Ritualism
4. Dawdling
5. Frustration often leading to temper tantrums

Dependence/Independence

The child's growing awareness of himself as a person brings about significant changes in his behavior. Previously, he maintained little conscious control over his actions. Now, as a person in his own right, he is beginning to understand that he has this power of control.

He hears "No, no" many times a day. Sometime during his development, he realized that he could disregard this "No, No" and that afterward, the world still stood. This is heady knowledge and he becomes intoxicated with power.

However, his mother's approval is still extremely important to him. What should he do—yield to that overwhelming urge toward independence, or seek his mother's praise? All too frequently, he finds that he cannot have both. It is a difficult decision.

A complicating factor is his lack of experience. How can he know the rules until he tries them out? He is like a stranger in a foreign land. He has to learn the laws, and he is quite willing to explore. He can explore and learn only if he has the comfortable knowledge that he can return to the tried and to the familiar if his new experiences tend to be overwhelming. He exhibits the same type of behavior that the well-known ethologist, Konrad Lorenz, found in the baby water-shrews he tried to raise in a large aquarium in his home. Lorenz wrote, "The water's edge seemed to exert a strong attraction; they approached it ever and again . . . the shrews interrupted their careful exploration of their new surroundings every few minutes to dash wildly back into the safe cover of their nest-box."*

* Lorenz, K. Z.: King Solomon's Ring. P. 100. New York, T. V. Crowell, 1965.

Negativism

Negativism quite naturally grows out of the toddler's growing sense of independence. He is comfortable with the background experience he has acquired, but the unknown is always frightening. He has two strong urges, to say "No" to every command, and to obey. Being caught between the two, he frequently tries both. It is not at all unusual to hear Johnny say "No" quite firmly when his mother calls him, at the same time moving in her direction. Add all this to the fact that "No" is the word he has heard more often than any other, and you have one basis for a negativism that is often more apparent than real.

Ritualism

The toddler also employs ritualism as a compromising device. If you have done much baby-sitting for this age group, you no doubt have encountered the child who must follow a certain pattern exactly, especially at bedtime. His clothes must be placed just so, and his toys must all be in a certain order.

This is important to the toddler for his security in what is familiar to him. The amount of security he has already developed determines his ability to go forward into the new and the unfamiliar. This ritualism can, of course, be carried to excess, and may indicate some deep-seated emotional disturbance. A certain amount, however, is normal in a young child.

Temper Tantrums

The child's urge to do it himself naturally results in many frustrations. Add to this the fact that he is reluctant to leave the scene for necessary rest, and you can see that frequently the frustrations become just too great. Even the very best of mothers can lose patience, showing a temporary lack of understanding. The only reaction Johnny can show to this is rebellion, which he is likely to employ with as much enthusiasm as he would use in any other situation. This too is a phase he must live through as he works toward becoming a person.

THE TODDLER IN THE HOSPITAL

When the toddler enters the hospital, he brings his own developmental patterns with him. If he is a normal child, he may show negativism and dependence as well as independence in the way we have just observed. In addition to this, his physical development is at the stage when his muscles must be used actively. All this makes this age a difficult period for hospitalization.

The hospital is an institution set up primarily for the treatment and the healing of the sick. At its best, it can never provide an adequate environment for a developing child. It cannot take the place of a child's home, even when that itself is far from ideal. At home, he gets some degree of recognition as a person, and some personal attention from his mother or someone in her place.

The goal of a hospital pediatric staff must be to get the child well and back into his home as quickly as possible. It must never be forgotten that despite our best efforts, we can never really take the place of the home, or become "mother substitutes."

While we do have the child in the hospital, however, we have a duty toward him. We must try to meet his needs here and now, under the existing circumstances. In order to meet his needs, we first have to understand them.

Naturally, a healthy child is not admitted to the hospital as a patient. He may have pain, or be uncomfortable and ill at ease. He may have little incentive to carry on with his previous zest for living.

His development continues, however. When his illness keeps him from obeying the demands of his nature, he becomes cross and irritable. If he must be confined to his crib, he becomes increasingly restless.

Disciplinary Problems

Whenever a nurse feels that she must punish a child for non-conforming, she forgets one basic fact. The child is already being punished pretty severely by his environment and by his discomfort. The nurse should think carefully before adding to this unpleasantness.

Certainly a sick child needs discipline. A sick child who is pampered and indulged, and is perhaps allowed to follow his own immature impulses, is just as unhappy as he makes others. He would be grateful for limits set, if it is done with love and understanding.

The disciplinary problems of this age group are many and varied. The answers are not so clear. No two children come to the hospital from the same environment. Some have been ill for a long time and have been overindulged. Others have been severely disciplined or even rejected. Every child has a different capacity to withstand frustration, depending on his personality, his background, and upon his state of health.

Emotional Support

The nurse must be constantly aware of all phases of the child's reaction to illness. She must try to avoid causing any unpleasantness, and must be reluctant to add to the child's unhappiness.

Suppose we take a representatve young person through a hospital admission. We should start before he reaches the front door of the hospital if we really want to understand him. Johnny is now a normal two-year-old, slightly below the average in height and weight. His mother is rather concerned about his poor appetite and has tried many devices to get him to eat. She has explained the hospital to him, and has tried to prepare him for this experience.

The mother as an aid to the nurse. Johnny has had a close, warm relationship with his mother. He has not been away from her for any length of time, and has never been away overnight. At two, he is not yet mature enough to enter nursery school. He plays contentedly in the fenced yard, coming to the house every half hour or so just to assure himself that his mother is still there. His growing independence and self-reliance are possible only because they are firmly rooted in a comfortable sense of security. His mother—his source of strength—is still there. (Fig. 78)

When Johnny enters the hospital, he comes along cheerfully enough with you, chattering and smiling, and holding his mother's hand. Your strange cap and apron may puzzle him, but his mother is right there, and he is clutching his favorite toy.

He enters a room with many cribs, is undressed and put into one. You say to his mother, "Mrs. Smith, please sit out in the office, the doctor wants to ask you about Johnny." His mother leaves, up goes the crib side and you hustle out.

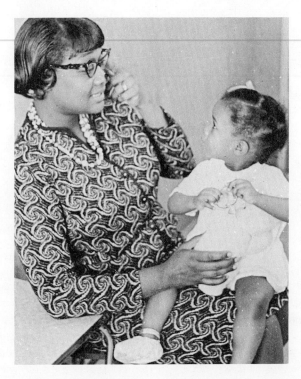

Fig. 78. Toddlers are content when their mothers can stay.

Now Johnny *is* frightened. Never before has he been completely undressed in the middle of the day, and put to bed; or perhaps his mother had thus punished him. If so, what has he done wrong now? So often he gets punished without any clear understanding of the "why." This must be such a time, but where is his mother?

Soon you come back and, turning him over, take a rectal temperature. This is uncomfortable as you well know if you have ever had a rectal temperature taken. He tightens up and becomes even more uncomfortable. This time, you leave him screaming with fright.

Is there any way you can make this introduction to the hospital more pleasant and set the stage for a happier stay? Suppose we examine this experience step by step.

Johnny has entered the hospital with considerable confidence. The building is big and strange, the elevator ride perhaps a new sensation. However, his feet are firmly planted in the old and the familiar. His stuffed animal, his shoes, his clothes, and most of all, his mother, are all part of his security. Now you proceed to remove that security. Is it any wonder that he is frightened?

When you bring him into the ward, must he be undressed immediately? Could he and his mother wander around a little, try out the toys, peep into the playroom, or speak to other small children?

Rules are rules, of course, and are set up for valid reasons. Sometimes, however, the nurse merely assumes that certain rules prevail, without actually finding out. Sometimes rules are enforced after the reason for their use is past. It never does any harm to ask.

If the hospital policy is such that Johnny must go to bed at once, think of other ways to make him feel more at ease. Let his mother leave some object intimately associated with her person in his hand, so that he can still feel her presence.

Little children are very possessive about some articles of their own clothing, especially their shoes. Some actually seem to feel that their shoes are an integral part of themselves. One little boy wore his shoes to bed, and another stamped manfully to his bath in his bathrobe and cowboy boots.

A bathrobe and a pair of slippers are usually left with the child and are comforting if in plain sight. His own pajamas are a big link with home. All of these articles give him a feeling that he has not been abandoned in a strange new place.

If his mother can stay with him until the strangeness has worn off, this benefits all concerned. Who can get the urine specimen easier than his mother who has just been training him in bladder control?

It is amazing that we persist in doing things the hard way. Johnny can nearly always "go" for mother, but tightens up and actually cannot urinate to please a stranger. What, then, can we do? We could wait until his mother has left, and try to make him urinate—without success. We could clap on restraints, and fasten a urine collector on him. Thus we build up resentment and fright, neither of these emotions being noted as conducive to good health.

One little fellow went for hours with a urine collector taped to him, afraid to urinate, until at last he could hold out no longer and flooded everything, bringing embarrassment to him and displeasure from the nurse.

Whenever possible, it is an excellent idea to let his mother take Johnny's rectal temperature. She has almost certainly done this before, and Johnny feels that he can trust her. Perhaps she has taught him to use an oral thermometer, but because toddler's wards in general employ rectal thermometers, it may be better to let his mother take the first rectal temperature and thus show him that although this may be uncomfortable, it is not painful.

If the nurse stays with Johnny and his mother for a few minutes before she leaves—if she must leave—and for 10 or 15 minutes after her departure, this would ease greatly the strain of separation. He will not feel quite so alone because you, his friend, are there with him. Perhaps a coloring book with large crayons might keep the two of you so engrossed that parting might be endurable.

Of course you are busy, but are you sure that you cannot spare enough time from your other duties to help a stranger feel at home? Perhaps the other duties seem so urgent because you yourself are uncomfortable in the situation, and cannot bear to see the child's distress. This, of course, is not helping the child.

Eating Problems

One problem that seems to loom large in nurses' minds is that concerned with the toddler's eating habits. How to get Johnny to eat? A worthwhile exercise for the nurse is to sit quietly for a moment, and let her mind wander back to a time when she was away from home, perhaps for the first time. Perhaps you can remember visiting your grandmother or other relatives, and were quite proud that you were big enough to stay without your mother. But after your mother left, things seemed very strange. You were lonely, perhaps homesick, or tired and confused. Perhaps even more recently, you can recall your first day away at school, or at college or at nursing school. You felt strangely alone; you sat down to a meal prepared differently from any your mother gave you. The foods were different, they did not even smell the same. How was *your* appetite?

Many small children are considered to have eating problems at home. They no longer need food with such intensity as they did during their first year, and this being the age for dawdling—they dawdle. A mother becomes anxious or frustrated or angry. In any case, Johnny quickly learns that this is an opportunity for a scene, and he dearly loves scenes. This is his big opportunity, such as he had never anticipated. Mother can urge, bribe, coax and scold, but the most she can do is to put food into his mouth. She cannot make him swallow it. If she does succeed, he can always bring it back again!

Mealtime thus becomes a hectic time in many households. Frequently a mother says to the nurse, "To make him eat, try giving one bite to his doggie then one bite to him," or "Pretend that the spoon is a steam shovel delivering down the little red lane," or even, "Be cross with him and he will eat." Food thus has assumed an importance out of all proportion to its value, and the nurse is left with an added problem.

Eating as a social function. In hospitals we frequently tend to forget that eating is a·social function in our culture. Many a toddler who sits in his crib playing with his food would eat with relish if he were placed at the table with his contemporaries. We know this, and go as far as to provide small tables and chairs, but again and again we see a little one still in his crib with his breakfast set up in front of him because someone found it easier to give him his tray there than to get him up.

Why can't he get up for breakfast? Would something serious happen to him if he were to get up before his bath? Few children have to stay in their cribs all of the time, but even if a child must be confined to his bed, he can be pulled over nearer to the more fortunate ones for companionship.

FAMILY-STYLE MEALS. Some pediatric wards serve meals family-style around a big table. A fortunate few allow the nurse to eat with the children. If this is not the case in your hospital, see if Johnny cannot be allowed to go into another ward where his friends are for at least some of his meals.

You say that you have tried all of this, and that Johnny still won't eat? What next? First of all, what do you mean that Johnny won't eat? Do you mean that Johnny won't eat *enough*? Enough for you, or perhaps enough for an inactive two-year-old? Did you give him a plate piled high with food or did you give him tiny portions? That mountain of food frequently seen on small children's trays is enough to discourage anyone. Dr. Lowenberg* says that a good rule to follow is to give him less than you expect him to eat, and let him ask for more.

Finger foods and table manners. Finger foods, if available, have considerable attraction for a young child. Perhaps this is a good place for a word about the child's manner of eating. Small children are great believers in do-it-yourself. You may find that he might get more down, and keep it down, if he puts it there himself. He has probably become quite adept with his hands, but table utensils may be another matter. When

---

* Lowenberg, M.: Food as Children see it. Film, 16 mm., sound, 17 min. Grand Rapids, Michigan, General Mills, 1952.

you see him struggling with the spoon, trying to get the contents into his mouth, don't interfere. He will soon put the spoon down, and use the utensils nature gave him.

The hospital, a sick child, and mealtime do not make a favorable situation for teaching table manners. If he is not deliberately turning his glass upside down, or overturning his plate, or throwing his food on the floor, leave him alone. What is your objective—to get him to eat or to teach him Emily Post?

A little calculated neglect at mealtime often works wonders. When you hover over him urging him to take just one more bite, the attraction of saying no becomes irresistible. If it appears to make no difference to you personally whether he eats or not, there is no need for resistance, because there is nothing to resist. He can then permit himself to be influenced by the attractiveness of the food. He is also free to fall under the influence of his peers at the table, one of whom, it is hoped, is a good eater. An adult at the table eating in a businesslike manner may be a beneficial influence.

Still, he doesn't eat. He is too sick, or not hungry. If left alone, he plays with his food or he ignores it. Along comes the doctor or the head nurse and tells you that you must make him eat. And the first thing his mother asks when she arrives is "How did he eat today?"

Now what?

Favorite foods. Does he like ice cream? Of course, but he must eat his meal first. Why? Remember that your objective is to get nourishing food into his system. What could be more nourishing than ice cream? Forget for a moment your own childhood inhibitions. You have a sick, unhappy child before you whose need for nourishment is greater at the moment than is his need for discipline. Which is better for him: to engage in a contest of wills, or to eat ice cream in peace?

It is frequently suggested that the nurse ask the mother about her child's likes and dislikes. This is fine and helpful, but all too often in a busy hospital there is little chance for the nurse to procure for the child any foods other than those being served. Be sure to find out if there are any other possibilities. Some hospitals allow a mother to bring in the child's favorite dish cooked the way he likes it. Many hospitals, however, do not allow any food to be brought in.

Small children frequently find it difficult to do quite ordinary things in front of strangers. It is common to find a child who has been eating well enough to refuse to eat if she has a new nurse. Sally is a good example.

Because of extensive burns she sustained when she was an infant, Sally had spent at least one-third of her three years in and out of hospitals. She adjusted as well as one could expect, but whenever there was a change in student rotation Sally was in trouble.

One day the instructor walked into the ward to find the student nurse nearly in tears. "I don't know what I am doing wrong," she said, "but Sally won't touch her breakfast." The instructor looked at the untouched food. "That seems to be a pattern with Sally whenever she has a new nurse," she remarked. "By the way, where is Sally?" Silently, the nurse pointed at the floor, and there was Sally crouched under the table.

They decided to go slowly and to let Sally make the advances. By the next day, she was eating happily with the others and telling her nurse about the proper way to clean her "pedicle."

Toilet Training Problems

When Johnny entered the hospital at the age of two, he had discarded his diapers and was wearing training panties. This helped him to stay dry, because everyone knows that diapers are for wetting.

Much of what happens to the child after his admission depends on the kind of attention he receives. In the face of pain and loneliness, he may regress to a more infantile level. If this occurs, he should be put back into diapers without comment. No attempt should be made toward bladder and bowel training while he is sick and away from his mother.

We expect little children who have only recently, or partially learned control, to regress during illness. This, however, is insufficient justification for putting all toddlers into diapers on admission to the hospital. Some children will be secure enough and maintain control if their needs are met promptly. Putting a child into diapers invites regression.

Many children who have achieved control try quite desperately to maintain it. They sit in their cribs calling "Potty" until they can hold out no longer. One or two times are sufficient to cause them to forget completely. It is unfortunate that we ever allow this to happen.

Control is too new to other children to enable them to remember to ask in time. Placing the child on a potty-chair at two hour intervals can help him to maintain his control. As we observed before, it is quite useless to train a child in bladder and bowel control if he is sick and away from home.

Marie stayed dry quite successfully during the day, but she wet her bed at night. This distressed the night nurse, who felt that Marie, at three years of age, should be able to indicate her need at night. She was put into diapers every night at bedtime, with the remark that this was done because she was acting like a baby.

One day, Marie's mother brought her a pair of bright, frilly panties. Someone forgot to remove them at bedtime, and in the morning Marie was still dry. She would not wet her beautiful new panties. Thereafter, Marie wore panties at night instead of diapers, and there was seldom an accident.

One curious phenomenon may be observed in a toddler's ward. The small child has learned that bed-wetting is socially unacceptable. When his mother has found his bed dry in the morning, she has praised him, as well as proudly proclaiming his accomplishment to the rest of the family.

After he enters the hospital, the situation is somewhat different. When the little girl makes known her need to urinate, a bed pan is slipped under her. It takes more maturity than most two- or three-year-olds possess to be able to differentiate between urinating into a bed pan and wetting the bed. Sitting her on a potty-chair at the bedside places her in a familiar situation, and enables her to function properly.

The little boy also experiences difficulty with the unfamiliar. The urinal is a strange device. He may not be able to understand its use, especially if he is set up in bed to use it.

Many children can be allowed to use a potty-chair at the bedside even if they are on bed rest. Permission for this must be obtained, of course.

When caring for a child who must wear diapers, either because he has not yet learned control, or because he has regressed, be sure that the diaper is securely fastened. It must be large enough to be comfortable, but secured with pins at the waist and at the legs as well. Many nurses fit diapers carelessly, leaving large openings at the legs. The first time that you come into the ward and find the crib, the bedside stand and the child himself thoroughly finger-painted, you will learn that four diaper pins are essential. This experience, both you and the child can well do without.

Force Fluids

The small child's need for fluids is usually more important than is his need for food when he is sick. Some of these fluids can be nourishing drinks and thus take the place of food. A diet of milk shakes, ice cream, fruit juices and jello water is not too bad nutritionally, at least for a while.

Remember that a little child has a small capacity, so it is best to offer small servings of liquids. A small child does not come to you and ask for a drink; you must anticipate his needs.

You have an order that reads "Push fluids to 1500 cc." For breakfast, Johnny takes 35 cc. It looks like a long bleak day ahead. You hopefully hold the cup to his lips, and he seems to sip away. Your heart sinks, however, as you note that the level of the fluid has not sunk at all!

The only answer seems to be persistence. Offer the drink in a small cup. A 1 oz. medicine cup is just the right size, and seems to empty quickly—if the toddler has not already been conditioned against a medicine cup.

A morning tea party with small cups and a pot to pour from provides entertainment as well as fluid. Taking turns pouring prolongs the party until everyone has had a turn. The pot may need many fillings, but the fluid chart is going to look much better. Often we find that it takes just a little imagination to help solve the problems of little people.

A child who must stay in bed has one overwhelming ambition: to see his mother. To have something to show her when she comes adds to his pleasure. A helpful device is a large picture of a drinking glass drawn by the nurse and pinned up in full view. The glass is marked off into sections according to the number of small drinks the child needs to fill his quota. Each time the child empties a cup, he chooses a crayon and colors a section. The object of the game is to have a beautiful multi-colored glass to give mother when she comes. It really works.

Whatever method you use to entice a child to drink is going to require a great deal of patience and persistence on your part. If every time you go to the child you offer him a drink, it may surprise you how much it will add up. You can take pride in your own sense of accomplishment when you go to the head nurse at two o'clock and say, "Johnny has had 800 cc. today."

Penicillin b.i.d.

Miss Ferris carefully laid out her syringes, her needles, and her skin antiseptic. With flawless technique, she filled her syringes and started her rounds. Her entrance into the ward was greeted with howls, screams, and cries of "Go away." When she left, she walked out on a most unhappy ward.

Every nurse has had a similar experience at some time. It is hard to take. She has made a persistent effort to win the affection of the children, and had thought that she had met with some success—but not now. The child who was sweet and loving this morning now declares "I hate you!"

In some hospitals, the student nurse gives total care to her patients. The same nurse who cares for the child plays with him and comforts him, also gives him his medication. That is ideal for several reasons. The child has learned to know and to trust her, and knows that she is not going to hurt him deliberately.

Other hospitals still use the functional method of giving medications, in which one nurse is the medicine nurse for the entire ward, or for the team. In either case, dispensing medications on the pediatric department presents problems.

Safety measures are always important. Some of them assume special significance in the toddler's ward because of the distinctive nature of the patients. A few may be considered here before we start out with the medicine chart.

Perhaps most of the errors in giving medications on children's wards are from incorrect identification. When you passed medicines on the ward and you took Mrs. Smith her medicine she may have said, "But I always get two yellow pills, you have given me three pink ones." Either you explained to her that this was a different brand of the same medicine, or you went back and checked. In any event, you respected her judgement. But when three year old Susy says "I want a red pill," you are apt to tell her to take the pill you are offering her. You do not expect her to have the judgement Mrs. Smith had, and you suspect her of just being whimsical.

Again, if you go into the ward and ask that mischievous Dennis to tell you his name, he may give you any name that suits his fancy at the moment. Nor is there anything to prevent him from climbing into another child's crib and answering to whatever name he fancies, Billy, Johnny, or whatever. Inasmuch as positive identification is essential, the responsibility rests entirely on you.

If the child has removed his identification band, it would be well worth your while to confirm the identification before you give out the medicine. Also, the rule of checking the medicine card with the patient each time becomes doubly important.

The age at which children can swallow pills varies greatly. Some quite small children down them readily, whereas other, much older children gag and choke. If you have given a child a pill, make sure that he swallows it before you leave. Usually he opens up so wide that you can see way back to his tonsils.

It usually is best, however, to give a small child his medicine in solution form. If you must use a tablet, dissolve it in water. Do not use orange juice for a solvent unless specifically ordered to do so. The child may associate the taste of orange juice with the unpleasant medicine for the rest of his life. If the medicine is bitter, honey or corn syrup can disguise the taste. He may come to dislike corn syrup, but this is not going to be important to him as the inability to take orange juice.

An interesting example of one person's use of imagination to help a child take medicine occurred with three-year-old Bobby. He was a co-operative child, but had great difficulty in taking his medicine. He absolutely refused the suspension form, and gagged over the pill. Medicine time became a time of trial. Finally someone crushed the pill, placed it between two layers of honey on a spoon, and told Bobby to take the spoon in his hand and lick it like a popsicle. Thereafter, twice daily, he sat solemnly licking his "popsicle."

If you do come up with some such solution to a problem, be sure to make note of it on the kardex. It is also a good idea to ask the previous medicine nurse about any successful tricks she has learned.

There seems to be little excuse for restraining a small child and forcing the medicine down. Even though it does go down the esophagus instead of the trachea, you run a good risk of having it returned to you. The danger of aspiration is very real.

Perhaps giving the medicine from a spoon instead of a cup, or letting him sip through a straw, is all that is necessary. Perhaps he has just awakened and feels bewildered and cross. Go quietly on to the others and return a little later. You may find he makes no protest this time.

If he still refuses in spite of all your efforts, however, notify the head nurse. The doctor may change the form of the medication, or some constructive advice may be forthcoming.

Children, of course, have the same fear of needles that adults have. Students are reluctant to hurt the child, and frequently cause the very pain they are trying to prevent by inserting the needle slowly. A swift, sure jab is nearly painless, but the nurse must be prepared for the child's squirming and stay calm and sure. She should avoid trying to give an intramuscular injection alone to a small child. Another person is essential if the child is to be held firmly.

Always take time to explain to the child what you are going to do when you give him the needle. He may be too small to understand all of the words, but tell him anyway.

Of course you never tell him that it will not hurt, or that he is a big boy and should not cry. It does hurt, he is *not* a big boy, and there is nothing babyish about crying over a hurt anyway.

Be careful, however, not to spend too much time on preparation. The child can sense your reluctance and is quick to take advantage of it with stalling tactics. He may also find it quite impossible to comply even if he wants to please you. He has a definite need for your firmness. Explain what has to be done, then go ahead and do it.

One scheme that has proved successful in helping to remove the fear from the procedure worked something like this.

Jimmy was understandably reluctant to leave his play and lie down for his intramuscular injection. The nurse told him that after she finished, he could give a "shot" to his boy doll. Immediately after she had finished, Jimmy sat up, took the syringe and gave the doll three really vicious jabs. Every day thereafter, Jimmy could hardly wait until the nurse had finished so that he could do the same to the doll.

Amazingly, this works with a good many children. A little girl will dry her tears, carefully wipe off the site on her doll, insert the needle, draw back the plunger, remove it and then comfort her doll. One little miss looked up solemnly and remarked that her dolly said 'ouch.'

In one four-bed ward, each little boy had to have a turn trying out this procedure, although only one of them had actually received an injection. Nearly every child succumbs to the fascination of this, always under the watchful eye and close guidance of the nurse. One boy decided to put the needle into his doggie's tail! (Fig. 79)

Treatments

One of the most difficult duties a pediatric nurse has to perform is that of assisting with, or performing, painful treatments on, a small child. Most nurses find satisfaction in perfecting their technique and carrying out a smooth, flawless performance. Their confidence, though, is shaken

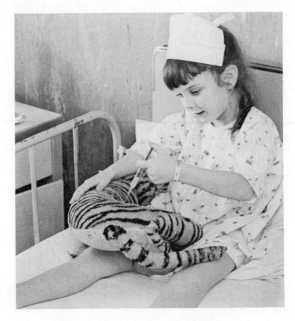

Fig. 79. Tiger gets an injection too.

when they realize that they are causing great discomfort, with the child understanding little of the the cause or reason for it.

The pediatric nurse on the toddler's ward has a greater opportunity to explain than she did on the infants division; but at best she will be imperfectly understood. Even if the toddler does grasp the words, they have little meaning for him. The big reality is that he hurts.

Sometimes the child's interest can be reached so that he can forget his fright. He must always be allowed to cry if he needs to do so. He should always be listened to, and his questions answered. It takes maturity and experience on the nurse's part to know exactly when the questions are stalling techniques, which call for firmness and action. Frequently, the nurse spends much time talking and reassuring the child, with the result that he senses the nurse's own insecurity. He needs someone to take charge in a kindly, firm manner that tells him that the decision is not in his hands. He is really too young to take this responsibility for himself.

Billy, age three, had to have daily treatments which were quite uncomfortable. He was told that he could cry as much and as loudly as he wished, but that he must lie still. Every day Billy marched into the treatment room, helped to arrange himself on the table, and never moved. As soon as the doctor appeared, he opened his mouth and yelled until the treatment was finished, but he did not move. When the nurse said, "You may stop crying now, Billy," he closed his mouth, climbed down from the table and went about his business. It was all a part of the treatment.

Nurses have conflicting feelings about the merit of giving some reward after a treatment. Careful thought is necessary about this. Whenever a child is given a lollipop or a small toy following an uncomfortable procedure, he tends to remember the experience as not wholly bad. This has nothing to do with his own behavior. It is not a reward for being brave, or good, or big. It is simply a part of the entire treatment. The unpleasant is mitigated by the pleasant.

An older person can supply his own reward by contemplating the improvement in his health, but the little child does not have the background for this.

Joy of Living

Perhaps what we have said above makes the task of caring for a small child in the hospital seem a rather unhappy affair. Actually, the opposite is true. It can be one of the most satisfying nursing experiences.

A toddler is such a delightful person. He can accept much physical discomfort and frustration and still continue with the business of living. Put a child of a year-and-a-half in Bryant traction, and in a very short time you will find him lying on his abdomen with his head and shoulders up and his body twisted in a position that you would never have believed he could assume.

Judy, with her enormous hydrocephalic head and meningocele was nearly helpless. She had been in the hospital since birth and knew nothing else. Seeing her, one was tempted to say, "What a pity that she had to live at all." Judy did not think so, nor did her adoring nurses. During her brief two years of life, Judy spread so much sweetness and light that everyone who knew her was grateful for the opportunity. The big smile that lit up her entire face, her eagerness to do everything she was able to do, made it fun to care for her.

This story could be repeated many times and in many ways.

It takes imagination, resourcefulness, and an enormous amount of patience to care for a toddler. You have heard before, and will hear again, the injunction, "Put yourself in the patient's place; use empathy." This can become just a glib phrase, but just for now, really try it. Actually—in your own mind—become two years old. It is not too hard. We all have imagination, only some of us have let it rust with disuse. Make a list of the developmental norms of a two-year-old. Really feel how it is to be this age.

Then, when you have assumed his thoughts, his feelings—the very essence of being a two-year-old—you will find that the answers come much more easily. After all, you really were this age.

BIBLIOGRAPHY

Lorenz, K. Z.: King Solomon's Ring. P. 100. New York, T. V. Crowell, 1965.
Lowenberg, M.: Food as Children see it. Film, 16 mm., sound, 17 min. Grand Rapids, Michigan, General Mills, 1952.
Mead, M.: A Creative Life for Your Children. Washington, U. S. Government Printing Office, 1962.
Murphy, L.: Widening World of Childhood. New York, Basic Books, 1962.
National Dairy Council: Feeding Little Folks. Chicago, National Dairy Council, 1963.

SUGGESTED READINGS FOR FURTHER STUDY

Brazelton, T. B.: A child-oriented approach to toilet training. Pediat., 29:121, 1962.
Breckenridge, M. E., and Murphy, M. N.: Growth and Development of the Young Child. 7th ed. Philadelphia, W. B. Saunders, 1963.
Kennell, J. H., and Bergen, M. E.: Early childhood separation. Pediat., 37:291, 1966.
Spock, B.: Dr. Spock Talks with Mothers. New York, Basic Books, 1962.

13

Accidents and Accidental Poisoning

ACCIDENTS

In the United States as well as in many other countries, accidents kill more children than any single illness. Throughout the entire world, deaths from childhood accidents appear third on the list of causes of child mortality. In the United States the most common cause of home accidents among children from the ages of one to five is accidental poisoning.

The nurse, as an educator and leader in public health practices, must be acutely aware of these facts. She must first examine her own conduct. What sort of example does she set in the home, in the hospital ward and in the community? Children under the supervision of nurses are by no means exempt from painful accidents caused by negligence or carelessness.

It is rather frightening to consider that whereas the death rate from disease among small children has been drastically reduced in recent years, the accidental death rate has not been. Motor vehicles appear first on the list as a cause of accidental death, and home accidents appear second. A short discussion of the various kinds of accidents that occur in the home and the hospital can help fix certain preventive measures in our minds. As has often been pointed out, the best treatment for accidents is prevention.

Incidence

The age group in which most accidents occur is that of the toddler and the preschooler. The toddler's urge to explore, coupled with his lack of experience, leads him into innumerable dangerous situations. Painful burns occur when he pulls the pan or the cup down to his level to discover the contents. That electric cord, dangling so invitingly, must have something at the other end; what can it be? Anyhow, electrical outlets are intriguing and meant to be poked (to the imaginative mind of an 18-month-old child). (Fig. 80)

A healthy toddler is constantly on the go during his waking hours. It is indeed difficult to keep up with him, or to foresee all possible dangerous situations. Warning a small child of potential danger is of little value, because his memory span is short, and he has had no background experience to reinforce the warning.

218

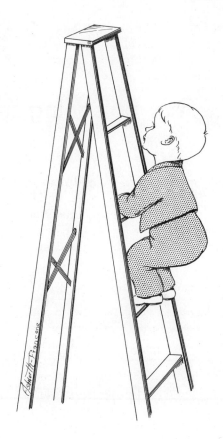

Fig. 80. Toddler climbing step ladder.

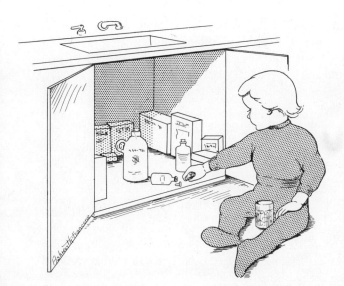

Fig. 81. Toddler playing with cleaning agents.

Much has been written about the hazards present in everyday living for the young adventurer, but it is not until a child comes into the hospital with a badly burned mouth from chewing on a electrical cord, or with some equally severe injury, that these warnings really take on serious meaning.

A short discussion of potential hazards for the toddler should help the nurse to be more alert herself, as well as to be better prepared as a health educator.

Common Accidents in the Home

The kitchen is the scene of many accidents. We are all aware that pans on the stove should always have their handles turned in. For that matter, it is a good idea to turn in the handles whether there is a child around or not. (Fig. 82)

A number of burns have occurred when a mother has stepped out for only a minute to answer the door bell or the telephone. Tiny tots have been known to push chairs over to the stove and climb up to see "what's cooking."

The bathroom is also a scene of tragedy. One well-informed mother put her preschooler and her toddler in the tub together, then stepped out to get towels and night clothes. The older child turned on the hot water tap, and the toddler was right under it.

Mothers are pretty well aware that they should never leave a small child alone in the tub, and should let the door bell or telephone go unanswered. Yet it is a hard thing to do, after all—it only takes a minute. In only a minute, toddler can slip under a few inches of water and drown, as has happened many times.

Probably the most important thing to remember is that most small children develop the ability to get into things much faster than their parents realize. Clever cats and dogs learn to open doors and to ring doorbells, so we should not expect less from our children.

Other Common Hazards

Electrical appliance cords and wall outlets offer temptations. Toddlers like to poke, and it is fun to poke something into the outlet just the way mother does. Safety caps on those outlets not in use can help. Appliance cords are pulled (or poked) and several severe mouth burns have occurred when little ones have chewed or plugged in cords. Cautioning helps not at all—it is apt to stimulate the child to find out for himself. (Fig. 83)

Tablecloths hanging just within reach are nice to pull on. Down comes the cup of hot coffee too.

Stairs are made to climb. Little Joe heard his mother upstairs, so he decided to creep up to meet her. She came to the head of the stairs, and

COMMON ACCIDENTS IN THE HOME

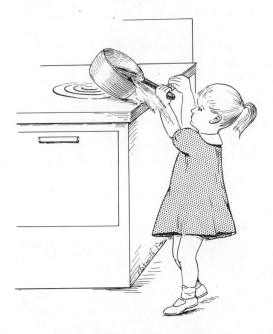

Fig. 82. Toddler pulling pan from stove.

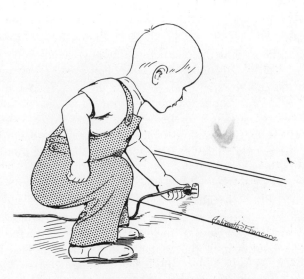

Fig. 83. Toddler playing with light plug.

Joey promptly raised his arms to be picked up, of course, toppling down backward. Here, the gate at the top of the stairs was not enough.

Many hazards have been so well publicized that it seems unnecessary to mention them, but accidents do still happen. Some of these hazards are plastic bags, discarded refrigerators, uncovered wells, ponds, and, of course, street hazards. Constant and intelligent vigilance seems to be required until the child reaches an age at which he can reason.

Two of the most common and most serious kinds of accidents are accidental poisoning and burns. Both of these need more detailed discussion.

ACCIDENTAL POISONING

Accidental poisoning during childhood brings a tragic toll in needless anxiety and even death to many homes. Many children die every year as a result of their own curiosity, and for every death there are scores of non-fatal poisonings.

When the nurse sees the child come into the hospital terribly frightened and frequently in pain because of someone's carelessness, she wonders how this can be allowed to happen. Yet doctors and nurses are far from blameless. Not only are they frequently careless themselves, but they are too often apt to forget their duty as teachers. Often it would take only a few words of caution to make parents more alert and thus avoid tragedy.

The commercial products of today bring an ever increasing supply of potential poisoners into the home. Mothers are accustomed to storing cleaners, polishes, deodorants and other housekeeping aids in cupboards, convenient for use. We are of course grateful for all of these materials that make the work at home easier, but we have not kept pace in our consideration of the dangers involved in their careless storage.

In the same manner, medications today have been of the greatest help to all of us; yet here again, we have not been alert to their potency in the hands of small children.

There is a strange phenomenon relating to medicines and small children. A person can coax, or bribe or threaten a small child in a vain attempt to get him to swallow some tasteless or even flavorful medicine, and only a short time later, find the same child stuffing a handful of pills into his mouth.

This is exactly what did happen to one small girl. She had been placed on routine barbiturates for mild seizures, but her mother had great difficulty getting her to take the medication. One day, however, when her mother was away, she climbed to the medicine cabinet and swallowed about half of the contents of the bottle. This was not discovered until several hours later when the baby sitter was unable to rouse her from an unduly long nap.

Many of these incidents do seem almost unavoidable, or at least so unlikely as to be totally unanticipated. In the light of the increasing complexity of materials in the home, and the known exploratory instincts of little children, one needs very nearly to anticipate the impossible.

Cardinal Safety Measures

There are a number of safety measures we all need to know and understand so thoroughly that they become part of our daily routine. Here are a few.

1. Use your prescription drugs only for the purpose for which they were ordered. This is difficult to do when you have paid a high price for the medicine. Perhaps his sister took this medicine last month for her cough, so let's give it to Johnny before we call the doctor. The prevailing practice in the United States of marking prescriptions by number only, and omitting the name of the drug from the label, increases the danger of giving the wrong medicine. Perhaps Johnny is allergic to the ingredients of this medicine, or possibly his cold is far different from his sister's. All too frequently drugs are removed from their original containers for one reason or another, even though correctly labeled—so it is possible that it is not even the medicine you gave his sister. It just is not safe. Keeping drugs in case they "come in handy" only adds to the store of potential poisons that children can get into.

2. Discard your unused drugs, but not in the garbage or rubbish. Many children, as well as pets, have been poisoned from eating pills or drinking liquids found in rubbish containers. Pills can be dissolved and flushed down the household drainage system, and liquids may be discarded in the same manner.

3. All medicines should be kept under lock and key. Even a locked cupboard may not always be safe from an active, exploring youngster, however. It is helpful if cabinets are high out of easy reach and locked, but a determined child can find a way. There are on the market cabinets that require considerable ingenuity to open. This is good, but another problem presents itself. If a medicine is being used routinely, it is quite a nuisance to unlock a cabinet for every administration, and, all too often, the medicine is left out in a convenient place while it is in use.

If grandmother comes to stay for the weekend, she might put her sleeping pills in the drawer by her bedside, just the way she does at home. Uncle John is a diabetic, so when he comes he puts his urine reagent tablets conveniently on the bathroom shelf. After all, who would want to swallow them? Johnny would.

Aunt Ruth comes to call and lets Susy play with her purse, completely forgetting the bottle of Dexedrine she carries with her, and so it goes. Here, even locking the medicine cabinet did not help.

4. Store all household chemicals such as cleansers, polishes, and insecticides, out of easy reach. Parents do not always realize that most cleaning agents (which are not meant for consumption) are potentially poisonous. They must sacrifice a measure of convenience for safety.

5. *Never* put any product not intended for eating or for drinking in a food or a beverage container. The temptation to do so is great, but the temptation to the toddler to eat or to drink from the bottle or the cup is greater. Always act as though anything in a food container carries a sign saying "eat me" or "drink

me" to the young explorer in Wonderland. After all, he has just learned the purpose of eating utensils and how to use them.

6. Tell your children honestly that you are giving them medicine and not candy. Every year, children come into the hospital after having eaten flavored or candied medicine, because the adults in their lives have told them in the past that it was candy in an effort to get them to take the medication.

The new method of flavoring children's drugs has been a great boon to mothers. Sweetened fruit flavors often disguise the taste to the extent that medicine becomes quite acceptable. Unfortunately, a small child has no compunction about helping himself to more.

These are only a few of the modern hazards of which we must be aware.

Internal Manifestations of Poisons

There is no place that sharpens this awareness as well as a hospital in which one sees children who have swallowed every imaginable substance. Parents need to know that many of the cleaning substances and furniture polishes contain kerosene, which can cause a fatal pneumonia if swallowed. Ant buttons, rat killers and insecticides contain arsenic, strychnine or other chemicals that are just as lethal to the child as they are to the pest one is trying to eliminate.

Esophageal Burns. Many children come into the emergency ward after having swallowed corrosive acids or alkalies, either in commercial form or in solution. The preparations for cleaning toilet bowls or for opening drains are often kept on the floor or in a low cupboard for easy access when needed.

A child who has been burned by a corrosive substance presents a most tragic figure. Two children were admitted to the same hospital one summer, each having picked up a pop bottle on a hot day and having rapidly swallowed its contents. Each bottle contained a considerable amount of lye solution that someone had placed in it.

Although separate incidents, both children suffered severe esophageal burns with almost complete occlusion of the esophagus. Both required extensive surgery with months of hospitalization and considerable follow-up. This story can be repeated over many times in numbers of children's wards throughout the world.

Any children who get a corrosive substance as far as the mouth need to be examined for burns. Most children who swallow such substances have some burning and scarring of the esophagus. Many children of five or six are still entering the hospitals for repeated dilatations following lye ingestion during the second year. Fortunately, the discovery that the use of corticosteroids early after ingestion markedly reduces the amount of scarring has resulted in widespread use of these drugs with less serious after effects.

Pulmonary Irritation. All petroleum distillates are irritants, the principal manifestation being pulmonary irritation. The resulting pneumonitis appears to be the result of aspiration either during ingestion or during the vomiting that follows. Vomiting should never be induced, although it is seldom possible to prevent spontaneous vomiting. If much of the substance has been ingested, the physician may elect careful gastric lavage. Children are usually kept in the hospital for a period following kerosene ingestion because of the extreme likelihood of pneumonitis. In a majority of cases, the petroleum distillate that has been ingested is kerosene, although cases of gasoline ingestion have been reported.

Poisonous Medications—Aspirin

If one moves on to consider the poisonings by medications, aspirin is found to be the chief offender. Many parents do not seem to recognize this particular danger, and because a majority of households contain aspirin, or compound analgesic tablets containing aspirin, children have ready access to it. The orange-flavored children's aspirin tablets are very tasty. Drug companies are now making safety caps for bottles of children's aspirin, but no cap can be entirely childproof. The bottles are still poor playthings for children.

Safe Dosages. The readiness with which parents give aspirin to their children for any disorder contributes to the hazards. Although a majority of aspirin poisonings are of acute origin, some of them are the result of accumulated doses given by parents who are ignorant of the safe dosage or of the cumulative effects. A safe dosage for the average child under the age of five is one grain of aspirin for each year of life, given not more often than every four hours. Thus a six-month-old child might receive one-half grain. Some children may be allergic to aspirin, however, and thus an average dose could have an extremely dangerous effect. This does not mean that the physician may not prescribe larger doses than the average for specific conditions, but it should be given under his guidance. All of this seems to point up the dangers inherent in giving even aspirin without a physician's order.

Emergency Measures

Miss White was enjoying a leisurely breakfast on her day off, when there was a frantic ringing of her door bell. "Oh Mary," panted her neighbor, "I just found Janie playing with my prescription medicine bottle; the cap was off, and the bottle was empty. Oh, what shall I do?"

"What was the medicine for?"

"Oh I don't know, for my nerves I guess—but then I had heartburn too, and pains in my side. The doctor said it would help me, but I don't know what it was."

"Were there many pills in the bottle?"

"Several, I don't know how many. Do something, quick!" Mary White had her car on the road in a matter of seconds, heading for the nearest hospital emergency room, with two-year-old Jane in her mother's arms in the back seat. As she drove along, Mary White instructed the mother to put Jane across her lap, to open her mouth and tickle the back of her throat to induce vomiting. Mary had remembered to pick up a dish on her way out of the house, in which she told the mother to save the emesis. She had also remembered to ask the mother to bring along the empty medicine bottle.

At the hospital the child received a gastric lavage at once. The doctor could not be located immediately, but the pharmacy at which the prescription had been filled was called and the drug identified, so that appropriate measures could be instituted.

Other neighbors were called and asked to go into Mrs. X's home and search carefully in the area where the child had been playing for any tablets resembling those which had been in the bottle. Several of these were found, so it was never determined whether any had actually been swallowed. In view of the possible fatal consequences of even a small number of these tablets to a two-year-old child, Janie was kept in the hospital for a few days and observed closely for any symptoms. Happily, none appeared, and she was discharged.

Now that the danger was over, Mary White decided not to miss the opportunity to do some teaching. She realized that Mrs. X would not be receptive to teaching when her concern over Janie's recovery was so great, but she believed that the time was now exactly right. Both Mr. and Mrs. X were eager to prevent any similar incidents in the future.

Mary explained things somewhat like this:

"Mrs. X, the first thing I did after I went home that day when I brought Janie to the hospital was to go through my own house to look for hazards there. Although we have no small children, many neighbor's children come in, and you sometimes bring Janie over. I found aspirin in the kitchen, my mother's pills in her bedroom, and hair spray in the bathroom, as well as household chemicals that could cause illness if they were swallowed.

"You told me yesterday that you have gone through your own house and put everything away carefully, and have thrown out a number of old medicines, ointments, and rubbing lotions.

"In spite of the greatest precautions, children do get into things. You certainly did the right thing when you brought Janie right to the hospital."

"You did that, Mary," said Mrs. X. "I keep wondering what I would have done if you had not been at home. George had the car, and I could not get him—and even if I had called the doctor's office it would have been some time before they could have located him."

"I am sure that his nurse would have told you to take Janie to the hospital. You could have called the police, and they would have seen that she got there promptly. You could have induced vomiting at home if you had had to wait, but it was right to get her started on her way to professional help first and then get her to vomit. If a mother has the time, she can give the child quantities of warm or salty water to drink to induce vomiting, but it is very difficult to get a small child to drink enough to make him vomit. It is usually easier and quicker to do this with your finger, and it can be done on the way to the hospital.

"If you know what the substance was, and have a ready antidote at hand, by all means give it. There is something called the *universal antidote* which can be given safely after any suspicious substance has been swallowed. This consists of tannic acid, charcoal and magnesium oxide. It is sold commercially under various trade names, or it can be made up by combining two parts of burned toast, one part of milk of magnesia and one part of strong tea. Unfortunately, today's chemicals are frequently quite complex, so the antidote may not be as universally effective as formerly. If it is convenient, it should by all means be given after the child has vomited, but time should not be wasted in sending to the store or in making the concoction. Getting the child to the hospital or to the doctor's office is the most important step of all.

"If the child does vomit, be sure to take all the emesis you can capture for analysis. Also, take the container of the medicine or other substance, even if it is empty.

"I am afraid that we became so excited that we forgot to look to see whether any of the tablets had been spilled. In Janie's case, we wouldn't have known even then whether she had swallowed any, because we did not know how many had been in the bottle, and even though we had found the tablets on the floor, we would have taken her to the hospital anyway.

"If you had known what the medicine was, you or your doctor could have phoned the Poison Control Center, and they could have told you what to do. This is a great help, because they would know about the effects of the substance, and you would have been safe in treating her yourself if they advised it.

"Of course, if an antidote is printed on the label, give it if possible, but do not waste any time in getting the child to the hospital. It might happen that you are too far away from any professional help to get immediate action. One is seldom far from the telephone, however, and all major cities in the United States have Poison Control Centers operated on a 24-hour schedule. It is a good plan, though, if you are taking a long trip with small children to include a package of the universal antidote as well as a handbook for dealing with emergencies, and to keep them handy in the first-aid kit.

"By the way, there are some occasions when you should not make the child vomit. If he has swallowed either a strong acid or alkali, such as the chemicals used in bleach, drain openers, or in toilet bowl cleaners, he should not be made to vomit. Of course he is pretty sure to vomit anyway, but the substances burn the mouth and throat coming up as well as going down. If the child is seen immediately by the doctor, he may decide to pass a stomach tube and to wash out the stomach, but he probably will not even do that if it is more than half an hour after the accident.

"If the poison was kerosene, the child should not be made to vomit because the greatest danger here is from the fumes the child inhales. Here again, the doctor may decide to wash out the stomach, although studies are still being done to determine if this is the best procedure.

"The other occasion when it would be unsafe to induce vomiting is when the child is discovered unconscious. Aside from these situations, vomiting is often a life-saver.

"Perhaps you would like to know about some of the other things found in the home that are toxic if taken internally. Oil of wintergreen, which can give considerable relief for rheumatic pains, is fatal if swallowed even in small doses. Most cosmetics, hair-dressings and toiletries contain toxic chemicals.

"One interesting possible source of toxicity is found at Christmas. Small children are entranced by the bright lights, and want to touch, or even taste them. Both holly and mistletoe contains powerful drugs. Fireplace color crystals contain lead, arsenic, thallium and other chemicals. These can be highly dangerous, and should be reported at once if they are swallowed.

"The fluid in bubbling lights is also a toxic substance. Snow-spray, if inhaled, can cause lung irritation that could result in pneumonia."

THE NURSE IN THE HOSPITAL

Teaching along these lines is very effective, and is the duty of all nurses, not just those concerned with public health. Perhaps one more word might be helpful to the hospital nurse. New medications are being produced rapidly as research discovers new methods for combating disease. It is difficult for the nurse to keep up with all of them. She has been taught never to dispense a drug without knowing its properties and its effects. Some of these she may not be able to find in the drug index on the department. She may have a heavy medication load and many interruptions, but she must not let this keep her from getting the information. There are still other sources; she can call the hospital pharmacy and ask, or she can ask the doctor who prescribed the drug. She certainly has an obligation to know what she is dispensing *before* she gives it, and not after she is finished.

In the rush and the hurry of the day, the nurse may find herself becoming tense and anxious. In this state, it is perfectly possible to give the wrong drug or to mistake a child. Even if she has observed all the rules, has not talked to anyone while pouring, has read the label three times, and has identified her patient, mistakes can happen.

If, however, she has bypassed a rule and made an error, she feels even more guilty. It may be hard to report an error in any case, but it is very difficult indeed to report an error that was the result of her own carelessness. The temptation becomes strong to save face and to "wait and see." Probably nothing will come of it, she is tempted to think.

The nurse must discipline herself in this respect. If there are to be adverse effects, a delay may be the difference between life and death. Let her consider how much greater her sense of guilt will be then, even if she is the only one to know. The temporary disgrace is naturally disturbing, but it can be borne far better than a lasting sense of guilt, and her prompt reporting may very possibly save a child's life.

ASPIRATION OF FOREIGN BODIES

The severe consequences following aspiration of a foreign body are well known, but nurses in the hospital and parents in the home may be very careless about this hazard. A small child in the hospital, kept in bed and suffering from boredom, may find pleasure in taking a toy car or a truck apart, or removing the eyes from a stuffed animal. Following this, the next move is to put the small wheels, the toy truck driver, or whatever, into his mouth. Sometimes the whole toy fits in, as when the nurse noticed that Jimmy had a big mouthful of *something*, and succeeded in removing a tiny motorcycle, complete with rider, just before it disappeared.

Parents are frequently inclined to give their hospitalized child a coin or two before they leave for the day; these are also convenient things to put in the mouth.

In the home (or in the hospital) safety pins, thumb tacks, or any variety of small metallic objects have been aspirated. Often this is not known at the time, and the object may be lodged in the trachea or the larynx for a considerable length of time. One child was admitted in acute respiratory distress with a probable diagnosis of laryngotracheobronchitis. The distress was so severe that an emergency tracheotomy was performed. The following day examination revealed a small open safety pin lodged in the larynx, which on extraction showed by its appearance that it had been there for some time. The mother then recalled two episodes of choking and coughing within the past two weeks, with increasing horseness, but no one knew about the pin.

Any child being seen for respiratory symptoms of wheezing, hoarseness, or croupy cough, should be examined with the possibility of aspiration in mind, even though there is no history of foreign body aspiration.

If the object is lodged in the larynx, a severe degree of dyspnea may make a tracheotomy necessary before a laryngoscopic examination is done.

Vegetable matter, such as popcorn, peanuts, seeds or pieces of raw vegetable are easily aspirated by a toddler. These are extremely difficult to remove because they swell in the moist atmosphere of the respiratory system, and crumble into fragments when grasped with an instrument for removal.

Objects that become lodged in a bronchus may cause complete obstruction, with inflammatory swelling, atelectasis and emphysema.

Objects that are not removed from the air passages eventually cause death in a majority of cases. Particularly tragic are those instances when small children have fed particles to the tiny baby in the home, entirely unknown to the parents. One such young infant died, despite every possible treatment for an unidentified respiratory difficulty, which an autopsy proved caused by a particle of vegetable material in a bronchus. Such accidents are so totally unexpected that they may never be considered.

Peanuts and popcorn are not safe food for toddlers. Children are fond of finger foods, and raw carrots or other raw vegetables are colorful and of pleasing texture to a child of three or four. Toddlers cannot be trusted to chew them well enough, and even a three-year-old should not be allowed to run around while eating chewy foods.

If an object has been aspirated, treatment consists in removal by direct laryngoscopy or bronchoscopy. Secondary infection is treated by antibiotic medication as indicated. The most effective treatment, however, is prevention.

FRACTURES IN CHILDHOOD

Childhood fractures differ from those of adults in that they are generally less complicated, heal more quickly, and usually occur from different causes. The child has an urge to explore his environment, but lacks the experience and the judgement to recognize possible hazards. In some instances, parents may be negligent in their supervision, but frequently the young explorer is just too fast for them.

Some Major Causes of Fractures in Children

Falls from high chairs and cribs
Falls from grocery carts in supermarkets
Rolling off beds or flat surfaces
Falling out of cars
Falls due to motor imbalance (cerebral palsy, convulsive disorders)
Birth injuries
"Battered child" syndrome

A mother telephoned the pediatric department of the hospital to ask where she could purchase a restraint jacket of the type they used on the ward. Her toddler had just learned to climb over his cribsides, and was inclined to practice his new skill while the rest of the household were sleeping. She was advised that such a jacket would not be safe to use on an unattended child, because toddlers easily become tangled in the ties. She was told to relax, that the child would soon outgrow this phase, but she remained unconvinced. She just wondered what to do until he did outgrow it, because he already had fallen twice. Another young child, looking for his favorite blanket, saw it under his younger brother, and promptly yanked it out. Unfortunately, his brother came with it, with the result of a trip to the hospital for Bryant's traction for a fractured femur.

Safety on the Toddlers Ward

The problem of giving adequate protection to the young children under our care in the hospital is ever present, and we must exercise greater care and vigilance than we would in our own homes. When a toddler is home, his mother is there to watch him; if he falls, she may blame herself, but she, or someone taking her place, assumes responsibility. When a young child is injured in the hospital, however, it would be an unusual mother who would not think "I wonder if they really watched him carefully enough." Nurses on the children's ward have many children to watch, so they must be unusually careful.

High chairs in the pediatric ward present one hazard for the young person just learning to stand. Nurses, and mothers too, may as well accept the fact that a toddler will try to stand in his high chair; therefore, the sensible thing to do is to prevent the accident before it happens. The simplest and most effective way is to abolish the use of high chairs in the hospital. Low chairs and tables are preferable for children who can sit steadily; a Baby-tenda is good for smaller ones. Of course, he may fall from a small chair too, but the consequences are usually not so severe.

Children love to climb, and an empty crib is fun to climb into and less fun to fall out of. A good rule is never to leave small children unattended while they are up. A familiar sight in many children's departments is to see one, two, or three children tagging along while the nurse goes to the linen closet or the supply cupboard; and when she takes one child to the tub room, one or two others go along and play happily beside the tub where she can watch them. Cribsides kept up, whether or not the crib is occupied, also removes the temptation to climb in.

No child in restraint, whether it is the jacket type, net crib-cover, or other, should be left unchecked for very long. Children have strangled

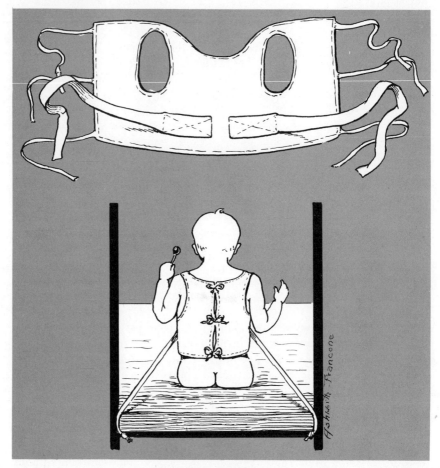

Fig. 84. Jacket restraint.

by getting their heads between the net edge and the crib, or by becoming
entangled in the jacket ties. (Fig. 84)

Typical Types of Fracture in Infants and Children

Fractures in the newborn. Fractures occur occasionally at birth, particularly during a hard delivery or a breech presentation. Fractures in
the newborn heal easily, requiring minimum care.

A fractured clavicle is probably the most common; it may be suspected by the nurse or the mother if the infant does not move one arm,
or if he cries when his arm is handled. Treatment may be by immobilization of the affected shoulder and arm. The body, the axilla and the arm
should be washed, dried, and the arm should be placed against the chest
wall, with the hand lying on the chest. A strip of stockinet may be used
to hold his arm in place, with cotton or some protective material placed

between his arm and his body. Frequently, this is not done, because the infant will not willingly move his arm in any event. If the arm is left free, care must be taken not to press the shoulder toward the midline of the body, nor should his arm be pulled through his sleeve.

A fractured humerus in the newborn is usually a transverse fracture, which heals quickly. The arm should be immobilized by being strapped to the side of the chest. Usually, an overgrowth of callus occurs after a fracture in a young infant, which is absorbed as the child grows.

Head Injuries. Because young children frequently land on their heads when they fall, head injuries are common. A fracture of the skull in itself is not of major significance, because there is no muscle pull; the important aspect is in the brain damage that may result from pressure or hemorrhage.

Older children also experience head injuries from playground, bicycle, or car accidents. A simple, linear closed fracture requires no specific treatment; parents are advised to keep the child quiet and to watch for indications of concussion or brain injury.

A depressed fracture may necessitate decompression or craniotomy. Subarachnoid hemorrhage is associated with nearly all cases of cerebral contusion or laceration, causing grave pressure symptoms. A child who has sustained a head injury must be watched for neurological signs indicating brain injury. Significant signs include the state of consciousness, either an increasing or a decreasing pulse rate, a rise or a fall in temperature, the kind of respiration, and restlessness. Eye signs, such as nystagmus or inequality of pupils, and bleeding from ears, nose or mouth, must be noted and reported.

A quiet environment is important; bed or crib sides should be padded to protect the child from injury, but mechanical restraints are generally considered harmful. A patent airway must be maintained, with a tracheotomy if it is necessary. While attending these needs, ordinary daily care should not be neglected. Diaper changes, mouth and skin care, and smooth bedding are all important comfort aids. The voiding pattern should be watched because the child's restlessness may stem from a full bladder.

Fracture of the clavicle. A toddler who sustains a fractured clavicle usually does well with a figure-of-eight flannel bandage for shoulder immobilization. The bandage should be tightened daily and changed frequently, with careful examination of the skin for breaks or abrasions. A small child usually recovers quickly (within approximately four weeks). An older child may require a cast applied in the same manner.

Fractures of the humerus or the elbow. These are relatively rare in children. They may be treated by a hanging cast, immobilized by a bandage, or at times, by traction. (Fig. 85)

Fracture of the femur. In children this is most frequently a transverse

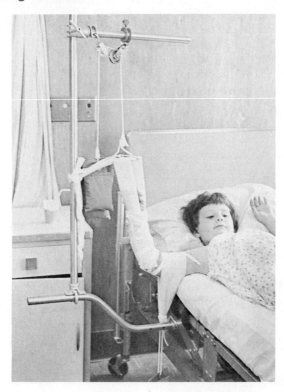

Fig. 85. This child has a transcondylar fracture
of the distal humerus.

or spiral fracture of the shaft of the long bone. A small child under the
age of three is placed in Bryant's traction for best results. The use of
Bryant's traction entails some risk of compromised circulation and may
result in contracture of the foot and the lower leg, particularly in an
older child.

For an application of Bryant's traction, two overhead bars are passed
horizontally over the crib, pulleys are attached to each bar, and the child's
legs are suspended from these at right angles to his body. Weights are
applied in sufficient amounts to keep the buttocks just clear of the bed.
(Fig. 86) The child's legs are wrapped with elastic bandages that must
be removed at least daily, the skin inspected, and the legs rewrapped.
Skin temperature and the color of his legs and his feet must be checked
frequently for circulatory embarrassment. Severe pain should not be
present; if it is noted, it should be reported because it may be an indication of circulatory difficulty.

An older child seems to respond best in Russell's traction. A child in
either type of traction tends to slide down until the weights rest on the
bed or the floor. He should be pulled up to keep the weights free, and the

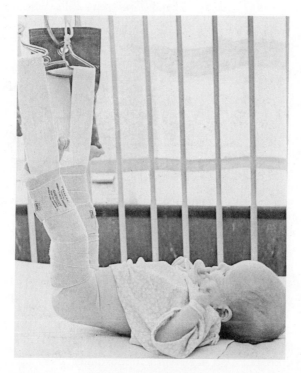

Fig. 86. Bryant's traction.

alignment should be checked frequently. An older child may coax his ward mates to remove the weights or the sandbags used as weights. When a child is in Bryant's traction, the nurse should be able to pass her hand between the child's buttocks and the sheet. A small child adjusts to this position with surprising ease. In fact, an infant cheerfully assumes the most unusual positions, such as turning over on his abdomen while he is still in traction. He is not the one who is likely to develop pressure areas on the back of his head or his shoulders, but instead an older child may do so. A child is not apt to complain of any specific pain, but becomes irritable, so that the adult in his life must seek the cause. A toddler is quite likely to regress to the use of diapers, especially if he has just completed toilet training. He may have great difficulty using a bedpan when he has just learned to sit on a potty-chair, so diapers are quite likely indicated. He may also regress to the nursing bottle again, especially in the hospital. It is not uncommon to see a two- or even a three-year-old child in the hospital carefully nursing his bottle. Just be sure that he has a plastic bottle.

The social, emotional and developmental problems need consideration if a child, regardless of his age, is immobilized by a cast or by traction.

It certainly interferes with his normal developmental activities. This same handicap can interfere with an adult's ability to earn a living, but a child may actually suffer impairment of normal growth and development. The child of two or three who must use his large muscles is definitely frustrated. Early childhood is a time for learning balance, motor coordination, and similar physical developmental skills. Socially, a deformity or a defect may bring ridicule or teasing from other children, causing a loss of self-approval.

An infant or toddler has neither developed a body image, nor is he inhibited by emotional barriers, so he may adapt more readily and make maximum use of any opportunities for development. In fact, he may accept his disadvantage as a normal way of life and go on from there. For instance, Bryant's traction may inhibit a small child so little that he may endanger his own recovery. It is an older child who is more likely to suffer emotionally from the inability to move freely and to control his own activities. Of course, a toddler brings along his own special problems to the hospital, which are so important that we must never overlook them. He still depends on his mother for ego strength, and is the poorest candidate of any for hospitalization if this means that he is separated from his mother.

The child may find overprotection and oversolicitude to be a problem as well. Parents and nurses tend to do those things for him that he could, and would, do for himself if given the opportunity and motivation. Children manage to feed and to help themselves in many difficult situations. They may need greater attention, understanding and approval for a time to sustain their ego, but this is not spoiling them, and the adult must watch for indications that a child is ready for a greater measure of independence.

ABUSED CHILDREN: THE BATTERED-CHILD SYNDROME

Within recent years, hospital personnel have been forced to face a most unpleasant fact. We have refused to believe it; we thought if we ignored it, or denied it, it would disappear. The fact remains, however, insistently demanding our attention. The plain truth is that we have, in apparently increasing numbers, infants and very young children on our wards who have suffered severe and repeated physical abuse at the hands of the adults in their lives—usually the parents.

Throughout history, the rights of parents over their own children have been unquestioned. Minor children have been at the mercy of cruel, neglectful, or indifferent parents, with a conspicuous lack of supervision or inquiry from any authority. The right of the head of the family to govern his household in any manner he saw fit has always been jealously guarded. Society was not child-oriented; indeed, society in general appeared indifferent to the rights of the child.

Eventually, as societies became more complex, the state stepped in to curtail or to limit parental rights when these did not serve the common interest. For instance, because it was economically unsound for large numbers of persons to grow up illiterate, laws were passed requiring parents to send their children to school, wherever the state provided the school and the teacher. Other absolute rights of parents over their children were curtailed as time passed. The belief persisted, however, that mothers instinctively loved and protected their children, and, if necessary, gave their lives for them. As our culture became more child-oriented, fathers no longer considered it necessary to show their authority by stern, uncompromising discipline. Society settled down into the comfortable belief that children were well protected, even pampered, except possibly a few from really depraved homes. It has come as a shock to our affluent society to discover that apparently respectable, ordinary people can be accused of mistreating their own children.

One of the earliest persons to focus our attention on this problem was Elizabeth Elmer, writing in a social work journal in 1960.* She cited several previous articles in which the possibility of skeletal trauma in inadequately explained conditions was discussed. In particular, she mentioned Silverman, who, in 1953, referred to physical trauma as "the most common bone 'disease' of infancy," and who also made note of the strong resistance of attending doctors to any implication of parental mismanagement.†

Professional interest was aroused, and many studies have since been conducted throughout the United States. The problem has been shown to be serious. In one study, 71 hospitals reported 302 cases of abuse. Of these children, 33 died, and 85 suffered permanent brain injury.* Similar findings have occurred in widespread areas throughout the country.

The term *battered-child syndrome* was used to characterize a clinical condition in young children who have received serious physical abuse at the hands of an adult, usually the parent. At present, the term is used to designate children who are the victims of passive as well as active abuse.

Active abuse is manifested in such conditions as:

1. Brain injuries, subdural hematomas, skull fractures.

2. Soft tissue injuries, such as bruises, lacerations, or burns.

3. Fractures of the long bones, rib fractures; X-rays frequently show multiple fractures in varying stages of healing.

Passive abuse includes:

---

* Elmer, E.: Abused young children seen in hospitals. Social Work, 5:98, 1960.
† Silverman, F.: The roentgen manifestation of unrecognized skeletal trauma in infants. J. Roentgenology, 69:413, 1953.
* Kempe, H., *et al.*: The battered-child syndrome. J.A.M.A., *181*:17, 1962.

1. Poor nutrition, failure to thrive, severe malnutrition.

2. Poor physical condition; neglected safeguards against disease, poor skin condition, lack of proper medical attention.

3. Emotional neglect; rejection, indifference, deprivation of love.

4. Moral neglect; allowing children to remain in an immoral atmosphere, particularly if the child is old enough to comprehend.

The Children

The majority of these children are young, under the age of three years. Frequently, one particular child is singled out for this type of treatment. The child may be a child with a behavior problem (whether he has a problem because of the treatment, or whether the abusive treatment occurs because of his behavior is usually uncertain). In any case, each kind of behavior intensifies the other, causing an exceedingly vicious cycle.

When an obvious injury has occurred, parents bring the child into the hospital with a vague history of accident. An older child has pulled a blanket out from under the baby; the child caught his arm or his leg in the crib sides; the child was climbing and fell on his head. X-rays of these children frequently reveal several older fractures in various stages of healing.

There are rarely any witnesses to the accident, and the child cannot speak for himself, or is too terrified to do so. Only occasionally does a husband or a wife admit to knowledge of abuse at the hands of the other.

In the hospital these children are not likely to look to their parents for protection or assurance. They "endure life as if they are alone in a dangerous world with no real hope of safety."*

The Parent

What kinds of parents are involved in these tragic situations? No particular level of society is exclusively involved. The child may come from a neat, well-kept home, or from a poor home.

The parents are frequently young, immature persons, unready to accept the responsibilities of parenthood. They may be interested in their own comfort and pleasure, rejecting a child who gets in the way. Their immaturity may manifest itself as jealousy, the abusing parent wishing all the love and attention for herself.

Other parents are aggressive and hostile, continuously angry and unable to control their anger. Usually such parents have a background of severe rejection and deprivation in their own early childhood, which in turn they inflict on their own children.

Another kind of parent is the dependent and timid person, wanting

* Morris, M. G., *et al.:* Toward prevention of child abuse. Children, *11*:55, 1964.

someone to tell them what to do, how to do it, and when to do it. They appear unable to direct their own lives, and are utterly helpless with their children.

Examples of abuse and neglect are numerous. Bobby, not yet three, was brought into the hospital with severe facial fractures, acquired, it was claimed, by climbing and falling. Much later it was acknowledged that he had been beaten for wetting himself. When a doctor, not knowing the background, stopped to look at his black eye, Bobby was observed to flinch as though expecting a blow.

Billy at nine months was thin almost to the point of emaciation. He gave a wide grin whenever he was spoken to, but then went back to his customary occupation of rocking. His appetite was ravenous, it seemed as though he could not be filled up. Unfortunately, rocking and pushing his hand back into his throat invariably brought the food up again. When carried, he clung in an aggressive manner, digging his fingers in sharply. However, he never cried when he was returned to his crib, seeming content to return to his self-absorption.

Because no organic lesion was found, a new regime was instituted. Instead of sharply limiting the food intake to control vomiting, he was fed all he wanted to eat. He was assigned to one nurse whose main duty was to give him quantities of loving attention. In addition, it became a common sight to see interns, medical students, and various staff members carrying Billy as they made their rounds.

Billy came from a middle-class home, where he had been kept clean and given all necessary physical attention. His intelligent mother, however, was too absorbed in her own interests and her career outside of the home to give him any warmth or love, thus Billy was forced to provide his own stimulation, which he did.

After several weeks of emotional support in the hospital, Billy had stopped his rocking and gagging, and no longer clung desperately to the person holding him, and he no longer showed passive acceptance at being placed back in his crib. Physically, he had gained weight. Whether he kept these gains depended largely on whether his home environment could be changed.

Another baby, found alone and in a filthy state, neither sat, smiled, nor responded to any show of friendliness. In his dehydrated, emaciated state, he gave the appearance of having less than normal intelligence. Here again, intensive physical and emotional support turned our Jimmy into a smiling, laughing and playing infant, apparently well on the way to catching up with his peers.

All stories do not end so happily. Many small children sustain permanent physical or emotional injuries. Many do not survive, and others go home only to return with fresh injuries, usually to a different hospital. What can be done about this?

Legal Action

In 1963, the Children's Bureau announced that the first step in a national program protecting children from physical abuse had been taken. The Children's Bureau proposed to supply to all states suggested language for laws requiring all cases of child abuse be reported to police authorities by the doctor who sees the child.

The purpose of the suggested law was not to punish parents, but to identify children in danger so they could be protected. Many doctors, although suspecting abuse in a child patient, were fearful of reporting such cases and thus face the possibility of lawsuit. Judges have been notoriously reluctant to remove children from their homes, especially if proof beyond reasonable doubt cannot be furnished. Too often these children have been restored to their homes to become the recipients of intensified fury from their parents because of the physician's report, making the physician understandably reluctant to cause added misery.

The proposed law would give the reporting doctor immunity from criminal or civil suit. Mandatory reporting also relieved the physician of the responsibility of deciding whether to report suspicious cases. Physicians were also reminded that privileged communication between patient and physician should not apply in these cases. Clearly the duty of the physician is to the child.

A few states had already enacted such laws, or were considering them. Acting with unusual speed, by the beginning of 1966, all but three states, plus the District of Columbia, had enacted laws whose aim was to increase the reporting of child abuse cases. Some states encouraged such reporting, but the majority made reporting mandatory for any physician who, on examination of a child, had strong suspicion of intentional abuse.

The laws differ in detail from state to state. Some require reporting to police authorities, others name child welfare or child protective agencies as the investigating persons. Excellent discussions concerning state laws protecting children are given in publications of the Children's Bureau and of the American Humane Association.*†

Helping the Family

The nurse who receives and cares for a badly neglected or abused child in the hospital faces a nearly impossible task in trying to remain impartial. As she sees the results of actions of adults on whom the child is utterly dependent, her rage mounts. When the mother of a child who died as the result of such treatment is declared "innocent" in court, the nurse relives the difficult days of caring for a small being with sad, hope-

---

* Paulsen, M. G.: Legal protection against child abuse. Children, 13:42, 1966.

† DeFrancis, V.: Review of Legislation to Protect the Battered Child: A study of laws enacted in 1963. Denver, the American Humane Association.

less eyes, who accepted pain and suffering without protest, and who, in her eyes at least, made no effort to live. This nurse feels only anger and resentment that such a mother could "get away with it"; she cannot calmly and reasonably see the whole picture.

Punitive measures, however, do nothing to diminish the number of cases of child abuse, nor do they change attitudes. Whereas the approach to the problem was formerly seen as an attempt to save the child from his home, we are now starting to see that the greater need is to save the home for the child, if at all possible. We are concerned for the welfare of the child and of his parents. We still believe that most parents want to be good parents, but find that many are unable to assume adequate parental roles without outside help.

A very good case can be made for the belief that child welfare or child protective agencies are best fitted by training and experience to be the agencies receiving reports of child neglect or abuse. These agencies, of course, must then have adequate means for receiving and investigating calls at any time, day or night. They must also have authority to remove a child from a dangerous situation, or they must work together with law enforcement officers when necessary.

Understanding, skillful case work may save the home for the child, even when temporary placement of the child outside of the home is necessary. Some homes, perhaps many, can never be made safe for the child without radical changes—changes that may not be possible.

An interesting use of homemaker services has been of value. Mature, friendly women with a real interest in people, working closely with child welfare workers, can frequently help parents by their understanding support and example. They can also evaluate family situations, and clarify the need for intervention in confused situations. Many of the inadequate parents are frightened by their own actions, and are asking to be protected from their own compulsive behavior.

As nurses, we must acquire a deeper understanding of the complex issues involved in this frightening aspect of life. We have a definite responsibility to these children to protect them from personality damage as well as from physical harm. If we are interested in preventing the child from growing up into an abusive, antisocial adult, we must recognize the need for help early, before there has been irreversible damage.

CARING FOR THE BURNED CHILD

Among the many accidents that occur in the lives of children, burns are the most frequent and frightening, exceeding even accidental poisonings in mortality rates. One tragic factor in this situation is that nearly all childhood burns are preventable, a fact which causes considerable guilt feelings on the part of the parents and the child. Failure to explain dangers to the child, carelessness on the part of an adult, the child's disobedience, all enter into the picture.

Common Causes of Burns

Scalds from Hot Liquids

This is a frequent type of burn in small children. Contributing factors may be:

1. A dangling cord from an electric percolator. The toddler pulls the cord to find out what is on the other end.

2. Pans of hot liquid on the stove. Handles are made for the purpose of pulling, or so the toddler reasons.

3. Cups of hot tea or coffee, and bowls of soup; all can cause painful burns if spilled on a child. An infant pulling on a tablecloth, or a toddler reaching for the teacup handle, may pull the hot liquid down over himself.

4. Small children left alone in bathtubs have frequently turned on the hot water tap, or older children have done it for them. Dangerous and fatal burns have occurred in this manner. It is never safe to leave a small child alone to play in the tub.

Burns from Fire or Heat

This type of burn is next in frequency. The contributing factors are:

1. Matches, which have an irresistible attraction for many children. Usually the child has been warned against playing with matches, so he will seek a place where he will not be detected—as a small closet or other place away from his mother.

2. Children's clothing. Many of the materials used in making children's clothing are highly inflammable and thus easily set afire. The child in panic runs for help, fanning the blaze.

3. Use of kerosene, gasoline or lighter materials for starting fires. Unfortunately, it is sometimes the adult himself who pours on the kerosene, or who is the model that the child copies when *he* tries to start a fire.

4. Burning buildings. This is not a common cause of childhood burns. Small children, however, left alone in a home are helpless if a fire breaks out, whether the cause was a child's mischief, an adult's carelessness, or some unforeseeable event.

Electrical Burns

Although not common in children, nurses do see infants or toddlers with severe facial or mouth burns requiring extensive plastic surgery, from biting on electric cords—unfortunately without first removing the plug from the socket.

Prevention of Burns

Regret and self-blame are almost always present for the parents of a burned child. If the mother had not gone to answer the phone or the doorbell while toddler played in the tub, if she had been careful to turn the pot handles in *always;* this would not have happened. The mother thinks she should have remembered how irresistible matches are to children, and should have tried harder to teach the dangers of playing with fire. If Johnny had not seen his father pour kerosene on the wood, how could he have known this method for making it burn?

As nurses, our primary task is to teach preventive practices, as well as to set proper examples ourselves. Generally, however, the first time a nurse in the hospital hears about a burned child is when she is asked to prepare a room for his reception as a patient.

The nurse caring for a burned child must be prepared to put into use some of the most specialized and precise nursing skills. In order to do this, she needs, first, an understanding of the principles of physiological action involved; second, understanding of complications to be watched for; third, and most important of all, principles of management and nursing care concerning the burned child.

Types of Burns

Burns are divided into types according to the depth of tissue involvement; whether superficial, partial thickness, or total thickness.

Superficial or first degree burns. The epidermis is injured, but there is no destruction of tissue or of nerve endings. Thus there is erythema, edema and pain, but prompt regeneration.

Partial thickness or second degree burns. The epidermis and underlying dermis are both injured and devitalized, or destroyed. There is generally blistering, with an escape of body plasma, but regeneration of the skin occurs from the remaining viable epithelial cells in the dermis.

Total thickness or third degree burns. Epidermis, dermis, and nerve endings are all destroyed. Pain is minimal, and there is no longer any barrier to infection, or any remaining viable epithelial cells.

Fourth degree burns. Some authorities list as fourth degree burns any burns with destruction of deeper elements than skin or subcutaneous tissue; that is, nerves, blood vessels, muscle, or bone.

The Type of Care Needed for Burns

Superficial burns are minor burns that heal readily unless they become infected. They can generally be treated on an out-patient basis; anesthetic ointment may be helpful if the area is not too large, or an analgesic may be given.

Partial thickness burns may be converted into full thickness burns in the presence of infection. It is not always possible to distinguish between partial and full thickness burns; also, with extensive burns, there is often a greater amount of full thickness burn than had originally been estimated. Partial thickness burns need to be kept free of infection, with hospitalization if they are extensive.

Total thickness burns require the attention, skill, energy and conscientious care of a team of specialists. Children with third degree burns or mixed second and third degree, involving 15% or more of body surface, require hospitalization.

Physiological Manifestations and Treatment in Severe Burns

First Phase—First 48 to 72 Hours

Hypovolemic shock is the major manifestation in the first phase of massive burns. As extracellular fluid pours into the burned area, it collects in enormous quantities, depleting the body. Edema becomes noticeable, and symptoms of severe shock appear. Intense pain is seldom a major factor.

The physician's primary concern is to replace body fluids that have been lost or immobilized at the burn areas. Because there is a distinct relationship between the extent of the surface area burned and the amount of fluid lost, the physician needs to estimate the percent of the skin area affected. The "rule of nines," which affords a rough guide, estimates body surface area in approximate areas of nine. For a small child, whose head surface area is larger, and whose leg surface area is smaller than that of the adult, modifications are made. The table gives an idea as to how percentages of burned areas are calculated.

Intravenous fluids for the maintenance and the replacement of lost body fluids are estimated for the first 24 hours, with one-half of this calculated requirement to be given during the first 8 hours. The patient's

TABLE FOR ESTIMATING PROPORTIONS OF BODY SURFACE*

Age	Head (%)	Trunk (%)	Upper Extremities (%)	Lower Extremities (%)	Total % of Body Surface
Birth	19	34	19	28	100
1 year	17	34	19	30	100
5 years	13	34	19	34	100
10 years	11	34	19	36	100
15 years	9	34	19	38	100
Adult	7	34	19	40	100

* Lund, C. C., and Browder, N. C.: The estimation of area in burns. Surg. Gynec. and Obstet., 79:352, 1944.

needs may change rapidly, however, necessitating a change in the rate of flow, the amount, or the type of fluid. The physician must check frequently and carefully the urinary output, the vital signs, and the general appearance of the patient. Frequent hematocrit and hemoglobin readings indicate needs for blood transfusion or plasma.

Adequacy of the patient's airway must be assessed in terms of a possible need for a tracheostomy, and an aseptic environment must be rigidly maintained.

Nursing Care During First Phase

Six-year-old Billy had been kept home from school because of a head cold. Billy, in his flannel pajamas, became bored because there was no one to amuse him. He did see one diversion: a book of matches on the table—and his mother, he knew, was at the store. What really happened after he lit that first match he never knew, but suddenly, his flannel pajamas were a sheet of flames, and Billy was running out of the door, screaming.

From that time on, things happened far too rapidly for a little boy to comprehend. He was in a hospital—he knew that—so many strange people around! Someone was talking about 60 percent burns, no one smiled, and everyone looked grotesque in masks and gowns.

For weeks, seemingly without end, one little boy existed in a nightmare world of total unreality, while many persons fought to bring meaning back into that world. Billy fought too: everyone and everything, frequently at the top of his lungs. Undoubtedly the stubbornness and rage he exhibited did more to save his life than any passive acceptance could have done, but there were many days when doctors and nurses were convinced that they were at the end of their endurance. Always, however, after a few hours of rest, they came back to take up their seemingly hopeless task. No one dared to predict the outcome: they "took each day as it came."

When the pediatric department was alerted to the impending arrival of a severely burned child, preparations to receive him were quickly begun. A private room, with a door that could be closed, and with running water, was chosen. The unit was set up for care of a burned child under aseptic conditions.

Following, in outline form, are supplies that should be in readiness for the care of a burned child.

Supplies to be Stocked for a Burn Unit

1. Sterilized sheets, towels, nurse's and doctor's gowns. "Burn packs" are usually available from central supply.
2. Sterile gloves. Sterile disposable gloves are useful, because many are going to be used.

3. Face masks and caps for personnel. Some hospitals include special shoe coverings.*

Clean Equipment to be Kept in the Room

1. Clinical thermometer, container, antiseptic solution.
2. Blood pressure cuff and stethoscope.
3. Intravenous pole.
4. Wall container of hexachlorophene soap for nurses' and doctors' scrub, orangewood sticks, and paper towels in rack.
5. Laundry bag or hamper, paper bag in wastebasket.
6. An antiseptic solution for damp dusting of furniture, and rags for dusting.
7. Routine equipment, such as a wash basin.
8. A large cradle to be covered with sterile sheets and placed over the child's body, keeping the covers away from his damaged skin.

Procedure Trays Ready for Immediate Use

1. Cut-down tray with intravenous fluids.
2. Blood plasma readily available.
3. Catheterization tray with a Foley catheter. For a child of six, size 8–10 Foley. Sterile water, a syringe and a needle for filling a Foley bag.
4. Emergency tracheotomy tray on a stand-by basis. Pediatric tracheotomy tube, the size according to age.
5. Nasogastric suction machine, clean and in working order. Nasal suction catheters, size 14–16 French.
6. Source of oxygen, pediatric-size face mask for emergency use.

Immediate nursing care is demanding, with many things to be done at once, a fact which makes it important that, if possible, more than one nurse be available. The nurse in a sterile gown, a mask and a cap, can help to place the patient on the sterile sheet spread over the bed, and can adjust the cradle over his body.

The room temperature should be kept around 80°F, because evaporation of water through the denuded areas, and even through the leathery burn eschar, proceeds rapidly, with a consequent thermal evaporative loss.

First, in order of importance, is the assistance in starting intravenous fluids, and assisting in performing the cut-down procedure. Temporary fluid, such as 5 percent dextrose in water may be started until the child's

---

* Hospital techniques and equipment for aseptic care vary, but the principles of asepsis remain the same.

needs have been calculated, then the ordered intravenous fluid must be prepared and hung. Aqueous penicillin or other antibiotic may be ordered for addition to the intravenous fluid.

Strict monitoring of all intake and output is essential, including the amount of fluid the child has received at any given time, the rate of flow, the time the present bottle was started and when it is due to be finished, and the contents of the present bottle. The bottle itself must be clearly labeled, with an indication of any additions to the original contents, as, for example:

250 cc. 5 per cent dextrose in water,
500,000 units aqueous penicillin.

A flow sheet, kept at the bedside, may be some variation of the following example.

FLUID BALANCE CHECK SHEET

Sol. #1	Gtt./ Min.	cc./ hour	time started	time finished	flow checked
250 cc. D/5/W					
50 cc. molar lactate					
500,000 units aqueous penicillin	12	48	9:00 AM		30 Min.

	INTAKE			OUTPUT		
Time Checked	Gtt./Min.	cc. in Bottle	cc. Given	Urine cc.	Emesis	Checked by
9:00 AM	12	250	0			S N
9:30	12	226	24			S N
10:00	12	202	48	20		S N
10:30	12	178	72			
11:00	12	154	96	25		
11:30	12	130	120			
12:00	12	106	144	25		

Urinary Output

After assisting with the insertion of a Foley catheter, the nurse should connect the catheter to a sterile drainage tubing and allow drainage into a sterile, closed, calibrated container. Urinary drainage is recorded every hour.

MINIMUM URINARY OUTPUT (NORMAL)

Age	24 hr. intake	Excretion/hr.
0–12 months	200–500 cc.	8–20 cc.
1–12 years	500–800 cc.	20–33 cc.

Vital signs should be checked and recorded at frequent intervals, ranging from every 15 minutes to every half to full hour, as the circumstances demand. Observation should include:

1. Patency of the airway. Check for difficult breathing, stridor, and sternal retractions.
2. Pulse rate, rhythm, and character. State whether it is rapid, weak, or irregular.
3. Body temperature, to be taken rectally if possible.
4. Blood pressure.
5. Restlessness, anxiety, excessive thirst, or presence of pain.

Oral Fluids and Medications

Oral fluids should either be omitted or kept to a minimum for the first day or two. Acute gastric dilatation is a common complication of burns, and can become a serious problem. The child's thirst, which is usually severe, should be somewhat relieved by the intravenous fluids, and sips of water may be allowed. The child needs considerable emotional support, however, to help him through this stage.

Antibiotics, if used, will probably be added to the intravenous fluids. Tetanus antitoxin or toxoid should be ordered according to the state of the child's previous immunization. If his inoculations are up to date, a booster dose of tetanus toxoid is all that will be required.

Emotional Support for the Child and His Parents

Immediately following such a traumatic accident, the child undoubtedly will be in a state of physical and emotional shock, to the extent that he is not acutely aware of what is happening around him. As his doctors and his nurses are going to be extremely busy giving him vital physical care, they may find it easy to forget the frightened child's emotional needs. A few minutes explanation of what is going to happen now, a kind and supportive attitude toward the child, is of great importance to him, even though he himself makes little response.

The parents probably need greater support than their child during the first hours, but they may get very little. No one has much time for them; they must stay out of the way. In fact, they will be quite willing to stay out of the way of such mysterious and frightening procedures.

Thoughtful concern for their comfort can be given by nurses not directly involved in the burned child's treatment, until the doctors can be free to explain and to counsel. A few friendly words from time to time, a smile in passing, an invitation to accompany some of the nurses on their coffee break, or just a willingness to listen—all this is welcomed by the parents, themselves in a state of emotional shock.

Continuing Care

After the initial fluid therapy has brought the burn shock under control, and after the extracellular fluid deficit has been made up, the patient faces another hazard with the onset of the diuretic phase. This occurs somewhere within the period of 24 to 96 hours after the accident. The plasma-like fluid is picked up and reabsorbed from the "third space" in the burn areas, and the patient may rapidly become hypervolemic, even to the point of pulmonary edema. This is the principle reason for the extremely close check on all vital signs, and for the close monitoring of intravenous fluids, which must now be slowed or stopped entirely.

The nurse needs to be alert for any signs of the onset of this phase, in order to notify the physicians at once. Clues to the onset of the diuretic phase include:

1. Rapid rise in urinary output. May go up to 250 cc. per hour, or higher.
2. Tachypnea, followed by dyspnea.
3. Increase in pulse pressure; mean blood pressure may also rise. Central venous pressure, if measured, will be found to be elevated.

If pulmonary edema becomes evident, vigorous action may be necessary, such as the use of rotating tourniquets, positive pressure respiration, and venesection. Morphine may be ordered.

Daily patient care through the first phases requires attention to positioning in order to help prevent contractures. This includes proper body alignment, the use of a footboard, keeping the head, the arms, and the legs in good position, as much as possible.

Frequent turning to prevent lung congestion and skin breakdown is extremely important, and extremely difficult. A Stryker frame, on which a child may be turned quickly and painlessly, may be used. Children are apt to become very frightened when being turned on the Stryker frame, requiring much reassurance and support.

Emotional Support for the Attending Staff

Constant nursing of a burned child is an exceedingly traumatic emotional experience, as well as a most exhausting physical one. The child needs to have one individual to give him the support so important to his welfare, and the explanation and demonstration of complicated procedures takes a disproportionate amount of time if these must be repeated to constantly changing nurses. The nurse on each shift who has the care of the burned child needs a great deal of support from the personnel on the department.

Frequent checking to determine her needs, whether it is some article from outside the room, help with a procedure, or a few minutes relief, is most welcome. She needs prompt relief for meals, and coffee breaks are of great importance in order to get her away from the situation for a short time. An occasional chance for her to ask advice or just to discuss her problems is also appreciated.

The high room temperature that must be maintained is a source of great discomfort to those attending the burned child, and the opportunity to change into a sterile nursery gown rather than putting a gown over her uniform would be welcome, if available. The odor, which invariably permeates the closed room of a burned child, adds to the nurse's discomfort.

SECOND PHASE (FROM 48–72 HOURS TO TWO OR MORE WEEKS)

Burns may be treated by the open method or by the application of pressure dressings. Many surgeons prefer the open (or exposure) method. The tough outer covering that forms over the burned area—called eschar —makes a satisfactory covering initially, but cracks between the eschar quickly provide a fertile breeding place for bacteria.

Infection is rarely a problem during the first 48 hours, if the proper aseptic environment is maintained. Normal skin bacteria invade the broken skin under the most careful management, however, so that every burn is potentially infected. Frequent incidence of *Staphylococcus aureus* and *Pseudomonas aeruginosa* infection are observed during the second phase in spite of stringent attempts at prevention of cross-contamination, followed too often by septicemia.[*]

Interesting new methods for limiting possibilities for cross-contamination in the hospital situation are described in current literature. These involve placing the patient in a self-contained unit, usually made of plastic, with treatment carried out through portholes, much in the same manner as the Isolette is used in caring for premature infants.[†] Shrine hospitals, designed to provide the latest concepts in the care of burned children, are in the process of construction. One such pilot project provides an entire patient care suite designed on an aseptic control concept similar to that provided in general surgical suites.[‡]

These methods do not, of course, control the problem of self-infection, nor do they appear to deal adequately with the emotional support needed so desperately by a hospitalized burned child.

Closed Method of Burn Treatment

Although the open method appears to be the method of choice in general, the closed method is still used, especially for hand burns, for purposes of splinting and for preventing edema. This may be done even if the open method is used for the remainder of the burn area.

[*] Haynes, B. W., and Hench, M. E.: Hospital isolation system for preventing cross-contamination of Staphylococcal and Pseudomonas organisms in burn wounds. Ann. Surg., *162*:641, 1965.

[†] ibid. p. 642. See also The Modern Hospital, *104*:76, (Jan.) 1965.

[‡] The Modern Hospital, *104*:81, (Jan.) 1965.

The closed method consists of the application of a pressure dressing to cover the burn areas. Sterile mesh gauze, impregnated with a bland ointment,* is laid next to the area, fluffed gauze is placed over the strips, and firm bandages, such as Kerlix, are used to hold the dressing in place. This is allowed to remain in place for several days, with dressing changes done in surgery if the dressing becomes odorous, or if the patient spikes an elevated temperature. These dressings may help protect the patient from the environment, but do not protect him from self-infection.

Débridement and Grafting

Early débridement of the eschar in order to allow early skin grafting is considered important in the control of infection. After the initial shock phase, tub baths may be given to assist the removal of eschar if the open method is used. Eschar requires approximately 7 days to two weeks to slough off spontaneously, so débridement is frequently done mechanically in surgery under light anesthesia. If the area is clear of infection, grafts may be applied at the same time. Blood for transfusion should be ready because there may be considerable bleeding, especially if large areas are debrided.

Skin grafts. Grafts may be either homografts or autografts. A *homograft* consists of skin taken from another person, and is eventually rejected by the recipient tissue, sloughing off after a period of three to six weeks. It provides a temporary dressing after débridement, and has proved a life-saving measure for children with extensive burns. Skin from cadavers is often used; it can be stored and used up to a period of several weeks, and permission for this use is seldom refused.

An *autograft,* consisting of skin taken from the child's own body, is the only kind of skin accepted permanently by recipient tissues, except for the skin from an identical twin. It is usually impossible to obtain enough healthy skin to cover a large area; therefore, homografts are of great value for immediate covering. If the donor site is kept free from infection, and grafts of sufficient thinness are taken, the site should be ready for use again in 10 to 12 days.

After grafting, donor as well as graft sites are kept covered with sterile dressings.

Nursing Care in Second Phase

Tub baths. The tub should be kept scrupulously clean, and preferably used only for burn baths. A child should be transported to the tub under aseptic conditions, and placed in warm water to which a soap solution has been added. This is a frightening, usually unpleasant, experience for the child, and requires gentle handling.

* Sold commercially as Adaptic, or under other trade names.

Soaks. Soaks may be used to help loosen the eschar, or in the treatment of an infection. They are applied as are any sterile, wet dressings, with the use of medicated solutions as ordered, or of normal saline.

Infection. The nurse must be constantly alert for any evidence of infection, which can quickly become systemic. Septicemia is still the cause of the large number of deaths that occur during this period.

Septicemia may be heralded by a sharp rise in temperature, but it must be kept in mind that one indicator of an overwhelming septicemia is a sudden *drop* in temperature to *sub-normal levels. Pseudomonas aeruginosa* and *Escherichia coli* are two frequent causative organisms in septicemia.

Other symptoms include a fall in blood pressure, a rising pulse, and possibly vomiting. Any suspicious symptoms should be reported at once.

Nutritional Needs

The child who has received extensive deep burns must receive special attention regarding his nutritional needs. The nutritional problem is much more complex than simply getting a seriously ill child to eat. He is in negative nitrogen and caloric balance from a number of causes, including the following:

1. Poor intake, from anorexia, ileus, Curling's ulcer, or diarrhea.
2. External loss, due to exudative losses of protein through the burn wound.
3. Thermal losses from the burn itself; heat loss from the radiation of heat and from water loss, responsible for large caloric losses.
4. Hypermetabolism, from fever, infection, and from the state of "toxicity."

A diet high in protein, for healing and for replacement, high in calories, and essentially bland in character, is an essential component of therapy. Great efforts must be made to interest the child in foods essential for tissue building and repair. Large servings are not acceptable because of anorexia as well as the physical condition of the child. This is one time when all the imagination and the ingenuity of the nurse and the dietitian are needed to the utmost degree. Foods rich in protein, high in caloric value, and easily digested are needed, but are going to be of no value if the child refuses to eat them. Colorful trays, foods with eye appeal, and any special touches to spur a child's appetite, should all be tried. A number of hints are suggested in the section The Care of the Chronically Ill Child.

Some kinds of useful food are:

Flavored milk shakes, ice cream shakes.

High protein drinks containing eggs and extra dried protein milk.

Hard candies, ice cream, milk and egg desserts.

Puréed meats, and vegetables.

With the best efforts of nurses, dietitians, and of the child himself, the burn patient can seldom eat an amount of food sufficient to meet his increased needs. Tube feedings are frequently necessary as supplements to the daily intake.

Great care must be used to avoid making tube feedings a threat—"Unless you eat, you will have to have a tube"—or a punishment—"You didn't eat all your food today." The child must understand what is to be done and why. For instance, "Johnny, you need extra food, more than you can eat by yourself, to help your skin heal and to help make you strong again. Let's put this tube into the doll's mouth (or nose) and watch. It goes right down into her stomach. See? Now, I'll pour some of this drink into the tube—down it goes! Do you want to try doing it? Now you know just what happens when you swallow the tube. It will make you gag a little bit, but it won't hurt."

Foods are "blenderized" into a liquid state for tube feedings. One such formula, containing 2,000 calories, is—

Cottage cheese	400 gm.
Soft cooked eggs	2
Ground cooked meat	180 gm.
Cooked potato	100 gm.
Cooked cereal	200 gm.
Canned carrots	200 gm.
Canned peaches	300 gm.
10% cream	200 gm.
Apple juice	200 gm.
Sugar	45 gm.

Complications

Curling's ulcer. Curling's ulcer is a gastric or duodenal ulcer that frequently occurs following serious skin burns. It can easily be overlooked when the attention of nurses and doctors is directed toward the treatment of the burn area and prevention of infection.

Symptoms are those of any gastric ulcer, but usually are rather vague, concerned with abdominal discomfort, with or without localization, or with relation to eating. Appearance of an ulcer, if it occurs, is during the first six weeks.

Blood may be present in the stools, an occurrence which, combined with abdominal discomfort, may be the basis for a diagnosis. If desired, roentgenograms can confirm the diagnosis.

Treatment consists of a bland diet, the use of antacids such as Maalox or Amphogel, and antispasmodics. Extensive hemorrhages are rare if the condition is recognized and treated.

Rehabilitation Phase

Occupational and physical therapy are frequently combined for the child in order to help maintain his normal functions, as well as to provide near normal situations for the child's continued growth and development.

One child's burns involved his chest, his axilla and his upper arm. It became essential for him to use his right arm in a variety of ways to prevent both contractures and permanent deformities, but Donny saw little sense in causing himself so much discomfort. Little by little, he was encouraged to use his arm for pushing along a wheeled toy, for crayoning, for cutting pictures, and for similar activities. The real inspiration was the solitary fish in a small bowl. Bright yellow stones came in a bag for Donny to drop in, one by one, to provide a foundation, and every day he raised his arm to drop food into the bowl. Soon he became proud that he could feed his fish with his right hand, and willingly gave the fish loving care. (Fig. 87)

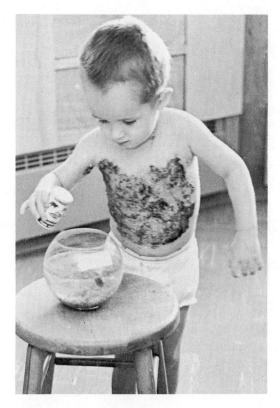

Fig. 87. Motivating the child to move his right arm after chest and axillary burns. Feeding the fish is fun.

BILLY'S STORY

Perhaps if we return to our original Billy, with his 60% burns, and watch his progress during the difficult months of hospitalization, we can feel the magnitude of the task for everyone concerned.

Six-year-old Billy's behavior in the hospital was quite characteristic of the behavior one may expect to find in a severely burned child of this age group. For many weeks, he was in a private room with constant attendance while it seemed that painful or unpleasant procedures were almost constantly being performed. He fought back with all of his ability. He screamed and raged at everything done in his room, and at everyone doing it. He was terribly afraid of being turned on the Stryker frame, turning pale and trembling whenever this was done. If the attendant was not accustomed to his care, he would assure her that the security straps were not to be used, or that he was not to be turned any more, and became enraged when he could not control his environment.

His voice, when he was not shouting with rage, became a whine almost impossible to understand, a circumstance that only made him more angry.

Long* remarks about the similar behavior found in many severely burned children. It makes nursing the child so difficult and so exhausting, both emotionally and physically, that the nurse assigned to his care needs a great deal of support. These children need the ministrations of some one person in order to build up confidence and security. It is considerably less traumatic to a child if the person entering the room in the morning is secure in her knowledge of the physical care needed, as well as in her knowledge of this particular child.

Billy's slow progress proceeded over a period of months, until the entire process became a way of life for him, although he never fully accepted it. His burned areas were temporarily covered with homografts, but there was extremely little skin to use for autografts, and much scar tissue and many adhesions with contractures resulted.

After many months, some of Billy's problems had been solved, but many others remained. One was of fluid intake. Imagination on the nurse's part helped. One day, Billy became so intrigued with being allowed to pour his own drinking water from a light pitcher into a one ounce medicine glass, and reading the amount on the calibrated side, that he spent an hour pouring and shouting, "Another 45 cc., now 30; here's 60 more. Did you write that all down?" His nurse spent many hours finding drinks that he would take, such as weak tea and carbonated drinks, and occasionally he would consent to drink some chocolate milk.

Billy was now in a four bed room, and here he had considerable difficulty adjusting. The necessity of almost constant attendance had made him extremely selfish. He could not share either his nurses, the television, or the playthings. He would ask other boys to show him their toys, and frequently refuse to return them if they took his fancy. Long, patient, loving discipline was necessary before this little boy could learn to live with the others. Sometimes his rage at life was turned against his roommates who could do so many things he could not, and he would destroy their possessions. Gradually, he learned. He still required many hours of daily care, with wet packs over certain areas, with elastic bandages to his legs, and special shoes whenever he was up, and he

* Long, R., and Cope, O.: Emotional problems of burned children. New Eng. J. Med., *264*:1121, 1961.

needed much help generally. The nurse still needed to check orders carefully because he would solemnly insist that certain procedures were no longer being done.

Physical and occupational therapists worked with Billy daily. In spite of his severe handicaps, he learned to do much. His arms were contracted in a fixed position, but his wrists were flexible, and he learned to feed himself with little difficulty. The therapists taught him the ability to raise himself from a lying position to a sitting one and to a standing one without the use of his arm muscles. He learned to put on his bathrobe by backing into it. These skills were not easy to acquire, and he never volunteered information concerning what he could do, while on the ward. His normal mischievousness began to assert itself, although it found little scope in his restricted surroundings. It seemed to his nurses that it consisted mainly in misleading about his treatments and routines. If he became bored with physical therapy, he would solemnly assert that he was not to go today, and was believed. When the messenger came for him, he was not ready. The gleam in his eye when she came told of his satisfaction in having for once "fooled the nurses."

Billy started schoolwork with the teacher before his discharge, although his attention span was short, and he had difficulty disciplining himself to any serious work. He was an intelligent boy and could probably learn quickly once he had established the necessary habits. His greatest thrill in the hospital came when he was transferred from his Stryker frame to a regular hospital bed, "just like normal people use," he said.

Eventually, it was time for him to go home. His mother came to the hospital to learn how to care for him, and to take him home. He had been home for short periods of two or three days before, but this time it was for "keeps," until he needed surgery at a later date.

Billy faced tremendous problems at home. A normally active little boy, with lively brothers and sisters, he would find life far different from the home life that he remembered. The problems must have seemed tremendous to his parents too, but they were willing to try. The nurse in the community would have to give them much support and help. Billy still has a long road ahead, but he is alive, and learning to adapt to new skills every day.

BIBLIOGRAPHY

American Humane Association: Protecting the Battered Child. Denver, American Humane Association, 1962.

Beal, C. B.: Plastic bubble isolates patient anywhere in hospital. Mod. Hosp., *104*:83, (Jan.) 1965.

Burke, J. F.: Boston concept uses air and plastic for burn isolation. Mod. Hosp., *104*:80, (Jan.) 1965.

Child Welfare Protective Service Issue: J. of Child Welfare League of America XLII, (March) 1963.

De Francis, V.: Review of Legislation to Protect the Battered Child. A Study of Laws enacted in 1963. Denver, American Humane Association.

————: The Court and Protective Services. Denver, American Humane Association, 1960.

————: Community Cooperation for Better Child Protection. Denver, American Humane Association, 1959.

Ellerbe, T. F., and Henslin, R.: O.R. asepsis is goal of Texas burn center plan. Mod. Hosp., *104*:81, (Jan.) 1965.

Elmer, E.: Abused young children seen in hospitals. Social Work, 5:98, 1960.

Haynes, B. W., and Hench, M. E.: Hospital isolation system for preventing cross-contamination of staphylococcal and pseudomonas organisms in burn Wounds. Ann. Surg., *162*:641, 1965.

How one hospital planned its burn center. Mod. Hosp., *104*:76, 1965.

Isolation unit in France is designed for care of burns. Mod. Hosp., *104*:78, (Jan.) 1965.

Kempe, C., *et al:* The battered child syndrome. J.A.M.A., *181*:17, 1962.

Long, R., and Cope, O.: Emotional problems of burned children. New Eng. J. Med., *264*:1121, 1961.

Lund, C. C., and Browder, N. C.: The estimation of areas of burns. Surg. Gynec. and Obstet., *79*:352, 1944.

Morris, M. G., *et al:* Toward prevention of child abuse. Children, *11*:55, 1964.

Mulford, R.: Emotional neglect of children. Denver, American Humane Association, 1958.

Nelson, W., (ed.): Textbook of Pediatrics. 8th ed. Philadelphia, W. B. Saunders, 1964.

Paulsen, M. G.: Legal protection against child abuse. Children, *13*:42, 1966.

Silverman, F.: The roentgen manifestation of unrecognized skeletal trauma in infants. J. Roentgenology, *69*:413, 1953.

Urciolo, C.: Disturbance of acid-base equilibrium resulting from salicylism in children. J. Amer. Med. Wom. Ass., *20*:1021, 1965.

Wald, M.: Protective Services and Emotional Neglect. Denver, American Humane Association.

SUGGESTED READINGS FOR FURTHER STUDY

Cowin, R.: Social factors in treating burned children. Children, *11*:229, 1964.

Delsordo, J.: Protective casework for abused children. Children, *10*:213, 1963.

Dreisbach, R. H.: Handbook of Poisoning, Diagnosis and Treatment. 4th ed. Los Altos, California, Lange Medical Publications, 1963.

Farmer, A. W.: Management of burns in children. Pediatrics, *25*:886, 1960.

Fontana, V., *et al:* The "maltreated syndrome" in children. New Eng. J. Med., *269*:1389, 1963.

Foresman, L.: Strengthening family life. Children, *12*:23, 1965.

Fowler, R. S., *et al:* Accidental digitalis intoxication in children. J. Pediat., *64*:188, 1964.

Jensen, G. D., and Wilson, W. W.: Preventive implications of a study of 100 poisonings in children. Pediatrics, *25*:490, 1960.

Miller, R., and Johnson, S. R.: Poison control—now and in the future. Amer. J. Nurs., *66*:1984, (Sep.) 1966.

Rubin, M.: Balm for burned children. Amer. J. Nurs., *66*:296, (Feb.) 1966.

Stringer, E.: A tool for case evaluation. Children, *12*:26, 1965.

World Health Magazine: Accidents. (Special issue). Geneva, World Health Organization, 1961.

Zollinger, R. W., *et al:* Trauma in children in a general hospital. Amer. J. Surg., *104*:855, 1962.

14

Illness in the Toddler
Age Group

CONDITIONS OF THE RESPIRATORY TRACT

Nursing the Child with Respiratory Difficulties

Respiratory infections are common to young children, occurring, in many conditions, as complications. The average child over the age of one year is extremely susceptible to the common cold, and loses a considerable amount of school time in the lower grades. Eventually, most healthy children develop some degree of resistance, and less time is lost.

The child in nursery school, in kindergarten or in the first grade, picks up respiratory infections from other children or from the adults at home, acting in turn as an agent himself.

Care for the Child with Acute Nasopharyngitis (the Common Cold)

The simple cold develops with a runny nose, a slight fever, sneezing, perhaps a slight sore throat, and mild cough. The child may not feel particularly ill. His mother may have some difficulty keeping him in bed. Some mothers believe they can prevent chilling if they dress the child and let him play on the bed or the davenport, rather than run the risk of finding him running about in his bare feet and his pajamas. Providing adequate playthings can help to keep him reasonably quiet, particularly if other distractions are put out of sight. Certainly the child recovers faster if he is kept quiet and warm while any fever is present.

Preventive measures. Small children need to be kept away from persons with respiratory infections whenever possible. Particular care must be used if the child has a chronic condition that may be aggravated by a superimposed respiratory infection.

A small child put out to play in cold weather needs some protection against prolonged chilling, which may lower his resistance to a respiratory infection. Telling him to avoid getting chilled or wet from playing in snow or water has no effect other than to prevent him from coming into the house for fear of a scolding or punishment. A more realistic approach is to teach him to come in for a change of clothing if he becomes wet or chilled.

Sniffles, or other signs of rhinitis, need to be watched somewhat more carefully in a small child than in an older one, because a cold can develop more rapidly into something serious. After being put to bed at night, he should be checked once or twice for respiratory stridor or for difficult breathing. The common cold should not be taken casually by anyone, of course, but small children are particularly susceptible to complications. Middle ear infections frequently occur in small children; bronchitis and pneumonia are also complications that occur more often in this age group than in any other. In addition, what seems to be merely a mild cold may blossom out in a day or two into one of childhood's communicable diseases.

Clinical manifestations and treatment. Probably no one needs to have the symptoms of the common head cold recited. Serous nasal drainage at first, changing to purulent drainage; sneezing, headache and low grade fever, loss of appetite; aches throughout the body—all are quite familiar. Colds are usually of viral origin, and no one has discovered a cure for the common cold.

An infant or a small child cannot blow his nose to clear his airway. When the child reaches the age at which he can learn, he should be taught to blow his nose, at the same time keeping both nostrils and his mouth open, to prevent forcing infected material into the eustachian tubes and the sinuses.

If the nasal congestion is particularly troublesome, nose drops help shrink the mucous membranes and bring relief. Neo-synephrine or ephedrine, in aqueous solution, may be used no more often than every three hours, for a period of not more than two or three days. Oily preparations must not be used for children because of the danger of lipoid pneumonia.

Fluids are offered frequently, and foods are given according to the child's appetite. If the child can be kept quiet for a day or two following the acute phase, his chance of developing complications is lessened.

Epistaxis

Nosebleeds are common in childhood; they may be caused by forcible nose blowing or picking, rhinitis, foreign bodies, or by external trauma. A nosebleed may accompany many organic conditions, such as blood dyscrasias, hypertension and rheumatic fever.

Nosebleeds are easily controlled in a healthy child, and rarely present a serious problem. If the child sits quietly in a semi-erect position, with ice applied over the bridge of his nose, most nasal hemorrhages stop spontaneously. If persistent, cotton moistened in epinephrine (1:1000), may be placed in the nostril over the bleeding membrane and left in place until it has stopped. Massive or prolonged hemorrhages need to be treated by a physician.

Foreign Bodies in the Nose

Small children frequently poke beans, peas, beads and other small objects into their noses, and this may not be noticed by their parents until an irritation of the mucous membrane has developed. Sneezing and obstructed nose breathing, with a chronic, increasingly purulent nasal discharge, may be an indication of the presence of a foreign body.

Occasionally, the object may be sneezed out, but unskillful efforts to remove it may push it only farther into the nasal passages. If the object is of the vegetable family, it will swell and cause considerable irritation. Metal objects may remain for many weeks without being discovered.

Examination by a physician (with use of a nasal speculum) is indicated if nasal obstruction persists without known cause. The object will need to be removed by instruments handled by a skilled physician. If the object is securely lodged, a local anesthetic may be used.

Cleft Palate Repair

The child born with a cleft palate (but with an intact lip) does not have the external disfigurement that may be so distressing to the new mother—but his problems are more serious. Although a cleft lip and a cleft palate frequently appear together, either defect may appear alone. In embryonic development, the palate closes at a later time than does the lip, and the failure to close is for somewhat different reasons. The manner in which the palate normally closes is interesting.

When the embryo is about eight weeks old, there is still no roof to the mouth: the tissues that are to become the palate are two shelves running from the front to the back of the mouth, and projecting vertically downward on either side of the tongue. The shelves move from a vertical position to a horizontal position, their free edges meeting and fusing in midline. Later, bone forms within this tissue to form the hard palate.* Exactly what happens to prevent this closure is not known with certainty. It occurs more frequently in near relatives of persons with the defect than in the general population, and there appears to be some evidence that environmental and hereditary factors may each play a part in this defect.

A cleft palate may involve the soft palate alone, or it may extend into the nose and into the hard palate. It may be unilateral or bilateral, an isolated defect, or in conjunction with cleft lip.

Management of the Defect

Plastic surgeons prefer to wait until the child is over a year old before they attempt surgical repair. The goal is to give the child a union of the cleft parts that would allow intelligible and pleasant speech, and to avoid

* Fishbein, M. (ed.): Birth Defects. p. 242. Philadelphia, J. B. Lippincott, 1963.

injury to the maxillary growth. Timing of surgery is individualized, according to the size, the placement and the degree of deformity. The optimal time for surgery is considered to be between the ages of one and five years. Because the child is not able to make certain sounds when he starts to talk, undesirable speech habits are formed, which are difficult to correct. If surgery must be delayed beyond the third year, a dental speech appliance may help the child develop intelligible speech.

Home Care Before Surgery

The infant with a cleft palate (but with an intact lip) can learn to suck without much difficulty. A rather large nipple, with holes that allow the milk to drip freely, makes sucking easier for this child, who does not get quite as much suction as a child with an intact palate. The activity of sucking is an important one for the development of speech muscles. Special cleft palate nipples, with a flange to cover the cleft, are commercially available. They are, however, expensive and unnecessary for the average infant with a cleft palate. Holding the baby in a partially upright position while he is fed reduces the possibility of choking and aspiration. An occasional infant who is unable to manipulate a nipple may need to be fed with a rubber-tipped Asepto syringe.

Strained foods are introduced at the usual time and in the routine manner, within the framework of a normal diet. A little food or milk may seep through the cleft and out through the nose, and the mother should be informed of this possibility.

Cleft lip and cleft palate centers provide teams of specialists who can give the professional services that these children need through their infancy, preschool and school years. Members of the professional team include a pediatrician, a plastic surgeon, an orthodontist, a speech therapist, a social worker and a public health nurse. The services of a child nutritionist are also available. Explanations and counseling concerning the child's diet, his speech training, his immunizations and his general health supervision can be given. Questions can be answered and misconceptions can be cleared up.

It may sound strange to speak about preparation for speech training for an infant only a few weeks of age. The babbling and cooing of a young infant is an important precursor of speech activity, and the stimulation that the parents normally give when they repeat the sounds back to him is essential. Parents normally do this, but they may be too disturbed and tense to behave in a natural manner before an infant with a palate defect. This child, however, needs to hear these sounds as a pattern for learning, even more than an infant who does not have to overcome a physical impediment.

Dental care for the deciduous teeth is of more than usual importance. The incidence of dental caries is high in children with a cleft palate, but the preservation of the deciduous teeth is important for the best results in speech as well as for appearance.

Hospital Care

The child should be in a good nutritional state and entirely free from respiratory infection when he enters the hospital for surgery. Because it is imperative that he keep his fingers out of his mouth after repair, he should have a chance to become accustomed to elbow restraints before his surgery. These restraints and a sore mouth are going to be frustrating, and because he should not cry any more than can be prevented—in order to avoid strain on the sutures—his mother should be allowed to stay with him, to hold and comfort him. If this is not possible, he should become acquainted with his nurse before surgery, and learn to accept her in place of his mother for the time being.

Directly after surgery a young child is watched with great care to prevent the aspiration of vomitus or mucus, and to prevent occlusion of the airway by his tongue. Elbow restraints are applied firmly and are checked frequently. Fingers, or any object put into his mouth, may irritate or infect the sutures, causing an imperfect repair—which may not be operable a second time.

The operating surgeon will have a routine for postoperative repair that he finds most successful. Generally, the patient is allowed clear liquids after nausea has ceased. Spoons and straws are usually forbidden, only drinking from a cup or a glass being allowed. Clear liquids that are usually accepted are Jello water, apple juice, and the synthetic, fruit-flavored drinks. Broth may be offered, but is not a popular drink with this age group. Clear liquids are allowed for a period of from three to five days, followed by full liquids for approximately ten days, after which semiliquids such as cereal, ice cream or Jello may be fed with a spoon. Some variations from this schedule may be desired by different plastic surgeons.

The sutures are not cleansed or manipulated in any way. Water, or a clear liquid after a milk drink is helpful to keep the sutures clean if the child will cooperate. In addition to vigilance in keeping toys or any objects out of the mouth, considerable care must be exercised to keep anyone with a suspicion of a cold or a cough away from the patient, whether it is a staff nurse, a family member, or some other patient. A cough or a nasal infection may well damage the best repair.

If all goes well, the child can probably be discharged about the tenth day, returning to the clinic or to his doctor's office for suture removal about the third week.

Orthodontic treatment is necessary for the majority of these children. There may be a distortion of the maxillary arch causing malocclusion, and interference with optimal growth and development of the upper jaw.

Orthodontic observation and treatment is continued until the permanent teeth are in good occlusion.

Speech therapy is continued after surgery to aid the child in correcting faulty sounds learned before the defect was corrected. Parents and therapists work together with the child to help him achieve clear speech without disagreeable nasal tones.

The Tonsils and the Adenoids

A brief description of the placement and the functions of tonsils and adenoids may be helpful before the difficulties of infection and the indications for removal are discussed.

A ring of lymphoid tissue, called Waldeyer's ring, encircles the pharynx, forming a protective barrier against upper respiratory infection. This ring consists of groups of lymphoid tonsils.

The palatine tonsils, the commonly known *tonsils,* are two oval masses attached to the side walls of the back of the mouth between the anterior and posterior pillars.

The nasopharyngeal tonsil, known as *adenoids,* is a mass of lymphoid tissue in the nasal pharynx, extending from the roof of the nasal pharynx to the free edge of the soft palate.

The lingual tonsils are two masses of lymphoid tissue at the base of the tongue.

There is a normal progression of enlargement of lymphoid tissue in childhood between the ages of two and eight or ten years, regressing during the pubertal period. If the tissue itself becomes a site of acute or chronic infection, it may become hypertrophied to the extent of interfering with breathing, causing partial deafness, or it may become in itself a source of infection.

Tonsillectomies and adenoidectomies are not done as frequently today as in the past; many otolaryngologists are of the opinion that too many are still being performed. The surgery is too frequently considered by nonmedical persons, as well as by some nurses, as a relatively minor affair. In the United States, the surgical mortality total for tonsillectomies is between 250 and 300 yearly, which takes the operation out of the unimportant class.

No conclusive evidence has been found that a tonsillectomy, in itself, improves a child's health by reducing the number of respiratory infections, increasing the appetite, or improving his general well-being. Studies tend to show that incidence of colds may increase following removal of the tonsils. It is generally agreed that absolute indications for removal of tonsils are: frequent attacks of acute tonsillitis; recurrent peritonsillar abscess (which has become rare); chronically infected tonsils with enlarged cervical nodes, which fail to yield to antibiotic therapy; and hypertrophy of tonsils to the extent of interfering with swallowing and breathing. Systemic disturbances, such as rheumatic fever or glomerulo-nephritis, are not considered as indications for tonsillectomy, unless the tonsils can be proved to be the source of an infection that fails to yield to antibiotic treatment.

Adenoids are more susceptible to chronic infection. Indication for adenoidectomy is hypertrophy of the tissue to the extent of impairing hearing or interfering with breathing. An increasingly common practice is to perform an adenoidectomy alone, if tonsil tissue appears to be healthy.

Acute Tonsillitis

Acute infections of the throat are rare before the age of one year. Nonbacterial tonsillitis is usually mild, and is of short duration. Acute tonsillitis of bacterial origin commences with a high fever, followed by an inflammatory infection of the tonsils, the pharynx and of the soft palate. There may be fiery redness and swelling with exudate. Cervical lymphadenopathy is usually present.

The child should be kept in bed until his symptoms subside, and other children should be kept away as long as his condition is infectious. Fluids should be pushed to the extent the child will accept: persistence in presenting fluids, with imagination to make them acceptable, may be necessary. If foods are desired, they should be soft and easily swallowed.

Cold throat packs may relieve pain, although small children are usually impatient with any type of throat pack. Aspirin is ordered to be given as needed for relief of pain, and an antibiotic, usually penicillin, is given.

Aspirin dosage for children is one grain for each year of age, up to the age of five, not more often than every four hours. A word of caution is needed for the parents. Aspirin is given rather commonly to small children for fever or discomfort. In view of the fact that aspirin poisoning is the most frequent type of poisoning, and also because a certain proportion of people have a severe reaction to aspirin, it should not be given indiscriminately. Aspirin may have a cumulative effect as well—children come into the hospital suffering from the effects of too much aspirin over a period of time, as well as from massive, single doses. Penicillin also may cause a severe, sometimes fatal, reaction. One does not use the leftover penicillin from the last illness without the doctor's permission. Preferably, any leftover medication should be promptly discarded after the need is over.

Care of the Child Admitted for Tonsillectomy

Tonsillectomy is postponed until after the age of four or five years, except in the rare instance when it appears urgently needed. Often, when a child has reached the acceptable age, the apparent need for the tonsillectomy has disappeared. When the decision has been made to remove the tonsils, a period of two or three weeks following an acute infection should pass, although this is not always possible. On occasion, a surgeon, after several cancellations of surgery because of new infections, may decide that it is safer to operate while the child is relatively free from infection, rather than risk any more acute episodes. This may be demonstrated on the ward when the nurse reports a mild temperature elevation during the preoperative period. Normally, surgery is cancelled, and the child is sent home. When the child has been unable to maintain a period of two or three weeks free from throat infection, however, the otolaryngologist may agree to remove the tonsils, provided that no evidence of present acute respiratory infection is found.

Preoperative Care. In many hospitals, the child has had blood and urine tests performed before admission; if this has not been done, the nurse should make certain that the ordered tests are performed and the results entered on the chart. Written permission for surgery is then obtained, and the parents are notified of the time surgery is scheduled.

One unfortunate occurrence in busy hospitals ought never to be—that of a failure to notify the parents of an advance in surgery time, so that the parent arrives to find her child has already left the ward. A concerned parent is justifiably angered, as she visualizes her child's fright and insecurity. A most graphic illustration concerns a mother who had been given a definite time for her child's surgery the previous evening by the surgeon. An earlier case was cancelled, however, before the schedule was sent to the ward, and so the ward personnel were entirely unaware that the mother had been told a later time. Notification of scheduled time by telephone, if the information is not available when parents are on the ward (with care to notify when changes in scheduling occur), will prevent this from happening most of the time; especially if parents are advised to come at least an hour before scheduled surgery time, to allow for the period when the child is under sedation.

Emotional preparation for surgery has been discussed throughout this book. Acting out the forthcoming experience, particularly in a group, with the use of puppets, dolls, and play doctor or play nurse material helps the child to develop security. The amount and the timing of preparation before admission depends somewhat upon the child's age. The nursing care study discussed later in this chapter is applicable to any type of elective surgery.

On the morning of surgery, the child is given no food or fluids, a fact that may well traumatize the child emotionally if he has to watch the others getting their breakfast trays. If surgery is to be late, there is no reason for keeping the child in his bed. He will be happier and better adjusted if he can spend this time in the playroom, with someone responsible for helping him resist the temptation to drink, if he should forget.

A Six-year-old Has a T and A

Dick, a six-year-old boy admitted for tonsillectomy, was met in the pediatric admitting room by the student nurse who was to care for him throughout his hospital stay. She introduced herself to Dick as Carol B., and explained that she would be his nurse. Dick was disturbed and reluctant when the admitting nurse attempted to take his temperature. After Carol explained the procedure and showed him the thermometer, he accepted this manner of temperature taking.

Following a preoperative examination by the admitting pediatric intern, Carol took Dick to the laboratory for the routine blood check, which included an RBC, a WBC, and tests for bleeding time and clotting time. She explained to Dick that the technician would stick his finger to get a little blood, and she told him why. His only question was, "How will she take the blood out?" He cooperated well, but felt the need to cry, and was comforted by the nurse and his mother.

On the way to the pediatric department, Carol and Dick discussed what the ward looked like, why he was to sleep in a crib, and the delights of the playroom. The first thing he wished to do on his arrival was to crawl into the crib to find out what it felt like, accepting it as a novelty. He delighted in the playroom, played with the other children, and accepted his mother's departure calmly.

Although Dick had been prepared for the surgery experience by his parents, Carol talked with him about the next day's routine. She explained about the preoperative sedation, telling him it would be like the "shot" he sometimes got in the doctor's office. She told him the ride to surgery would be on a stretcher, showed him the stretcher and let him lie down on it. They examined a face mask together; Dick pretended to be a doctor, put the mask on, and listened to his own heartbeat with a stethoscope. Miss B showed him an oxygen mask, and explained that tomorrow he would wear one like it; there would be a sweet smell of ether, and he would get sleepy. Dick tried on the mask, and wanted to know where the ether would come from. After supper, Dick got into his crib, and Carol read him stories until bedtime.

In the morning Dick's mother arrived early, and shortly after her arrival he received his preoperative medication of Demerol 50 mg., atropine 0.2 mg., and Seconal 25 mg., given intramuscularly. Dick was invited to give a doll an injection, which he did with considerable vengeance. Rather than becoming drowsy, he reacted by becoming overactive and noisy, which embarrassed his mother. Carol assured her that sometimes children were stimulated in this manner, and that her son was not being naughty or uncooperative. Nevertheless, there was some difficulty in keeping him on the stretcher.

In surgery, Dick quieted and responded to the anesthiologist's explanation of the mask and the stethoscope by saying, "I know all about that; the nurse told me already." After the initial inhalation, anesthesia was given by intubation, and surgery was carried out smoothly.

In the recovery room Dick was placed in Trendelenburg's position. Carol noted that his color remained good, his skin was warm, his pulse was about 120, and that there were no signs of bleeding. In about two hours, he had recovered sufficiently to be returned to the ward, where he climbed into his crib and immediately went to sleep. Carol watched him carefully, checking his pulse every hour. The postoperative course was uneventful; Dick wakened at intervals, showed no signs of bleeding, and had only a small amount of dark brown emesis. He took fluids in satisfactory amounts, but he refused ice cream.

The night nurse reported an uneventful night, and in the morning Dick seemed glad to see Carol. He talked freely, recounting the events of the previous day until he "went to sleep," and asking in detail what happened after that. He particularly wanted to know, "What did they do with my tonsils after they took them out?" and, "What did my tonsils look like?"

Carol stayed with Dick until his parents came to take him home, reading to him and answering his many questions. Dick said goodbye with a smile, seeming to feel that he had made friends, and appeared not to have found the experience emotionally damaging.

Postoperative Care. Immediately following a tonsillectomy, the child is placed in a partially prone position, with his head turned to one side, until he is completely awake. This position can be accomplished by turning the child partially over and by flexing his knee on which he is not resting to hold him in position. Pillows placed under the chest and abdomen may embarrass respiration, and so are usually forbidden. A recovery room is generally available for patient care until recovery from anesthesia, but if the patient must return to the ward immediately following surgery, he should be carefully observed until fully reacted; after which, he may be placed in a semiupright position.

Vital signs are checked every 10 to 15 minutes until the child is fully reacted, then every half-hour or every hour. The nurse should be aware of the normal rate of pulse and respiration for the child's age, in order to interpret the vital signs correctly. Any unusual restlessness, frequent swallowing, or rapid pulse may indicate bleeding and should be reported. Vomiting of dark, old blood may be expected, but bright, red-flecked emesis or oozing indicate fresh bleeding. A tracheal suction machine, ready for use, should be at the bedside. Suctioning by the nurse must be performed with great care, and not extend beyond the front of the mouth.

Fluids are encouraged as soon as the child's nausea has subsided. The thirsty child may be eager to drink, but the painful swallowing will probably quell his enthusiasm, and encouragement will be needed. Jello water, fruit-flavored, uncarbonated drinks are allowed, with the oft-promised dish of ice cream in the afternoon.

The child is discharged on the day after surgery if no complications are present. Parents are advised to keep him in bed for two days, and fairly quiet for about a week. Soft foods and nonirritating liquids should be given during the first few days. The parents are advised that a transient earache may be expected about the third day. If bleeding should occur, the pediatrician or clinic should be notified at once.

Conditions of the Larynx and Bronchi

Spasmodic Laryngitis (Spasmodic Croup)

This condition may occur in children between the ages of two and four years. The cause is undetermined; it may be of infectious or of allergic origin, but certain children seem to develop severe laryngospasm with little, if any, apparent cause. The attack may be preceded by coryza and hoarseness, or by no apparent signs of respiratory trouble during the evening. He awakens after a few hours sleep with a bark-like cough, increasing respiratory difficulty, and stridor. The child becomes anxious and restless, and there is marked hoarseness. There may be a low grade fever and mild upper respiratory infection.

This condition is not serious, but is quite frightening, both to the child and his parents. The attack subsides after a few hours; little evidence remains the next day when an anxious mother takes him to the doctor. Attacks frequently occur two or three nights in succession.

Treatment. Humidified air is helpful in reducing the laryngospasm. Taking the child into the bathroom and opening the hot water taps, with the door closed, is a quick method for providing moist air—provided that the water runs hot enough. The pediatrician may prescribe syrup of ipecac in a dosage sufficient to produce vomiting, which usually gives relief. If repeated attacks occur, phenobarbital at bedtime may relax the child enough to prevent a recurrence.

Acute Laryngotracheobronchitis

Laryngeal infections are not uncommon in small children, and they frequently involve tracheobronchial areas as well. Acute laryngotracheobronchitis may progress very rapidly and become a serious problem within a matter of hours. The toddler is the most frequently affected member of the two to four age group. This condition is usually of viral origin, but bacterial invasion may follow the original infection. It generally follows an upper respiratory infection with fairly mild rhinitis and pharyngitis.

The child develops hoarseness and a barking cough, with a fever which may reach 104° or 105°F. As the disease progresses, laryngeal edema becomes marked, and the child's breathing becomes difficult. The pulse is rapid, and cyanosis may become marked. Congestive heart failure and acute respiratory embarrassment may result.

Treatment. The child is placed in a supersaturated atmosphere, such as that obtained in a croupette or some other kind of mist tent. The older croup tents, using hot steam, are rarely used. Greater relief is obtained from the use of a cold mist, and the danger of burns is avoided. The mist may be used with air under pressure, or with oxygen.

Close and careful observation of the child is important. Observation includes checking his pulse, his respiration, his color, listening for hoarseness and stridor, and noting any state of restlessness.

TYPE OF RESPIRATION. Pull down the covers, and watch the child breathe. Observe the amount of chest movement, shallow breathing and retractions. Listen with a stethoscope for breath sounds. Listen for the amount of stridor, indicating difficult breathing.

HEARTBEAT. Listen for the rate, quality, strength, and regularity of the pulse. A rapid, weak pulse may indicate impending cardiac difficulty.

VOICE AND COLOR. Increasing hoarseness should be reported. Cyanosis of the extremities or an increasing pallor should be reported as well.

Difficult swallowing, which may limit the airway, as well as prevent sufficient fluid intake.

Increasing restlessness and anxiety, are frequently signs of impending heart failure.

Intravenous fluids are usually needed, but they must be carefully monitored to prevent overloading the circulation and placing additional strain on the overworked heart.

Not all children with this type of infection become as acutely ill as their symptoms imply, but the possibility is present, and it should be understood. The majority of these infections are of viral origin, and do not respond to antibiotics.

If a tracheotomy becomes necessary because of any respiratory difficulty, the surgeon will try to perform this in the operating room, under more ideal conditions than can be obtained at the bedside. The decision as to when to perform a tracheotomy is a delicate one. Tracheostomy is a procedure not to be performed lightly or for insufficient reasons. The waiting period becomes a difficult one for the nurse, especially because her observations are used as partial basis for decision. The parents' anxiety, and her own feeling of helplessness add to her concern.

The nurse who is watching the child needs support from the other members of the nursing staff as well as from the physicians. She should not try to demonstrate her self-sufficiency or worry about the picture she may present to others. Her concern is for her patient, and she should seek help and advice without hesitation.

An emergency tracheotomy set is kept readily available for use if it is necessary, but because much better results can be obtained if the surgery is performed in the operating room—without the pressures of a last minute emergency procedure—the child will be taken there if possible. When the child is in surgery, the nurse will prepare his room for his return. The bed can now be changed completely, the mist apparatus cleaned and checked for maximum efficiency, and the plastic tent may be checked for tears or holes.

The tracheal suction machine is set up at the bedside, checked for working order, and equipped with suctioning materials.*

An adequate supply of linen, as well as all nursing equipment, is then brought into the room, because a child who has had a tracheotomy should never be left alone.

Nursing Care of the Tracheotomized Child

Directly following surgery, excessive secretions in the trachea can be

---

* The procedures for tracheal suctioning and for tracheotomy suctioning are to be found in the appendix.

troublesome. The tube will need frequent aspiration, and this can be quite frightening to the child. A second person to hold him, or a mechanical constraint may be necessary, particularly at first, when the tube is aspirated. As the secretions become less troublesome, aspiration is not so frequently needed. (Figs. 88a and 88b)

The nurse caring for the child must remain in a position from which she can observe his face at all times when the tracheotomy tube is in place, and she must not occupy herself with any duties that might distract her. When the child is turned, she should place her own chair at the other side of the crib, or turn the crib around. It is generally considered unwise to allow the child to lie on his abdomen, because of the danger of occluding the airway. (Fig. 89)

This constant vigil can become monotonous and tiring, and she may find it difficult to maintain her alertness. She should be relieved at intervals of two hours or less, for a period of relaxation.

The child seldom needs continual restraint while under constant observation, and certainly will be more comfortable if he can move about. His mother's presence may be soothing and comforting, depending on whether the mother can respond in a satisfactory manner, or is herself too frightened to give support.

As the child improves, he can be allowed to sit in his crib or up in a

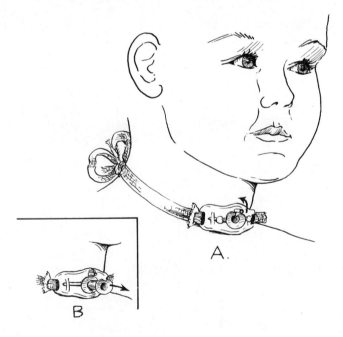

Fig. 88a. Tracheotomy tube in place.
Fig. 88b. Inner cannula unlocked and partially removed.

chair, and he should experience no difficulty eating. If no complications arise, recovery is generally rapid and the tracheotomy tube may be removed without difficulty.

Mortality rate has been considerably lowered during the last few years, with prompt treatment, antibiotic therapy to prevent secondary infection, and careful management.

CONDITIONS OF METABOLIC IMBALANCE

The Celiac Syndrome

Intestinal malabsorption with steatorrhea is a condition brought about by various causes, the most common being cystic fibrosis and gluten induced enteropathy, the so-called idiopathic celiac disease. In 1889, the condition of malnutrition, abnormal stools, distended abdomen and retarded growth was described and named *celiac disease*. Not until the late 1930's was it recognized that several distinct entities were being described, with cystic fibrosis and celiac disease as two conditions of

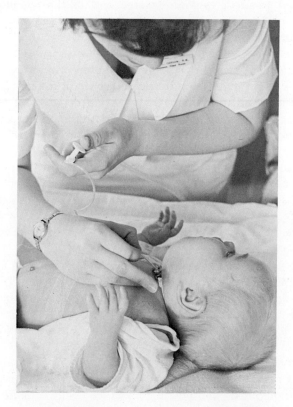

Fig. 89. The nurse is suctioning the tracheotomy tube.

differing etiology. The term *celiac syndrome* is now used to designate the complex of malabsorptive disorders.

Gluten-induced Enteropathy (Celiac Disease)

The "idiopathic celiac disease" is a basic defect of metabolism precipitated by the ingestion of wheat gluten or rye gluten, leading to impaired fat absorption. The exact etiology is not known; the most acceptable theory is that of an inborn error of metabolism with an allergic reaction as a contributing factor; or possibly, an allergic reaction as the sole factor.

Severe manifestations of the disorder have become rare in the United States and in western Europe, but mild disturbances of intestinal absorption of rye, wheat, and sometimes oat gluten, are not uncommon.

Clinical manifestations. Signs generally do not appear before the age of six months, and may be delayed until a year or later. Manifestations include chronic diarrhea with foul, bulky, greasy stools, and progressive malnutrition. There is anorexia, and a fretful, unhappy disposition is typical. The onset is generally insidious, with failure to thrive, bouts of diarrhea and frequent respiratory infections. If the condition becomes severe, the effects of malnutrition are prominent. Retarded growth and development, a distended abdomen and thin, wasted buttocks and legs are characteristic symptoms.

Diagnosis and treatment. At present the only way to determine if a small child's failure to thrive is from this disorder is to place him on a trial gluten-free diet and to evaluate the results. Improvement in the nature of the stools and general well-being, with a gain in weight should follow, although several weeks may elapse before clear-cut manifestations can be confirmed.

Response to a diet from which rye, wheat and oats are excluded is generally good, although probably no cure can be expected; and dietary indiscretions or intercurrent respiratory infections may bring relapses. The omission of wheat products in particular should continue through adolescence, because the ingestion of wheat appears to inhibit growth in sensitive persons.

Dietary program. The young child is usually started on a starch-free, low fat diet. If his condition is severe, this will consist of skim milk, glucose, and banana flakes. Bananas contain invert sugar and are usually well tolerated. Additions to the diet of lean meats, puréed vegetables and fruits are made gradually. Eventually, fats may be added, and the child can be maintained on a regular diet with the exception of all wheat and rye products.

It is not always recognized that commercially canned creamed soups, cold cuts, frankfurters, and pudding mixes, generally contain wheat products. The forbidden list also includes malted milk drinks, some candies, many baby foods and, of course, breads, cakes, pastries and biscuits,

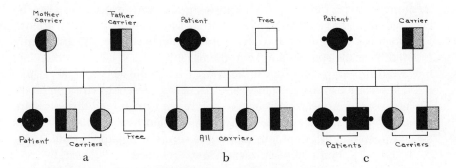

Fig. 90. Autosomal recessive pattern of inheritance.

a. Both parents carriers—ratio of one patient, two carriers, one free from disease.

b. One parent patient—one parent free from disease, all children carriers —no clinical disease.

c. One parent carrier, one parent has disease—ratio of two children with disease, two carriers.

unless the latter are made with corn flour. The list of ingredients on packaged foods should be read before purchasing.

Cystic Fibrosis of the Pancreas (Mucoviscidosis)

Cystic fibrosis is a generalized disease affecting many different organs of the body. The major organs affected are the lungs, the pancreas and the liver, and the sweat, tear and salivary glands. Cystic fibrosis is an hereditary disease, inherited as a recessive trait. When both parents carry a recessive gene for this condition, the expectation is that two out of four children will carry the trait, one will be free of it, and one will have the disease. (Fig. 90) There is, however, no way to predict the sequence, that is to say, it is possible for two or three children with the disease to be born in succession. When cystic fibrosis is present, the tears, the saliva and the sweat contain abnormal amounts of electrolytes, and the submaxillary salivary glands are enlarged in a majority of these children. These manifestations appear to be without significance, but are useful in the establishment of a diagnosis. In hot weather, the loss of sodium chloride and of fluid through the sweat produces frequent heat prostation in these children, so that additional fluid and salt in the diet, or salt tablets, should be given as a precautionary measure.

Pulmonary involvement. The severity of pulmonary involvement differs in individual children, a few showing only relatively minor involvement. The degree of lung involvement determines the prognosis for survival. Present figures show that 50% of affected children die before the age of 10 years, as the result of respiratory complications. Abnormal amounts of thick, viscid mucus clog the bronchioles and provide an ideal medium for bacterial growth. Staphylococcus aureous coagulase can be cultured from the nasopharynx and from the sputum of most patients. Pseudomonas aeruginosa and Hemophilus influenzae are also frequently isolated from the sputum and from the nasopharynx. The basic infection, however, appears most often to be caused by staphylococcus. (Fig. 91)

Complications arising from severe respiratory infection are numerous. Atelectasis may appear early in the disease, and small lung abscesses are common. Bronchiectasis and emphysema develop, with pulmonary fibrosis and pneumonitis, eventually leading to severe ventilatory insufficiency.

In the past, cystic fibrosis was a disease confined to children, because no one with respiratory involvement was known to live past adolescence. At present, with improved knowledge and methods of treatment, an increasing number are living through adolescence and into young adulthood.

Pancreatic involvement. The pancreatic ducts are obstructed by a thick, tenacious mucus, causing the flow of pancreatic enzymes to be diminished or even absent. This achylia or hypochylia leads to intestinal malabsorption and to severe malnutrition. The children with a moderate insufficiency do tend, however, to have a greater reduction in function as they grow older.

Because of the malabsorption of fats, the stools are bulky, greasy, foamy, and have a distinctively foul odor. Other malabsorption defects have this kind of stool however, so that this is not in itself diagnostic of fibrocystic disease. Rectal prolapse is a frequent complication if the pancreatic condition remains untreated.

Meconium ileus. Meconium ileus is the presenting manifestation of fibrocystic disease in approximately 5% to 15% of the newborns who later

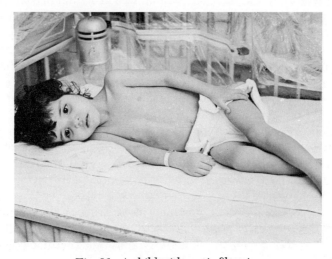

Fig. 91. A child with cystic fibrosis.

develop additional manifestations. Depletion or absence of pancreatic enzymes before birth results in impaired digestive activity, and the meconium becomes viscid and mucilaginous. The inspissated meconium fills the small intestine, causing complete obstruction. Clinical manifestations are bile-stained emesis, a distended abdomen, and an absence of stool. Intestinal perforation with symptoms of shock may occur.

Treatment is surgical resection, employing one of several methods, but the mortality rate is high in spite of skillful surgery. The majority of infants who survive develop cystic fibrosis of varying degrees of severity.

Diagnosis and Diagnostic Tests

Diagnosis is based on family history, evidence of elevated sodium chloride in the sweat, demonstration of hypochylia or achylia, the patient's past history of failure to thrive, and on roentgen findings. A combination of high levels of sweat chloride, malabsorption or pulmonary manifestations, and a suspicious clinical history is considered sufficient evidence for a definitive diagnosis.

Sweat test for elevated levels of sodium and chloride. The sweat of affected children contains high levels of potassium, sodium and chloride. In a majority of affected children, sodium and chloride levels are elevated two to five times above normal, with a lesser degree of potassium elevation. Laboratory determination of sodium and chloride levels in the sweat provides a useful diagnostic test.

The formerly used, thermally-induced sweating method has been largely replaced by the safer and more reliable pilocarpine iontophoresis method. Formerly, a small gauze patch was taped on to the child, out of his reach, usually on his upper back; a plastic sheet or bag was wrapped around his body, and he was covered with a blanket. Sweating was induced by keeping the child thus wrapped in a warm room for a period of three-quarters of an hour to an hour.

These children, however, have a particular sensitivity to heat, and they rapidly lose fluids and electrolytes. Several fatalities from hyperthermia have followed the use of this method on ill children. If this method is to be used, the child must be carefully watched and constantly attended.

The safe, reliable pilocarpine iontophoresis method of inducing sweating utilizes a small electric current that carries topically applied pilocarpine into a localized area of the skin. Because this method is widely used, it is briefly described here.

Pilocarpine iontophoresis method. An area on the child's forearm is washed with distilled water, dried, and is covered with a 2 x 2 inch gauze square that has been saturated with a measured amount of 0.2% pilocarpine nitrate. A positive copper electrode is applied over the gauze, and a negative electrode is placed elsewhere on the same arm, and both are attached with rubber straps of the type used for electrocardiography. Lead wires are connected, and low current is applied for five minutes.

Following iontophoresis, the electrodes are removed, the gauze is discarded, and the area is again washed with distilled water. Dry gauze, which has been weighed in a glass flask, is removed from the flask with forceps, placed over the area that has been iontophoresed, and covered with a plastic square, firmly secured around the edges with adhesive tape. After 30 to 45 minutes, the gauze is removed with forceps, placed in the flask, weighed and analyzed in the laboratory for its sodium and chloride content.

Duodenal aspiration for trypsin activity. An index of pancreatic activity may be ascertained by measuring the tryptic activity in aspirated duodenal fluid.* This is an uncomfortable procedure, quite unpleasant for the small child who must be immobilized, in a fasting state, for several hours. The tube also has a tendency to curl up in the stomach, or to become plugged with thick mucus, necessitating manipulation. Tests are frequently unsatisfactory and must be repeated. This test is important for diagnosis and treatment in a child with a positive sweat test, however. The nurse performing the aspiration should be free from other duties during the period when the tube is down, in order to give emotional support and comfort to the child.

Stool examination. The presence of tryptic activity is ascertained by the ability of a small portion of stool to digest the gelatinous coating of X-ray or photographic film. This test has only a limited value, because false, positive values may be obtained as the result of the bacterial activity.

A more useful study is made by determining the total fat content in the stools collected over a 72-hour period, during which time the child is on a diet containing a minimum of fat. When steatorrhea is present, the fecal loss of fat is greater than 5% of ingested fat. This test may be unreliable in certain circumstances.

Roentgenograms. Generalized obstructive emphysema is highly suggestive when associated with other clinical manifestations. Later in the disease, other pulmonary changes may be noted.

Treatment for Pancreatic Deficiency

The administration of commercially prepared pancreatic enzymes aid digestion and the absorption of both fat and protein. Pancreatic enzymes are given during meals, either in the form of granules, which can be sprinkled on the food, or in capsule form for older children. The pancreatic preparation should be given to all affected children, in a prescribed dosage, even if the pancreatic insufficiency appears minimal.

---

* The duodenal aspiration procedure for collecting duodenal fluid is described in the appendix.

DIAGRAMMATIC REVIEW OF CYSTIC FIBROSIS*

Note: Since 1963, it has been discovered that achylia is not always present, although some degree of pancreatic insufficiency is always found.

The generalized disease *Cystic Fibrosis of the Pancreas*—
unknown basic defect,
genetically transmitted
↓
Exocrine gland dysfunction—
electrolyte abnormality of sweat, saliva, and tears,
chemical and physiochemical abnormality of mucous secretions,
increase in parotid secretory rate
↓
Organ involvement—
lungs, pancreas, liver, eccrine sweat glands and others
↓
Clinical Symptoms—
chronic pulmonary disease,
intestinal malabsorption (from pancreatic achylia),
occasionally, heat casualties (due to massive salt loss through sweat)
Cirrhosis of liver
↓
Diagnosis—
elevated sweat electrolytes—main test,
obstructive emphysema and chronic bronchopneumonia on X-ray of chest,
absent pancreatic enzymes,
family history
↓
Prognosis—
pulmonary involvement dominates clinical picture and determines fate of patient,
chronic lung disease frequently progressive and often leads to
fatal termination in the pediatric age group

Dietary treatment consists of giving a diet high in carbohydrates and protein, with a moderate restriction of fats. These children have large appetites unless they are acutely ill, but they can receive little nourishment from food without a pancreatic supplement. If these children are properly treated with diet and with enzyme supplements, the stools become relatively normal, and their nutrition improves. A restriction of foods such as ice cream, peanut butter, butter, french fries and mayonnaise is advocated, but the child and his parents should not be made to feel that meals must be drab and unenjoyable. Advice similar to this might be given:

"Dick should start gaining weight and feel more peppy now that we have started his medicine. Suppose that one day a week, we let him choose his own meals, let him have anything he wants, and give him extra digestive enzymes. Then during the rest of the week he won't mind so much waiting for his peanut butter and ice cream."

* After P. A. di Sant'Agnese: Ann. N. Y. Acad. Sc., 93:495, 1962.

A positive approach makes the whole regime appear brighter.

Because of the increased loss of sodium chloride, these children are allowed to use as much salt as they wish, even though onlookers may think it is too much. Provision for additional amounts of salt in hot weather may be made by supplying pretzels, salt bread sticks and Saltines in liberal quantities.

Vitamins, in water-miscible preparations, are needed in amounts double a daily dose.

Treatment for respiratory involvement. Treatment for respiratory involvement is much more difficult. Treatment is aimed at providing respiratory drainage by thinning the secretions, and by mechanical means, such as postural drainage and clapping to move the secretions outward. Antibacterial drugs for the treatment of infection are necessary as indicated. Physical activity is beneficial as well, and should be restricted only to the extent of the child's endurance.

Inhalation treatment for thinning secretions. Prophylactic and therapeutic use of aerosol treatments is necessary for all children with cystic fibrosis. Intermittent inhalation by nebulizer of 10% propylene glycol in water or in saline, in addition to a bronchodilator drug, is necessary three or four times daily. The addition of a mucolytic agent, such as Mucomist, is especially useful during periods of acute infection.

The majority of these children profit by continuous aerosol therapy during their naptime and through the night, using a 10% solution of propylene glycol.

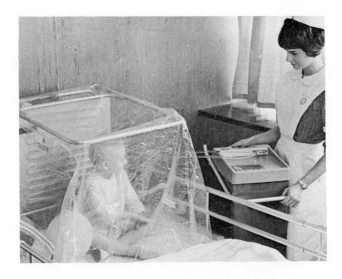

Fig. 92. Naptime for Bobby in his mist tent.

Humidified atmosphere. A mist tent for use during sleep is needed for every affected child. A heavy mist, raising humidity above 50%, is essential. Various types of mist tents are on the market that function through the use of a compressed air pump, but they may also use oxygen if it is necessary. An attachment for a nebulizer is provided. Children become quite accustomed to crawling inside their tents for sleeping, and in times of acute distress, the use of a mist tent becomes a necessary full-time treatment. (Figs. 92 and 93)

Postural drainage. Postural drainage is performed routinely three or four times daily, even if little drainage is apparent. Clapping and vibrating of the affected areas, if done correctly, helps to move the secretions upward and outward. The nurse should become quite proficient at performing this procedure; and also needs to be able to demonstrate it to the parents. Parents should watch and practice it until they, too, become proficient. (Fig. 94)

Additional treatments. Antibiotics for the treatment of respiratory infections are used as indicated. Whether these are given as preventive medicine, or are reserved for the treatment of acute infections, is not uniformly agreed upon at present.

Immunization against childhood communicable diseases is of extreme importance for these chronically ill children. All immunization measures may be used, and should be maintained at the appropriate intervals.

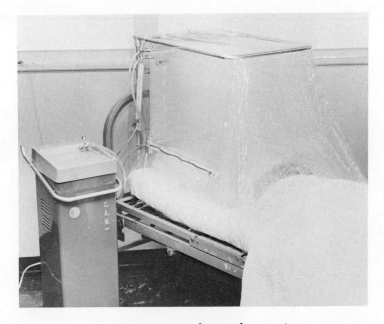

Fig. 93. CAM tent showing heavy mist.

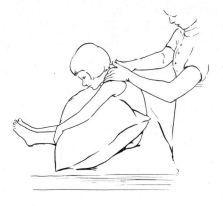 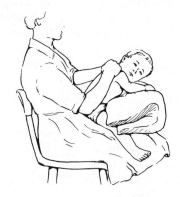

a. Upper lobes—posterior segments.   b. Upper lobes—posterior segments.

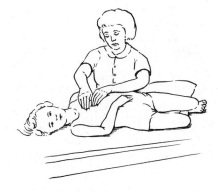 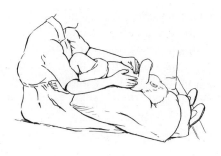

c. Left upper lobe—lingular segment.   d. Left upper lobe—lingular segment.

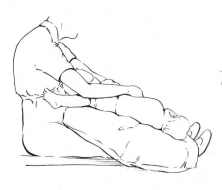 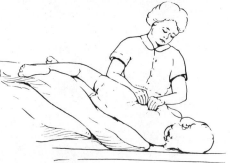

e. Left lower lobe—lateral segments.   f. Left lower lobe—lateral segments.

Fig. 94. Cystic fibrosis—postural drainage.

Home Care

The home care for these children places a tremendous burden upon the concerned families. This is no one-time hospital treatment, nor is there a prospect of cure to brighten the horizon. This, of course, is true of many chronic ailments, but in the daily care of a child with cystic fibrosis, a large amount of time is spent in the performance of treatments. Parents must learn to manipulate the mist tent compressor and the nebulizer, perform postural drainage and clapping techniques. The child's diet must be planned, with the regulation of additional enzymes according to need. Great care is needed to guard against exposure to infections.

In addition to all this, the parents must guard against over-protection and against undue limitation of their child's physical activity. Somehow, a good family relationship must be preserved, with time allowed for attention to other members of the family. This all adds up to a pretty big task.

Physical activity is an important adjunct to the child's well-being, and is a necessary help in getting rid of secretions. The child soon learns his capacity for exercise, and can be trusted to become self-limiting as necessary, especially if he has had an opportunity to learn the nature of his condition. Small children may find postural drainage fun when daddy raises their feet in the air and walks them around "wheel-barrow" fashion.

Hot weather activity should be watched a little more closely, with additional attention directed toward increased salt and fluid intake during periods of exercise.

The financial cost to the family is indeed formidable. It is unrealistic to quote prices, but the cost is high.

Parent groups, organized in most cities, help in morale building, fund raising and educational projects. The Cystic Fibrosis Foundation is presently active in research, with established centers in a number of cities.

EYE CONDITIONS OF INFANCY AND CHILDHOOD

Eye conditions in infancy or childhood that require treatment or surgical intervention are varied. Fortunately, certain conditions no longer appear, or are so rare that the average young nurse may confidently expect never to see them. One such condition is the dread gonococcal ophthalmia neonatorum which once was one of the major causes of blindness in newborn infants. Caused by a gonorrheal infection of the eyes, acquired by the newborn in the birth canal, it is characterized by an acute swelling of the conjunctiva, and a profuse, purulent discharge. Corneal ulcer, perforation and blindness commonly follow if specific antibody treatment is not promptly given. In the United States, all states have compulsory prophylactic treatment for newborn infants; the majority require instillation of 1% silver nitrate solution in the eyes shortly after birth. A few states allow the use of a stable, effective antibiotic such as penicillin ointment. This condition still remains an important cause of blindness in those areas of the world in which preventive measures are not in use.

Another, more recent cause of blindness is the condition of retrolental fibroplasia. It was a major problem in the United States in 1942, and not until several years later was it discovered to be a form of oxygen poisoning. New cases are now rare, but there were still an estimated 8,000 blind or partially sighted young persons in special schools because of this condition in the early 1960's.*

The nurse in the hospital situation today most often sees children who have entered for strabismus correction. Cataracts are prevalent among those who show complications of congenital rubella or galactosemia. Eye injuries bring still other children in, while a condition such as glaucoma is less frequently encountered. The most serious of any—though fortunately rare—is retinoblastoma, a malignant tumor of the retina which extends into the optic nerve with rapid metastasis by way of the bloodstream. Early enucleation, with removal of as much as possible of the optic nerve is necessary, but prognosis is doubtful.

A brief description of the more common conditions requiring treatment or surgery will help the nurse in her understanding of child care.

Eye Conditions Requiring Treatment or Surgery

Congenital Impatency of the Nasolacrimal Duct

Before birth, a thin membrane occludes the nasal end of the nasolacrimal or tear duct. In a majority of instances this membrane disappears just before, or shortly after, birth, but in some infants, the membrane persists. The tears pool in the lacrimal lake region, and spill over the infant's cheek. When the condition persists, some degree of infection occurs in both the eye and the lacrimal sac.

Treatment. Gentle massage of the lacrimal sac, by placing a finger on the nasal portion of the lower lid and massaging downward toward the nose may correct the condition. If surgical treatment is indicated, it is carried out by the insertion of a probe into the nasolacrimal duct, with or without light anesthesia. When infection is present, antibiotics are used prior to surgery. Eye surgeons prefer to probe the duct before the age of six months for best results, because permanent cures are less likely in older children.

---

* Scheie, H.: Disorders of children's eyes: notes on early recognition of disturbances. Clinical Pediatrics, 2:91, 1963.

Cataracts

Congenital cataracts are common complications of congenital rubella. Cataracts may also develop later in infancy or during childhood from an eye injury or from metabolic disturbances such as galactosemia or diabetes. The degree of opacity determines whether surgery should be performed. If the cataract is small and does not significantly impair vision, it is not usually removed. Nystagmus and strabismus which accompany cataracts may threaten visual acuity, and can be considered cause for cataract removal before further impairment of sight. Surgical results are not so successful as are those in the adult patient; 20/20 vision is rarely attained. The child may need to attend sight-saving classes.

Glaucoma

Glaucoma may be of the congenital infantile type, occurring in children under three years of age; juvenile glaucoma, showing clinical manifestations after the age of three; or secondary glaucoma, resulting from injury or disease. Increased intraocular pressure causes the eyeball to enlarge, the cornea to become large, thin, and sometimes cloudy. Untreated, the disease slowly progresses to blindness. Pain may, or may not, be present. Goniopuncture, which provides drainage of the aqueous humor, is effective in relieving intraocular pressure in a large number of cases. Goniotomy may improve the function of the filtration angle if it is defective. If persistent pain in connection with blindness is present, enucleation is indicated.

Strabismus

Strabismus is the failure of the two eyes to direct their gaze at the same object simultaneously. Binocular (normal) vision is maintained through the muscular coordination of eye movements, so that a simple vision results. In strabismus, the visual axes are not parallel, and diplopia (double vision) results. In an effort to avoid seeing two images, the child suppresses vision in the deviant eye, causing a condition of amblyopia ex anopsia (dimness of vision from disuse of the eye).

A wide variation in the manifestation of strabismus exists; there are lateral, vertical, and mixed types. There may be monocular strabismus, in which one eye deviates while the other eye is used, or alternating strabismus, in which deviation alternates from one eye to the other. The term *esotropia* is used when the eye deviates toward the other eye; *exotropia* denotes a turning away from the other eye.

Treatment is dependent on the type of strabismus present. Occlusion of the better eye in monocular strabismus, to force the use of the deviating eye should be carried out early, and should be continued constantly for a period of weeks or months. The child should be stimulated to use the unpatched eye by such occupations as puzzles, drawing, sewing, and similar activities.

Glasses can correct a refractive error if amblyopia is not present. Exercises (orthoptics) to improve the quality of vision may be prescribed to supplement the use of glasses or surgery.

Surgery on the eye muscle to correct the defect is necessary for those children who do not respond to glasses and exercises. Many children need surgery after amblyopia has been corrected. Early detection and treatment of strabismus is essential for a successful outcome.

Eye Injury and Foreign Objects in the Eye

Eye injuries are fairly common, particularly in older children. These are generally painful enough to bring the child to the physician or the clinic promptly. A penetrating wound is potentially serious—BB shots in particular are dangerous, and require the attention of an ophthalmologist. With any history of an injury, a thorough examination of the entire eye is necessary.

Sympathetic ophthalmia may follow perforation wounds of the globe, even if the perforations are small. Sympathetic ophthalmia is an inflammatory reaction of the uninjured eye, showing photophobia, lacrimation, pain and some dimness of vision. The retina may finally become detached, and atrophy of the eyeball may occur. Prompt and skillful treatment at the time of the injury is essential to avoid involvement of the other eye.

Small foreign objects such as specks of dust that have lodged inside the eyelid may be removed by rolling the lid back and exposing the object. Cotton-tipped applicators should not be used for this purpose because of the danger of sudden movement and of possible perforation of the eye. If the object cannot be easily removed with a small piece of moistened cotton or soft clean cloth, the child should be taken to the physician.

Eye Infections

A condition called properly *external hordeolum*, but known commonly as a *sty*, is a purulent infection of the follicle of an eyelash, generally caused by Staphylococcus aureus. Localized swelling, tenderness and pain are present, with a reddened lid edge. The maximum tenderness is over the infected site. The lesion goes on to suppuration, with eventual discharge of the purulent material. Warm saline compresses applied for about 15 minutes three or four times daily give some relief and hasten resolution, but recurrences are common. The sty should never be squeezed. Antibiotic ointment may help prevent accompanying conjunctivitis and recurrences.

Pink eye is an acute bacterial conjunctivitis, most commonly caused by Haemophilus aegyptius (Koch-Weeks bacillus); but may be produced by other bacteria such as pneumococcus, Influenzae bacillus, streptococcus and staphylococcus. It is an infectious condition that may be transmitted through fingers, clothing or other material contaminated with conjunctival secretions. Irritation, vascular congestion, photophobia, and a mucopurulent exudate are clinical manifestations. Children under five years of age are most often affected. Many instances of conjunctivitis are supposed by parents to be "pink eye," but the actual condition is relatively uncommon. Treatment consists of cool compresses and eye irrigations, with local instillation of ophthalmic antibacterial preparations.

Hospital Care for Child with Eye Surgery

A person suffering from any kind of sensory deprivation may experience difficulty in keeping contact with reality. A child who must have his eyes covered is particularly vulnerable. The implications of not being able to see are not always appreciated by nurses who have not themselves experienced this. A young child who wakens from surgery to find himself in total darkness may well go into a state of real panic. If one observes such a child closely as he is returned to the ward, the panic may be quite evident; he trembles, and starts nervously if he is touched or spoken to. In hospitals that still limit visiting hours, eye surgery is seldom considered a condition serious enough to allow a mother to stay continuously. His mother may be at the bedside when he returns from surgery, but who is there beside him when he hears strange voices the next morning—but sees no one?

Preparation for the event, should, of course, be carried out as well as it is possible to do so, but the small child has no background experience to help him understand what actually is going to happen. The darkness, the pain and the discomfort, and the total strangeness of the situation, can be overwhelming.

Restraints should not be used indiscriminately, but the majority of small children do need some reminder to keep their hands away from the sore eye, unless someone is beside them to prevent them from rubbing or from removing eye dressings. Elbow restraints are useful, although they do not prevent rubbing the eye with the arm. Flannel strips applied to the wrists in clove-hitch fashion can be tied to the cribsides in such a manner as to allow freedom of arm movement, but to prevent the child from reaching his face.

Special care should be taken by the nurse to speak to the child before touching him, and thus to make him aware of her presence. The child does need tactual stimulation though, so after speaking and identifying herself, the nurse would do well to stroke or to pat him, to pick him up, if this is allowed, or in some other way let him feel her presence.

If a nurse expects to have the care of a blind person, or one who must have sight covered, it becomes important that she find out from first-hand experience what the loss of sight means. She should cover her eyes for a period and learn the difficulties involved in finding her way about, or in ordinary self-care.

The reasoning for, and application of principles outlined in the nursing care study presented here show quite clearly the manner in which the experience can be handled to minimize the trauma so frequently associated with strangeness and loss of sensory perception.

A THREE-YEAR-OLD HAS EYE SURGERY

This résumé of a nursing care study carried out by a nursing student during her clinical experience in child care, is included here for three reasons. First, it illustrates the kind of experience that many students find to be of value in furthering their understanding of children; it shows, through the eyes of the child and of his nurse, the responses to hospitalization that are evoked in a small child; and finally, it attempts to illustrate the ways in which the traumatic effect of sensory deprivation, (in this case, a temporary loss of sight because of eye dressings) may be minimized. The study has been put into a compressed form, with names and details slightly changed.

This was a nursing care study concerning a child's response to hospitalization and surgery for the correction of exotropia of the right eye. The purposes of the study were outlined:

1. to observe the effects of hospitalization on the child,
2. to attempt to make the experience a maturing one for the child.

The reasons for choosing a patient having eye surgery took into consideration the fact that deprivation of sight, even though temporary, is frightening to a young child who cannot understand its temporary nature. The strangeness of the hospital environment may further intensify this fear, and lead to a feeling of abandonment. Therefore, this kind of patient should profit from pre-hospital preparation and from intensive care during the hospital experience.

The manner in which the patient was chosen. The nurse, Gail, spent a morning in the pediatric eye clinic observing eye examinations. Upon discovering that appointments for elective surgery were made three or more months in advance, it appeared unrealistic to choose her patient from among those in the clinic at that time. Therefore, with the assistance of the clinic personnel, she chose a three-year-old boy, Gary D., from the list of eye surgery cases scheduled for the following two weeks.

The preliminary planning. Gail called Mrs. D., Gary's mother, by telephone, and explained the purpose of her proposed study. Mrs. D. appeared interested and pleased; together, they made an appointment for Gail to visit Gary at home. Mrs. D. had told her son about the hospitalization, but welcomed the opportunity for Gary and herself to become acquainted with his future nurse.

She also had several worries about the forthcoming experience that she wished to discuss.

Following the telephone call, Gail spent several hours in the library, reviewing the norms of growth and development for a three-year-old, and read articles about the effects of hospitalization on a young child. She also familiarized herself with the condition of exotropia and its surgical correction.

Gail wished to discuss her participation in the home visit with someone qualified to make meaningful suggestions. For this, she chose the mental health instructor.

Further preparation included a visit to both surgery and the recovery room to familiarize herself with the physical setup, in order to feel at ease in her support of the patient. She also observed anesthesia induction in a young patient. Gail had no previous surgery experience, and she felt that this was very important.

The home visit. In preparation for the visit, Gail had made drawings that she thought would be of interest to a small boy about to enter the hospital. They included a boy on his way to the hospital, riding to the ward in an elevator and being admitted, and also pictures of a nurse and of a doctor. She believed that explanations to a three-year-old should be limited to a consideration of immediate events; therefore, she did not, at that time, depict hospital experience beyond admission.

Keeping all of this in mind, she made plans for the home visit as close to admission date as possible; this was to be two days before admission. Realizing that a small boy would be shy, Gail spent the first several minutes chatting with the family—his brothers and his sisters and his mother; then she invited Gary to look at her pictures. Gary, who preferred to be called Buddy, quickly overcame his shyness and chatted freely about his tricycle, a television program that he had been watching, and his red fire truck. He told Gail that he was "going to the hospital to get my eyes checked," and looked at her pictures with mild interest.

Gail had brought her nurse's cap, which she now showed him, and told him she would be his nurse. Then she put the cap on her head and wore it throughout her visit. She also showed him a patient gown and slippers similar to those he would wear. Gail had taken a blindfold along, intending to play "blindfold" with him, making a game of trying to identify objects and voices. She now decided, however, that this could be played more naturally with his family, and after explaining her purpose to Mrs. D., it was agreed that the entire family would play the game with him during the next two days.

Hospital admission. Gail met Buddy and his mother at the admission desk, and took them in the elevator to the pediatric department. Buddy was at ease with her, and was able to identify the surroundings from the pictures he had been shown. She showed him around the ward, making a point of taking him to the toilet room, because his mother had felt he would be too shy to ask, and might regress to wetting himself.

Buddy was called to the eye clinic, so his mother and Gail took him in a wheel chair, which he greatly enjoyed. Upon their return, Gail put on a surgical gown, a cap and a mask to show him how she would look tomorrow in surgery and in the recovery room. She told him she would go with him "to get his eye fixed," but he would be asleep when it happened. She worried over the "sleep" concept, not wanting to make him afraid of sleep, but she could not think of any way to avoid it. Buddy played with his toys, and accepted all of this quite casually—perhaps because of the casual way in which it was presented. Surgery was scheduled for the early morning, otherwise she might have chosen to wait until morning for this part of the preparation. After being tucked in, however, he slept through the night without waking.

Operative day. On the morning of surgery, Buddy was happy and full of energy, playing peek-a-boo with Gail and apparently enjoying the novelty of his surroundings. Just before the time for his preoperative sedation, she told him about it, saying it would hurt a little. He was cooperative and did not appear frightened. He did cry, however, and Gail picked him up, holding him for a little while.

In the surgery department Gail left him to change into surgery garb. She found him asleep, and unconscious of her return. She knew, however, that some children do not respond to sedation this quickly—in which case her precaution of showing Buddy how she would look in operating room garb could be helpful.

Anesthesia induction was by endotracheal tube, and Buddy relaxed smoothly. Surgery consisted of a shortening of the medial rectus muscle and a lengthening of the lateral rectus muscle of the right eye; an intricate process which took two hours. Both eyes were covered, and Buddy was taken to the recovery room.

When Buddy wakened from anesthesia, Gail recorded that he was "very irritable, nauseated, and sleepy." He was returned to his room where his mother waited, anxious to know his condition and the results of the surgical procedure. The eye surgeon described the surgery in some detail, and Gail was able to report Buddy's good condition.

An injection for the relief of his nausea made Buddy very angry, but he soon relaxed and slept most of the remainder of the day, secure in the presence of his parents and his friend, the nurse. He again slept through the night.

First postoperative day. When Buddy wakened, Gail was at his bedside and, putting her hand on his arm, said "Buddy, this is Gail." He smiled and stretched out his arms to her, and she "gave him a big hug, and told him I loved him." She felt that her preparation had been helpful and furnished a link between a frightening experience and the outside world.

Buddy was eager for breakfast, drinking his milk so fast "his tummy didn't like it." This disturbed him, but after Gail explained that his stomach was empty and that food would make it feel better, he ate all his breakfast, accepting the necessity of having to be fed, although Gail thought he did not like it. Gail told him the doctors were coming to remove the dressing from the unaffected eye, only minutes before they came. They removed both dressings, checked the operated eye, and replaced that dressing. He accepted the procedure well, but his eye was sore and he cried for a while after they left.

Gail had prepared a box of toys of a variety of shapes, sizes and textures for sensory satisfaction, for him to manipulate while his eyes were still covered. Buddy had not wakened sufficiently for this, but Gail now produced it, and he enjoyed playing with the toys, stringing the large beads to show her how well he could do. She stayed with him throughout the day, reading to him, giving him necessary physical care, and playing with him. His parents were with him during the evening and tucked him in for the night. Again, he slept well.

Second postoperative day. Gail had told Buddy she would not be with him until the evening. When she came, he jumped down from his mother's lap, showed Gail his toys and strung some beads for her. His mother said that he had sat on her lap since she had come, cried because Gail had not come, and had wet his bed during afternoon nap (a most rare occurrence for him). Gail felt that he had interpreted her absence as rejection, although she had tried to prepare him. She stayed with him through the evening, and put him to bed for the night, staying until he went to sleep.

Day of discharge. Buddy was discharged shortly after breakfast on the third morning. Before leaving, he and Gail made arrangements to visit at his home about 10 days later. Gail wished to discover if there was any noticeable change in his behavior, how he would react to her, and what parts of his experience he remembered, as well as how he interpreted the experience.

Second home visit. Buddy was playing outside when Gail arrived. He ran to the car, greeted her, and immediately started telling her about what he was doing. Buddy's mother and his older sisters thought that he was much more active than he had been before his hospital experience. They thought he was more forceful, and played more roughly with his younger sister. Gail wondered if this might be interpreted as a release of emotions built up during his hospital experience.

Gail found that Buddy's parents were greatly pleased with the interest she had shown, and with the results of their son's surgery. He had not talked much about the hospital experience, but frequently referred to "my nurse." He appeared to remember very little about his discomfort or the nausea following surgery.

Buddy sat on Gail's lap during her visit, gave her a present, and asked her to come again. A few weeks later, she visited him in the eye clinic, finding him friendly and cheerful, happy over her visit, but casual in his manner, showing his ability to put the entire experience into proper perspective.

The meaning of the experience to the nurse. This can best be expressed in Gail's own remarks.

"With a three-year-old, it is a very difficult task to explain an operation as a health-giving device. Instead of explaining the operation to Buddy, I told him the strange and new things he would see. I feel this worked out satisfactorily. He didn't have any severe emotional reactions to the operation, and he established a new relationship outside of his family group.

The most important result for me is the truly satisfying relationship that has been established between Buddy and myself. It is something I have never had with a young child before. I feel a relationship like this can help children through a traumatic experience. They must have this constant feeling of security and love, because everything is strange and frightening to them."[*]

BIBLIOGRAPHY

Barbero, G. and Sibinga, M.: Enlargement of the submaxillary glands in cystic fibrosis. Pediatrics, 29:788, 1962.

Bellam, G.: Tonsillectomy without fear. Amer. J. Nurs., 51:244, (Apr.) 1951.

di Sant'Agnese, P. A.: Diagrammatic review of cystic fibrosis. Ann. N. Y. Acad. Sci., 93:495, 1962.

Doershuk, C. F., *et al.*: A five year clinical evaluation of a therapeutic program for patients with cystic fibrosis. J. Pediat., 65:677, 1964.

Fishbein, M. (ed.): Birth Defects. p. 242. Philadelphia, J. B. Lippincott, 1963.

Gellis, S. S., and Kagen, B. M., (eds.): Current Pediatric Therapy. P. 90. Philadelphia, W. B. Saunders, 1964.

————: Current Pediatric Therapy. Philadelphia, W. B. Saunders, 1964.

[*] Original nursing care study carried out by Gail Womack, junior nursing student at the University of Oregon School of Nursing.

Matthews, L., *et al.:* A therapeutic regimen for patients with cystic fibrosis. J. Pediat., *65:*558, 1964.

Nelson, W., (ed.): Textbook of Pediatrics. 8th ed. Philadelphia, W. B. Saunders, 1964.

Scheie, H.: Disorders of children's eyes: notes on early recognition of disturbances. Clin. Pediat., *2:*91, 1963.

Schwachman, H.: Therapy of cystic fibrosis of the pancreas. Pediatrics, *25:* 155, 1960.

Silver, H., Kempe, C. H., and Bruyn, H. B.: Handbook of Pediatrics. 6th ed. Los Altos, Cal., Lange, Medical Publications, 1965.

SUGGESTED READINGS FOR FURTHER STUDY

Andersen, D.: Cystic fibrosis and family stress. Children, 7:9, 1960.

Kurihara, M.: Postural drainage, clapping and vibrating. Amer. J. Nurs., *65:* 76, (Nov.) 1965.

Mahaffy, P.: The effects of hospitalization on children admitted for T and A. Nurs. Research, *14:*12, 1965.

Milio, N.: Family centered care for cystic fibrosis. Nurs. Outlook, *11:*718, (Oct.) 1963.

Roche, A. F.: The influence of tonsillectomy on growth and caloric intake. J. Pediat., *65:*360, 1964.

Schwachman, H., *et al.:* Studies in cystic fibrosis: a report on sixty-five patients over 17 years of age. Pediatrics, *36:*689, 1965.

White, H., and Rowley, W.: Cystic fibrosis of the pancreas. Pediat. Clin. N. Amer., *11:*139, 1964.

Whyte, B. B.: After tonsillectomy. Nurs. Times, *58:*1280, 1962.

UNIT 5

THE PRESCHOOL CHILD

15

Normal Growth and Development

There is no firm demarcation line between the toddler and the pre-schooler. He does not change markedly between the ages of 3 and 3½. There is, however, a marked difference between the ages 2 and 4. Although growth and development proceeds in a continuum from birth to adolescence, the course is nevertheless marked by plateaus and spurts of growth.

The first year of life is marked by the child's rapid physical growth. During the second year, his growth slows down a little while he perfects his muscular control and learns his identity.

By the age of 3, the average healthy child has become a fairly independent person. His weight gain continues to be slower than that of the first year, but his gain in height is somewhat faster, so that he changes from a chubby toddler to a thinner child. During this period of his life, he probably averages a gain of five pounds a year.

Physically, he is losing his baby look and is maturing into the kind of person he is going to be in later life. His incessant activity keeps him too busy to show much interest in food. His mother has no need to worry about this if he is gaining slowly, is healthy and manages somehow to get his required nutrients. His appetite will pick up as he nears school age.

The child of three has developed motor control with increasing skill in finer movements. He is less often frustrated in his efforts to control his environment, and this adds to his self-confidence.

If the child has a consistently warm, accepting relationship with his mother, he can now begin to move away from her into a larger world. No longer do objects cease to be if they are out of his sight. Now he can go away from his mother, secure in the comfortable knowledge that she will be waiting for him when he returns. At three, he should be quite secure, absorbing his world and making it a part of himself. He is friendly and cheerful, and is learning to play with others.

One evidence of his increased maturity is his ability to attend nursery school. The two-year-old was too close to his mother to stand the separation, but a three-year-old lives in a larger world. He is not yet ready for an abrupt and prolonged parting. At first, his mother needs to go along with him and stay for a time until the surroundings have acquired a familiar, homey atmosphere. He is not yet mature enough to stay away overnight. The dark is frightening and filled with mysterious sounds and objects. He needs his old and trusted friends and belongings, each in its proper place.

All three-year-olds are not necessarily ready for nursery school or for separation from their mothers. Each child has his own rate of maturation and growth, which may be slower or faster than that of the average.

Three and four are interested in everything, and spend their days exploring and learning. In fact, the day is not long enough for them; they would prefer not to go to bed. Their endless calls for drinks, their numerous trips to the bathroom, the slipping downstairs to the living room to tell mother something "very important" are all evidence of their reluctance to leave the scene of living. They just might miss something!

The three- or four-year-old's appetite for living exceeds his capacity. He refuses to admit that he is tired and resists taking a nap. He frequently needs the firmness of an older person who knows that he has reached the limit of his endurance. The adult knows that he has long since reached his.

Our three-year-old, because of his increasing ability to understand is eager to learn. His eagerness ushers him into a more turbulent phase of life as he nears the age of four. At three or four, he is likely to be one big question mark. His curiosity grows as it is fed, until one thinks that he is never quiet. He has the ability to construct sentences and to formulate ideas. Because he has achieved the power to vocalize, he must use this power to the limit. Not only that, but the sound of his own voice is pleasant to him. His muscles, his intellect, and his voice must all be constantly active.

His world continues to expand during kindergarten until at last, the day arrives when he can enter what to him is the truly grown-up world of the schoolboy.

AVERAGE DEVELOPMENTAL LEVEL OF THE PRESCHOOL CHILD

Three to Four Years

The three-year-old has matured in a number of ways, although he has a nearly complete ignorance of the world outside his home. Evidence of his maturing skills and perception include the following.

> can go upstairs alone, alternating his feet,
> can run smoothly, jump with both feet together,
> is able to pedal a tricycle,
> likes to feed himself and to pour from a pitcher—seldom spills,
> is able to string large beads, work a very simple puzzle,
> builds a tower of 9 or 10 blocks,

can copy a circle, and fit circle, square and triangle into a form board, even if their positions are reversed.

The three-year-old is developing a color sense, and loves to paint or crayon with bright colors. His perception has advanced so that now he sees you as a person, and he has developed a desire to please and to conform—usually.

He likes people, and is able to wait his turn and to share toys if he is not taxed too severely, but he still likes parallel play. He can be reasoned with, within the limits of his understanding.

At three, he is in love with words, trying out sounds for their melody or humor, and indulging in chants and soliloquies.

The three-year-old is beginning to sleep through the night without wetting, and can begin to attend to his own toilet needs. He still needs a long afternoon nap of an hour or two.

His sense of belonging to the family group is evidenced by his

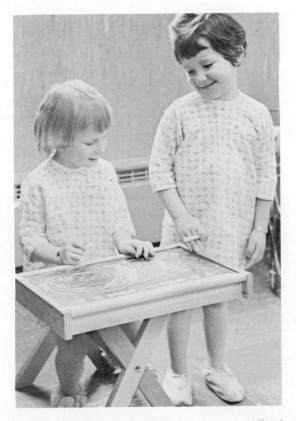

Fig. 95. Four is a wonderful age, especially if there is a congenial playmate.

pleasure in doing small errands around the house, in putting silverware on the table, or perhaps in carefully drying a dish. He is indeed becoming a person.

Four to Five Years

Four-year-old has increased self-confidence. He can tell you his age, he can adapt more easily to change of routine, and has powers of generalization and abstraction. (Fig. 95)

His powers of imagination are high; so high that he cannot make a clear distinction between reality and fiction. When his father tells a remarkable story about events of the day, four-year-old will tell sociably about his adventures, which though fantastic, seem no more so to him than his father's story. He is in no way consciously "lying," and should not be told that he is. His mother may be able to help him by casually remarking "That is a good pretend story," if she is able to do so without implying criticism or rejection.

Physical and motor maturation are shown in these areas. He can walk upstairs without grasping a handrail, he can walk backward, he is able to cut out pictures, to copy a square and make a better circle than he could at three, he can dress himself, and can manage large buttons, and he may no longer take an afternoon nap, although many still do.

Intellectually, his questioning is at a peak—largely to validate his own understanding rather than to gain new information—but it seems that he never stops. At this age, he may have an imaginary companion to whom he talks and appears to treat as a real person.

Five-Year-Old

At five, a child is about ready to join the larger world outside his family. He enjoys kindergarten and may even appreciate the short, daytime separation from home. His abilities include:

jumping rope, skipping, good motor control,
can brush his teeth and wash his face,
knows primary colors, can count to ten, can copy a triangle,
has a sense of order, likes to finish what he has started—can carry a project over from one day to the next, and his questions are now more meaningful.

The five-year-old tends to be obedient and reliable, is protective of younger children, and tries to comfort the unhappy ones. He now prefers group play and co-operates in projects. Playing house, dressing up, and playing at various adult roles is his specialty. He is beginning to develop an elementary conscience which has some influence in governing his actions.

THE PRESCHOOL CHILD IN THE HOSPITAL

The small child may enter the hospital well prepared for the experience. Perhaps he has a need for some corrective surgery that has been postponed until he has grown some more and until his capacity for understanding was greater. Now he needs this surgery, either to make him look like others, or to improve his health, or to avoid unnecessary absences from school later.

Although these children have had ample time for adequate preparation for the hospital experience, many others do not have this opportunity. The toddler and the preschooler are frequently victims of their own curiosity. Most cases of poisoning occur in children under the age of five years. Accidents also bring many children into the hospital, including that most dreaded of all accidents, severe burns.

When the preschool child moves out into the larger world and enters into neighborhood activities, he encounters several risks to his health and well-being. His lack of experience leads him to take risks that frequently cause painful accidents. He is exposed to the common childhood diseases, and is quite susceptible to infections. One of these experiences may bring him to the hospital.

The child who enters the hospital in a routine manner has had advantages that the child who comes in on an emergency basis cannot have. There has been ample opportunity to prepare the non-emergency child for this experience. Many pediatricians carefully explain hospitalization to the child, but the responsibility for adequate preparation rests with his parents.

Parents, however, are not always too well informed about hospital procedures. Rumors and tales are spread around about misunderstood hospital experiences, causing anxiety among those whose task it is to reassure the child. A mother is poorly equipped to handle a situation about which she herself has serious misgivings. Her words may *sound* confident, but the child senses the uncertainty behind them. Such a situation occurred when four-year-old James was being prepared for tonsillectomy. He had been cheerful and pleasant since admission, but when the nurse prepared to give him his preoperative medication he went into panic. No one, including his mother, could calm him. He was a husky boy, and he put up a truly remarkable resistance. He fought and kicked. His mother repeatedly remarked that she could not understand it, because she had told him exactly what was going to happen, and he had seemed to accept it well.

After a thoroughly frightened, exhausted little boy had gone to surgery, his mother showed her own anxiety in the following words: "I have been dreading this. Are you sure he's going to be all right? A little boy in our neighborhood just died from an operation like this, and I have been worried."

One can only imagine what bits of gossip and half-understood talk the child had heard. Unfortunately, no one on the staff knew or understood the cause of his fear. James returned in good condition and was later discharged, but the emotional trauma must have been considerable.

Could a more perceptive nurse have avoided this episode? It is difficult to say. Small children do not readily voice their fears and imaginings. It would seem worthwhile to assume that every child has at least some misgivings about the forthcoming experience. Direct questioning profits little, but the nurse might borrow from play therapy techniques and let the child play out his feelings.

The Nurse's Role in Preparing the Child for a Hospital Experience

Such a technique could be carried out using hand puppets. If a group of children are admitted at the same time for surgery, they might have a short period together with the nurse; even an individual child could profit from this puppet play.

The nurse can have a doctor or nurse puppet on her hand, while the child wears a boy or girl puppet. A dialogue can be worked out so that the child is able to tell what he knows and voice any concern that he may have. The nurse can reinforce any teaching that the child has received, straighten out misunderstandings and generally put the child more at ease. It is much easier to put ideas into the mouth of a puppet than to voice them as your own, and the puppet can ask questions that the child may shrink from asking as his own.

One precaution must be kept in mind. Too much preparation, with too much lingering over details, may frighten the child rather than reassure him. Letting the child participate in role-playing is a manner of providing him with an opportunity to bring out his own apprehensions, and to straighten things out in his own mind.

One group of students devised a plan that worked very well. They made a two-room hospital from a carton, papered it with shelf paper and furnished a ward and an operating room, using cardboard, pipe cleaners, paper cups, small containers, pictures, and plenty of imagination. Small dolls represented Johnny, his mother, the nurse and the doctor, with one or two patients for atmosphere. A nursing student acted out a trip to the hospital, making the doll-patient go through an admission and an entire stay. The entire play lasted about 20 minutes, and attention never wavered. In fact, there were always calls of "do it again."

Another group of nursing students asked the hospital carpenter to build a doll's house. They then had a student party at which they papered, painted, hung curtains, knitted rugs, and furnished the entire house. It was kept on the ward for any child to play with, and proved a big attraction to children waiting for surgery. The project would have been even more valuable if some of the older children had been allowed to help decorate the house, and to make some of the doll clothes.

As has been said before, one needs imagination when caring for children. Expert physical care is not enough.

Relieving the Child's Anxiety

George was a child with an obsessive fear of needles. His one anxiety from admission onward concerned the injections he might receive. He did indeed receive an injection of vitamin K shortly after admission, and the nurse was unable to promise that he would not receive another in the morning.

At bedtime, George was missing. A thorough search did not reveal any George, and eventually the alarmed nurses were considering calling his mother, when someone noticed a slight shadow behind the ward door. George had been crouching there for nearly an hour, not making a sound, and quaking with fear.

In the morning, George asked incessantly, "I don't have to have a needle, do I?" As surgery was to be quite late, George was brought out to the nurse's station and was encouraged to draw pictures. One picture after another was rapidly drawn and pinned up on the bulletin board as a prized picture. Each time he asked the question "Do I have to have a needle?" the answer was a firm "Yes, George, you will have to have a needle before you go to surgery." Eventually, George accepted this fact enough to change his question to, "I will only have to have one, won't I?" When the time came to get ready for surgery, he went willingly enough, and although he could not find enough courage to hold still, he accepted the intramuscular medication without protest.

It is not necessarily the openly terrified child, however, who is afraid. The child who is good, who makes no protest, is frequently as terrified, but is able to suppress his fears. This child may be facing a greater psychological emergency than the one who overtly (and loudly) expresses his distress.

Helping the Child Develop Sense of Trust

The nurse who has learned to respect the child as a person, and who has developed the ability to sense his needs, and who can meet those needs with kindness and firmness does much to develop a sense of trust in the child. Such experiences help the child grow to maturity rather than hinder his progress.

In practical terms, what does respecting the child mean? It does not mean that Johnny must run when I say run, or must eat when I say eat. It does not mean imposing your will on the child. Some young nurses, and perhaps older ones too, find it difficult to listen to a child. The nurse says, "I was brought up to obey without question, and I expect these children to do the same." Why does she expect this? Could it be because she would like to make someone else feel small and insignificant the way she was once made to feel?

Certainly the adult has, or should have, more mature judgment than the child has. There are many things in the hospital that have to be done in a certain way and at certain times, and it is not always possible to make thorough explanations to the child. Many of these things are unpleasant or uncomfortable. Johnny must take his medicine, and the nurse must know if Johnny is testing her to find out how far he can go with his delaying tactics. Johnny will not respect her if she allows him to delay indefinitely, but he will sense her weakness. Johnny needs a strong person from whom he can draw strength for meeting unpleasant situations.

However, if you respect Johnny as a person, you listen to him and treat him with the respect you would give any person. Do you *have* to interrupt his lunch to give him that medication? Could a little thought on your part have made the interruption unnecessary? Billy likes apple juice but not grape juice; he likes ready-cooked cereal but not hot cereal. What excuse do you have for not allowing him to have the food he likes?

Billy is marching around the ward doing nothing but singing to himself. You say, "Billy come *now* and brush your teeth, or have your bath, or take your nap." Would you like to be told that "You must do as I say, *now?*" Or would you be more inclined to respond graciously if you were told "Lunch will be ready in five minutes," or "It will be nap time in ten minutes," or even "Which of you two would like to have your bath first?"

It is true that some children have been treated in such an inconsistent manner at home that they do not know where the limits are, or even whether there are limits. Even the well brought up child rebels occasionally. When the five or ten minutes are up, and Billy shows no signs of conforming, then firmness must be shown. Billy may not like it, but he learns that you are fair and that you keep your word.

Some of these children are admitted for diagnostic purposes. The convulsive child may come in for electroencephalograms, blood tests, and perhaps for more strenuous neurological tests. The child who has failed to grow properly may be tested for fibrocystic disease, or celiac disease. Perhaps the child has been admitted because of an exacerbation of a long-term illness.

These children may have been prepared for admission, but still find it very difficult to adjust to the necessary tests and procedures. Little can be done by way of explanation before admission. The nurse must play a supportive role during the unpleasant times.

Two little sisters were admitted for tests to determine the presence of fibrocystic disease. The six-year-old was permitted to stay in the same ward with her three-year-old sister to help her adjust. Both girls were subjected to the extremely uncomfortable duodenal drainage test for the presence of trypsin. At mid-morning they lay in their beds "draining," while between the two beds, their nurse sat quietly reading to them, turning the book from time to time to show them the pictures.

This nurse showed her understanding of what nursing really means. The ward had not been tidied up, and the girls had not been bathed, but the nurse had been able to communicate her understanding and sympathy. Anyone coming into the ward could feel the confidence and trust they had in their nurse. She rightly understood that the other tasks were secondary to the main problem of providing support and understanding in time of stress.

Additional, much needed support is provided if the familiar nurse accompanies her patient when he has to leave the department for various diagnostic procedures or treatment. Any patient appreciates the presence of a familiar person when he encounters new and potentially frightening situations, but for the young person who cannot understand what is happening, a familiar person to comfort and—he reasons—to protect him, becomes an essential part of his nursing care. This kind of support is not always given the serious consideration it deserves, but it holds importance equal to any other essential procedure. Of course, in the ideal situation, the familiar person is mother—and why shouldn't she be? When free visiting hours are a reality, this usually can be accomplished.

In *The Widening World of Childhood,* the implications of injury and hospitalization to the small child are brought out with keen insight.* Three-year-old Sam, having lost the tip of his little finger in a slammed door, is helped through the subsequent hospital and surgical experience with the understanding support of his mother, his doctors and his nurses. Sam's reaction to separation from his mother during surgery and at the surgeon's office, his use of "Woody," an imaginary elf to take his mother's place, as well as the positive aspects of the experience, are brought out in a manner that provides guidance for the nurse which is probably unequaled elsewhere.

What about the child who comes into the hospital on an emergency basis? Jimmy found a peanut can in a cupboard under the sink. He hardly had time to sample the contents before his mother came and immediately began to act very strangely. He knew that he was not allowed to eat peanuts, but his mother acted as though he had committed some crime. She snatched the can away from him, spanked him, then grabbed him up and called the doctor. In no time at all, he was being sped to the hospital where more strange and terrifying things happened to him. His stomach was thoroughly washed out, a most uncomfortable procedure. He struggled manfully against this indignity, but many big hands held him firmly and his mother never did a thing to interfere. She must have been really angry.

The next thing he knew, he was undressed, taken on a sort of rolling bed up in the elevator and put to bed in broad daylight. People in white gowns and caps came with further indignities, needles to jab into him, unpleasant medications, jackets tied on to him to keep him in bed, strange

---

* Murphy, L. B.: The Widening World of Childhood. Chap. 6, pp. 115–144. New York, Basic Books, 1962.

food on trays, thermometers, stethoscopes, doctors who punched and probed. When would this nightmare end and when could he find out that it was all a bad dream?

Not right away, because Jimmy had to stay in the hospital for days and days, each day followed by a scary night away from home. For the "peanuts" Jimmy had eaten were mole pellets that contained arsenic. Fortunately, treatment was prompt and thorough, and he went home still wondering why such a little act should have brought about so much punishment.

The independence of the young child, coupled with his lack of experience, leads him into many dangers. He does not understand what these dangers are, and instead, quite innocently eats or drinks a substance not meant for human consumption. Soon he feels ill, and perhaps he becomes extremely ill. If he has swallowed lye or a strong acid, his mouth and throat are burned. He finds little support in his mother who is far more frightened than he. He is rushed to the hospital and treated in a way that does nothing to strengthen his sense of security.

Dealing With the Sense of Guilt

If this child is three, or four, or five, he has other problems. Quite likely, he has been told not to touch, or not to go into the street, or some other prohibition has been made. Being at the stage of development where the forbidden is glamorous, he did touch, or eat, or run into danger. So now, he has strong guilt feelings to add to his misery. Anything that you, as a nurse, may have to do to him undoubtedly is understood as punishment.

We hear of parents who threaten their children with the policeman or the doctor in order to get them to obey. That this is true is evidenced by the words one hears during visiting hours. "If you don't leave that alone, I will tell the nurse and she will tie your hands down," or "Drink that or the nurse will come and give you a needle," and so on. The reaction of the parents can be better understood if one can feel their anxiety; procedures are frightening to parents too. All too often, no one has bothered to explain them. Picture how an oxygen tent or gastric suction must appear to someone who has never seen them before.

Then also, the mother may feel as guilt-laden as the child. She knows that many, perhaps most, accidents could be avoided. Over and over again she thinks, "If I had only done so-and-so, this wouldn't have happened." Perhaps the father, distraught, and not entirely free from guilt himself, adds to her distress. All too often, the parents catch snatches of conversation on the ward in which they hear themselves condemned for their carelessness. One would suppose that the burden of guilt that a parent has to carry, perhaps throughout life, would be great enough without adding to it.

Neither are nurses always guiltless in this respect. One group of students who overheard the doctors discuss the possibility of an insecticide spray as a causative factor in a blood dyscrasia, accepted this as a proven fact, and discussed it so freely that the parents heard the discussion. Another group severely criticized a mother for neglect of her infant because of a doctor's free, but indiscreet, diagnosis. In both cases, the assumptions were false, but the damage was done. We are apt to forget to put ourselves in another person's place.

Accepting Regression

The child who has been admitted because of an emergency, or the child who has come in without preparation for the experience, is almost certain to regress to a more infantile level. He seeks comfort and reassurance from those things that memory tells him have brought him satisfaction in the past. He may regress to thumb sucking or bed wetting. He may pick his nose, or rock himself. None of this behavior needs any comment from the nurse. She can, however, do much for him by providing him with some of the comfort he is seeking. It is sad to see little children sitting alone and idle in their cribs hour after hour, and a good nurse does not allow this to happen.

When nap time comes, many small children find it quite difficult to quiet down and to relax, yet this is extremely necessary for them. Of course, each child takes his cuddly toy or his security blanket with him, while other toys are removed from the crib. It is an excellent plan for the nurse to sit quietly in the ward for a few minutes after the children are all tucked in. Perhaps she may tell a short bedtime story, or sing a quiet song. If she wishes, she may play a lullaby on the record player. She will find that the few minutes so spent pay dividends not only in quiet, relaxed children, but in her own peace of mind. She will find that the trips she needs to make to the ward to quiet restless children are drastically reduced, and the calls are less frequent. Also she finds happier, better rested children at the end of the rest period.

The preschool department is a delightful place for the nurse to work. Children are inclined to make the best of a bad situation, and ignore much physical discomfort if they become absorbed in play.

BIBLIOGRAPHY

Breckenridge, M. E., and Murphy, M. N.: Growth and Development of the Young Child. 7th ed. Philadelphia, W. B. Saunders, 1963.

Gesell, A., *et al:* The First Five Years of Life. New York, Harper & Brothers, 1940.

Murphy, L.: The Widening World of Childhood. New York, Basic Books, 1962.

Plank, E.: Working With Children in Hospitals. Cleveland, Western Reserve University Press, 1962.

Strang, R.: An Introduction to Child Study. 4th ed. New York, Macmillan, 1959.

United States Department of Health, Education and Welfare: Your Child from One to Six. Washington, U. S. Government Printing Office, 1964.

Watson, E. H., and Lowrey, G. H.: Growth and Development of Children. 4th ed. Chicago, Year Book Publishers, 1962.

SUGGESTED READINGS FOR FURTHER STUDY

Dombro, R., *et al:* The child in a hospital environment. Int. Nurs. Rev., *11*:19, (May–June) 1964.

Fraiberg, S. H.: The Magic Years. New York, Scribners, 1959.

Gruenberg, S., (ed.): The Encyclopedia of Child Care and Guidance. 2nd ed. Garden City, New York, Doubleday, 1963.

Heavenrich, R. M., *et al:* Viewpoints on children in hospitals. Hospitals, *37*:40, (May) 1963.

Hurlock, E. B.: Child Development. 4th ed. New York, McGraw-Hill, 1964.

Mayer, J.: Reaction of children during hospital admission. Ment. Hyg., *48*:576, 1964.

Outland, C. A.: A Child is hospitalized. Amer. J. Nurs., *64*:135, (Jun.) 1964.

Potts, W.: Dispelling fears of the hospitalized child. Hospital Topics, *41*:77, 1963.

Smith, M.: Ego support for the child patient. Amer. J. Nurs., *63*:90, (Oct.) 1963.

Stuart, H. C., and Prugh, D. G.: The Healthy Child: His Physical, Psychological and Social Development. Cambridge, Harvard University Press, 1960.

Wu, R.: Explaining treatments to young children. Amer. J. Nurs., *65*:71, (Jul.) 1965.

16

The Mentally Retarded Child

The term mental retardation is used freely, but not always with a clear understanding of its meaning. Definitions formulated within the past few years have done much to clarify our concepts of mental retardation.

"Mentally retarded are children and adults who, as a result of inadequately developed intelligence, are significantly impaired in their ability to learn and adapt to the demands of society."[*]

Another definition is equally helpful.

"Mental retardation refers to subaverage general intellectual functioning which originates during the developmental period and is associated with impairment in adaptive behavior."[†]

Impairment in adaptive behavior is reflected in maturation, learning and in social adjustment. Actually, mental retardation is a relative concept that depends on the prevailing educational and cultural standards of society. A person who may function adequately in a society that demands proficiency in certain skills, may be utterly unable to cope with the demands of a complex culture.

Intelligence itself is measured in terms of ability for abstract thinking. It includes causal reasoning, spatial comprehension, verbal expression, visual and auditory memory, and other adaptive adjustments.

Methods for attempting to measure intelligence were first formulated in France in the early 20th century, in an effort to screen out mentally deficient persons from the general population. Alfred Binet and his colleagues developed tests for measuring intellectual levels that have been modified and revised by Terman and others. These tests measure one aspect of intelligence, but do not necessarily indicate the degree of social adjustment or the maturational level. Other measuring devices, such as the Bender-Gestalt, or the Draw-A-Man tests, attempt to reach

[*] from: A proposed Program for National Action to Combat Mental Retardation. A Report of the President's Panel on Mental Retardation. Washington, U. S. Government Printing Office, 1962.

[†] Heber, R. I.: Modifications on the manual on terminology and classification in mental retardation. Amer. J. Ment. Defic., 65:499, 1961.

305

a *gestalt,* or organized pattern of experience.* All of these tests have real value, particularly if no one test is relied upon for the total measure of a child's ability to adapt to his environment. No test has been able as yet to solve the problem of innate intelligence versus social deprivation, the so-called nature-nurture problem.

NORMS OF INTELLECTUAL ABILITY AND ADAPTIVE BEHAVIOR

While keeping the limitations of predictive tests in mind, some idea of what to expect from a person in terms of intellectual ability and social adaptation is necessary. Labels are important insofar as they affect the education that a child is offered. A label has negative value if it is used to hold a child within a given area, such as severely or moderately retarded, without frequent attempts to discover whether he can make further progress. His developmental level must take into account his mental, physical, emotional and social adjustment.

TERMS USED FOR MEASURING EXTENT OF MENTAL IMPAIRMENT

The older terms of moron, imbecile and idiot carry high emotional import, and are no longer in good usage. Preferred terms are mildly, moderately, severely and profoundly retarded. Terms such as educable, trainable and dependent are still in common use, but these terms tend to set limits that may influence attempts to help the child reach a higher potential.

The Mildly Retarded Child (Educable). This child is a slow learner, but is capable of acquiring basic skills. He may learn to read, to write, and to do arithmetic to a 4th or 5th grade level. He is slower than the average child in learning to walk, talk, and feed himself, but his retardation may not be obvious to casual acquaintances. With support and guidance, he usually can develop social and vocational skills adequate for self-maintenance as he grows to childhood. He has a mental age of 6 to 10 years; his intelligence quotient is 51 to 70.

The Moderately and Severely Retarded Child (Trainable). The moderately retarded child has little, if any, ability to attain independence and academic skills. He has a noticeable delay in motor development and speech, but is capable of responding to training in self-help activities. He may be able to learn repetitive skills in sheltered workshops. Some may learn to travel alone, but few rarely become capable of assuming complete self-maintenance. Mental age range is from 2 to 6 years. I. Q. score, 20 to 50.

The Profoundly Retarded Child (Totally Dependent). This child has a minimal capacity for functioning, and has need of nursing care. He

* For a description of types of educational and psychological measurements, a good source is: Thorndike, R., and Hagen, E.: Measurement and Evaluation in Psychology and Education. 2nd ed. New York, John Wiley & Sons, 1961.

may eventually learn to walk, and develop a form of primitive speech, but is not capable of self-care and needs continued nursing care. Mental age range from 0 to 2 years. I. Q. score, 0 to 20.

As our understanding of mental retardation progresses, and as newer teaching methods develop, fewer persons need to remain at this level. Exciting results have occurred in terms of learning some degree of self-help, such as toilet training and self-feeding. There remain those, of course, so severely damaged that even this amount of learning appears to be unattainable.

ETIOLOGICAL FACTORS IN MENTAL RETARDATION

Prenatal Causes

INBORN ERRORS OF METABOLISM. For example, phenylketonuria. Very early detection may lead to measures preventing serious mental damage.

PRENATAL INFECTION. For example, toxoplasmosis. Microcephaly, hydrocephalus, and other brain damaging conditions may result from intrauterine infections.

INTRAUTERINE GROWTH RETARDATION. The cause is not clear. A higher incidence of mental retardation is found in this group than in the general population.

TERATOGENIC AGENTS. For example, maternal irradiation or drugs. It appears that most drugs pass through the placental barrier, and that some of them may have an adverse effect on a developing fetus.

GENETIC FACTORS. For example, Down's syndrome. Inborn variations of chromosomal patterns result in a variety of aberrations, the most commonly known being mongolism (Down's syndrome).

Perinatal Causes

Birth injuries, anoxia, and difficult birth, have all been etiological factors in brain damage. It is possible, however, in some instances, that prenatal factors were already present.

Postnatally Acquired Mental Deficiency

POISONING. For example, lead poisoning. Children who develop encephalopathy from chronic lead poisoning usually suffer significant brain damage.

INFECTIONS AND TRAUMA. For example, meningitis. Convulsive disorders, hydrocephalus, and other brain damage, are frequent sequelae of central nervous system infections.

IMPOVERISHED EARLY ENVIRONMENT. The degree of stimulation the infant receives in early life is an important factor in intellectual development. It is generally accepted that irreversible impairment to a child's ability to respond to his environment may result from complete emotional rejection in early life. Certain physical disabilities may so hamper a child that he cannot respond normally to his environment. The child severely affected by cerebral palsy who cannot talk, walk, or care for himself, may have no damage to his intellectual capacity, but his motor disabilities effectually hinder his ability to learn.

MEETING THE NEEDS OF THE MENTALLY HANDICAPPED CHILD

The most important need of any child is for understanding parents, and the mentally handicapped have this need in at least as great a measure as do normally bright children. Perhaps the greatest change we need to make is in the way we view these children. These are not children set apart or different; they are our children, just as all the others are. An unfortunate condition makes them slower to develop, and places a limit on their learning, but they are still our children. Not until we really grasp this point, both intellectually and emotionally, can we be of help to them.

As we examine our own feelings, can we honestly say that we have no tendency to recoil from a defective child, regarding him as "something other" than a child, a slow child—perhaps rejected by society—but still a child? When we have faced our own feelings and have resolved them, we are ready to offer our counsel and assistance to the child and to his family.

Counseling the Family

One of the meanings of counseling is "Interchange of opinions as to future procedure: consultation: deliberation."* This is just what the nurse hopes to do. She accepts the parents as they are, and she starts from there. This implies that she understands what happens when the knowledge comes that their child is mentally retarded.

The first reaction of most parents to this tragedy is one of disbelief: this cannot be, there must be a mistake. When forced by obvious facts to accept the condition, a search for a reason begins. Sometimes the concept of punishment enters in; perhaps this pregnancy had been rejected. Probably all women have a few moments of unhappiness over their thickening figure, curtailment of previous activity, morning sickness; but if the result of pregnancy is an imperfect child, there are apt to be feelings of guilt. Many other presumed causes, frequently unrealistic, are found, because the shame of not being able to produce a perfect child must be dealt with in some manner.

Some rejection of this child is nearly inevitable, but this is also unacceptable. It may be compensated by over-protection or over-concern to the point of making the child unnecessarily helpless, with perhaps some of the anger and frustration taken out on the normal children.

* The American College Dictionary. p. 276. New York, Random House, 1964.

Another method of coping with this intolerable problem is to set the child apart as someone special, someone sent to teach them love, humility and charity. If parents are to become effective, they have to face their reactions, until they can accept the child as a member of their family, to be helped, loved, disciplined and accepted just as the others.

The nurse, however, should not expect the parents to pour out their feelings to her, nor should she expect to assume the role of a professional counselor—a role for which she has neither the training nor the experience. She should be ready to listen, to observe, to help formulate a plan of care, and to use her knowledge and skills as they are desired and accepted. As she works with the family, her acceptance of them makes her an understanding partner, a partner in whom one can confide and with whom one can discuss problems. If the family and the nurse find the problems are beyond their ability, the nurse should know where they can seek expert help.

The Nurse's Role

In practical, everyday terms, what is the nurse's role? She may go into the situation prepared to discuss long-term goals and overall plans, but she is quite likely to find that the immediate, practical problem of getting the child to eat is absorbing the mother's attention, and that the mother is impatient with abstract goals until she has been able to cope with today's problems. Therefore, the nurse must begin with the problem at hand.

All but the most profoundly retarded children go through the sequence of normal development, with delays at each stage and a leveling off of ability much earlier as they reach the limits of their capacity. A retarded child, however, proceeds according to his mental age rather than according to his chronological age. Thus, a six-year-old retardate may be functioning on a mental level of two years, and the expected behavior must be, essentially, that of a two-year-old.

The most important requirement for the nurse is an adequate knowledge of the important landmarks of normal growth and development, in order to understand the progressive nature of maturation. One of the first expectations of normal development is that the infant's nervous system will have matured sufficiently at six or eight weeks to enable him to smile purposefully: that is, he smiles in response to pleasure and refuses to smile when he does not wish to do so. Failure to have developed this far is a cause for concern. Whether the abnormal maturation is the result of environmental conditions or from a lack of intellectual ability, there is still cause for concern. The next section makes some suggestions about helping the child to cope with the basic skills of everyday living.

TEACHING SELF-HELP TO THE CHILD

Teaching a mentally retarded child the basic self-help skills does not differ in principle from teaching any young child. If we can accept the fact that this child is "anychild," and not just a strange creature, we can free ourselves of all fanciful imaginings, and set about meeting his needs according to his present stage of maturation. In actual fact, one should not need any particular set of rules for this child, but because the physical image *does* distort our judgment, a reinforcement of the application of knowledge of growth and development usually proves helpful.

First Steps

1. Study the child for the effects of any superimposed physical handicaps. The incidence of muscular disability, a physical anomaly or cardiac disease, is higher than in the average child population. The presence of these handicaps modifies the child's rate of development whether or not he has limited mental ability.
2. Estimate the child's present stage of mental development. If, at the age of six, he shows the developmental level of two-year-old, be prepared to start at a two year level.
3. Know the average development expected of the various age groups. It is difficult to start from a two year level unless you have a good understanding of the normal development of a two-year-old.
4. Keep in mind the one factor that makes this child different from the average child: his lack of ability for abstract reasoning. This prevents him from transferring learning, or applying abstract principles to varied situations. He has to learn by habit formation.
5. Remember the three Rs of habit training—Routine, Repetition and Relaxation.
6. Watch for any signs of readiness, and take advantage of them.

Helping the Child Learn Toilet Control

Looking for signs of readiness. The average child shows this progression in toilet training:

AGE	
One year	regular time for bowel movements.
15 to 18 months	can achieve bowel control.
about 18 months	intervals between urination of one to three hours.
1½ to 2 years	can achieve daytime control—must be reminded.
2 to 3 years	asks for toilet usually, may lose control in unfamiliar surroundings.
3 to 4 years or later	night control for many, but not all.

The attempt to assess the child's maturational level does, of course, take into consideration all of the developmental skills, as well as the child's environment. Has he made any attempt to walk, or has he been kept in his crib with no opportunity or encouragement?

If the mother is uncertain of the child's urination pattern, it might be helpful if she keeps a "wetting" chart for a few days.

Habit formation. Place the child on the toilet at regular intervals of approximately two hours during the daytime. It may be best to do this according to his "wetting" pattern, or it may be more effective to establish a habit before and after meals, in mid-morning, mid-afternoon, and at bedtime. Taking the child to the toilet should always be accompanied by a verbal explanation—simple, direct and friendly.

Establishing a *place* is important. If the toilet chair is moved from room to room, or if the child is placed on it while he eats, or plays, or watches television, he is not learning toilet habits. He also needs to learn that society accepts the toilet room only, as the proper place for elimination.

Routine and *repetition* are obvious factors. *Relaxation* is not so easily attained. It is very easy for the procedure to assume undue importance until it becomes an obsession, making everyone tense, including the child. It undoubtedly will be a long time before he succeeds in urinating at the proper time, rather than directly after he is taken off. Expressed appreciation when he has achieved, a relaxed "better luck next time" when he has not, helps keep this experience in proper proportion. About five minutes is long enough for an individual try, but if child resists, it is better to put this off for a while longer.

As with the average child, the proper clothing helps. Diapers are associated with wetting and soiling, whereas keeping training pants dry can be a source of pride. Keeping in mind that even the profoundly retarded child may reach the mental age of two, we may find that we are setting our sights too low for a particular child.

Helping a Child Learn Dressing Skills

Readiness. Any child learns to *undress* before he learns to *dress*, because manipulation of clothing is a complex skill. Records of attempts to teach aborigines who have never worn clothing to put arms and legs in the proper openings, to manipulate buttons or zippers, show how incredibly difficult this type of learning is.

The first task is to teach the child how (and when) to remove clothing, which may be more difficult than it sounds if he has formed the habit of removing shoes or clothes whenever he fancies.

When ready to teach dressing, make the experience as simple as possible. Clothing that is easy to put on, and that is placed in a predetermined order for dressing facilitates learning. Perhaps a brightly colored label to show which is the back might be useful. He probably

MENTAL AGE GUIDE FOR DRESSING SKILLS

AGE

1 year	Tries to help by co-operation, such as holding out an arm or a leg. Can remove socks.
1½ years	Removes easily accessible clothes. Tries to put on shoes.
2 to 3 years	Puts on simple clothing, perhaps backwards, shoes on wrong feet. Tries to button large, easily accessible buttons, manipulate zipper.
3 to 4 years	Can dress self except for help with difficult clothing. Can button and use zipper.

will learn more easily if practice is with clothing itself, rather than with especially designed material for learning buttoning, tying, and so forth, because the transfer of learning from the form to his clothing may prove to be a difficult step.

It is important to remember that most mentally retarded children do increase in mental age, slowly, and to a limited level. Therefore, every child needs to be watched for evidence of readiness for a new skill, regardless of the label of mental ability.

Motor Skills

Motor abilities for retarded children follow normal developmental curves at a lower level and higher chronological age.

Norms for acquisition of motor skills in the general population:

AGE

1 month	Exhibits tonic-neck and startle reflexes.
4 months	Grasps objects if placed in his hand. Holds head and chest up when on abdomen.
6 to 7 months	Transfers objects from hand to hand—sits with some support—rolls over.
9 to 10 months	Transfers self to sitting position, usually pulls himself to his feet, can creep.
18 months	Walks alone, pushes chairs or objects around.
2 years	Runs, although unevenly. Turns pages of book.
3 years	Rides tricycle, climbs. Walks up and down stairs in adult manner.

Teaching the acquisition of motor skills is largely concerned with the provision of opportunity, enrichment of the environment, provision of approval of attempts, and acceptance. A child placed on the floor finds it easier to roll over than when he is lying on a soft mattress. A bright, attractive object, just out of reach, may some day catch his eye and provide an incentive to move toward it. An opportunity to observe other children attempting new motor skills sometimes provides inducement toward trying similar feats.

Providing an Enriched Environment

Environmental stimulation is essential for everyone's development. If we think that the retarded child does not need this enrichment because "he could not learn anyway," we are discouraging further development. As a matter of fact, the retarded child needs much more environmental enrichment than does the average child who can help provide his own stimulation.

Things to look at: Attention Getters

Mobiles, moving gently in the air, are attention catchers. Bright-colored paper butterflies or birds, or more complex objects such as airplanes or boats, strung on wires or on heavy strings of varying lengths—these can be simple for the nurse to make, or may even become an absorbing hobby for her.

Cradle gyms can be made by stringing all sorts of objects on heavy cord: painted spools, plastic lids, painted toilet paper rolls, large wooden beads. (Fig. 96)

Pictures, large, simple, brightly colored, pasted in cloth scrapbooks, on cardboard, or pinned up in easy sight.

Bright and interesting stuffed toys, large enough to be noticed.

Things to handle, hear and manipulate

A *sensory box* can be made up from everyday objects that can be handled for texture, form and size.

Furry object, smooth plastic, velvet, silk or satin, burlap.

Large smooth stones, sponge, sand, soap.

Small horn, bells on string, music box.

Small cars, planes.

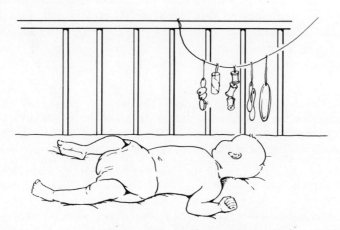

Fig. 96. Homemade cradle gym.

Active manipulation

Painted tin cans of various sizes, colors.
Colored spoons to pick up and to lay down.
Hand puppets.
Bongo drums, made from coffee cans with plastic tops.
Clothes pins to drop into large plastic, cut-down bleach bottles.
Clay, play dough.
Water play. Funnels, squeeze bottles, cups.
Gum drops for learning to chew.
Cereals such as Cheerios for hand, eye coordination.

This list grows easily with a little imagination and practice.

DISCIPLINE FOR THE RETARDED CHILD

Discipline, in the sense of teaching acceptable and unacceptable behavior, is as important for the retarded child as it is for any other. There are some special considerations for dealing with these children, because of their limited ability to adapt behavior to varying circumstances.

Discipline should always be consistent, and should enable a child to know what to expect. Language should be simple, direct and concise.

A positive approach, relying heavily on example and demonstration, gets much better results than a constant "don't touch" or "stop that." Obedience is an essential part of discipline, especially for the child with faulty reasoning ability, but the objectives of discipline should be considerably broader if peace and happiness are to be achieved.

One way to help prevent resentment and stubborn behavior is to set up a daily schedule and adhere to it as nearly as possible. Because of his impaired ability to reason and transfer learning, the child needs routine for his support. Reminders of the next item coming up on the schedule are frequently needed, such as "After you put your blocks away, we will have dinner;" at the same time, giving a hand to get him started. Laura Dittmann, in her excellent writing about discipline for these children, tells of three-year-old David, a mongoloid child.

"Even at 3 he can be as stubborn as a ton of cement when it comes to leaving one thing and starting the next. He twinkles and smiles, but won't budge. . . . When his mother insists that he get out of the bathtub he . . . howls and hits at her arms as she reaches for him. . . . She lifts him out, singing a song about bedtime and slippers. And David gets absorbed in rubbing the soft fur of his slipper and forgets all his objections. If his mother became confused about her requests and let David win, bathtime the next night might be even more difficult. By the time David is 12, possibly no one can get him to do anything."*

* Dittmann, L.: The Mentally Retarded Child at Home. P. 36. Washington, U. S. Government Printing Office, 1959.

If firmness and consistency are essential, so are kindness, love and understanding. Time out for a kiss for the hurt finger, rocking for a tired child, understanding of hurt feelings; these are part of the day as well.

If punishment is needed, it is important that it follows the deed directly, with cause and effect made as clear as possible to the child. Taking him away from the group for a short time, quietly but firmly, may help him quiet down and gain self control. Retaliation can confuse and anger him. If he is using "bad" behavior in order to get more attention, more praise and approval for good behavior may take away the need for misbehaving.

THE OTHER MEMBERS OF THE FAMILY

What happens to the siblings of the retarded child? The problems created by the presence of a retardate in the family can be severe, even in well-adjusted families in which the slow one is accepted, with allowances made for his inadequacies.

Undoubtedly, the proper care and training of a slow child take a disproportionate amount of his mother's time. It is natural for the others to feel some neglect, wishing that they could get the same sort of attention, and could themselves be helpless once in a while instead of always being called upon to be the responsible ones.

Some children do, in fact, regress to the behavior level of their retarded sibling in an attempt to get their share of attention. Parents, in turn, find it difficult to understand why the normal children cannot consistently feel the same amount of concern for the slow one's progress.

In homes in which shame is felt over the retarded child, social life is frequently sharply disrupted. The children cannot bring friends home, the older siblings hesitate over their dates. Even in homes in which the retarded child is accepted, his irresponsible behavior may create embarrassment for the rest of the family and their guests.

The nurse working with the retardate needs to be aware of these various natural reactions, showing herself friendly and interested in the other children. As she becomes familiar with the family, she should be able to help by her understanding and acceptance, as well as friendly counsel.

HOME CARE VS. INSTITUTIONAL CARE

Today, there is a tendency to keep these children at home rather than place them in institutions. As more and better opportunities for help, education and guidance arise in the community, more families gain confidence in their ability to care for their retarded children in their own homes.

There is much to be said for home care for the retarded child. The individual attention, security, and the sense of belonging, of being a member of a family, are all important factors in the child's progress toward a higher level of adjustment. No institution, however progressive and expertly staffed, can entirely supply the experience a child gets in his own family.

The solution—home or institution—is not this simple, however. The profoundly retarded child may indeed take too much time and strength from the mother to allow her to give even adequate attention to the rest of her family. The retarded child may be uncontrollable, and become a great nuisance in the home and neighborhood. Parents may feel that any benefits received by the child by staying in his own home ask sacrifices entirely out of proportion for the other family members.

Each family must, of course, make its own decision. The nurse can listen, can present facts, and help find necessary information, but she should never attempt to persuade or push her own views. Such a situation is emotionally charged, and whichever way the family decides, there are undoubtedly going to be moments when they are going to wonder if their decision was the right one. Their regret can only be intensified if they believe that they made a decision against their better judgment.

Institutions in general are moving away from accepting children before the age of two, many waiting until the child is five or six. An infant is a fairly helpless person, requiring considerable care whether he is bright or dull. Therefore, the burden on the parents grows heavier as the child grows older.

Whether the child is cared for at home or not, parents may be greatly encouraged over the intense interest being shown for these children. Research centers are exploring new possibilities, homes for the retarded are receiving money for newer appliances, better surroundings and, most important, are attracting well-trained, sympathetic personnel intent on applying newly understood principles and practices.

CONTINUING CARE

Mental disability is becoming the first cause for institutionalizing children, according to statistics provided by the Children's Bureau.* These are children who are handicapped emotionally and physically; however, the number of children in institutions for the mentally retarded increased nearly 15% between 1960 and 1964. It is hoped that our newer emphasis on programs for the mentally retarded can bring about a decrease in the child population in mental institutions.

Among the general population of the mentally retarded, it is estimated that not more than 10% to 25% are in the profoundly, severely and moderately handicapped group, with an I.Q. below 50. The trainable mem-

* America's Children and Youth in Institutions—1950–1960–1964. Washington, U. S. Government Printing Office, 1965.

bers can benefit from special education in schools in which it is provided. The profoundly retarded become increasingly difficult to handle as they grow older and larger, because they still need total care. Most of them must eventually be institutionalized, but there have been attempts to train even these children. Training includes placing the children on flat surfaces on which they can roll about, or in supported sitting positions for a period each day, providing sensory stimulation such as using a few certain words to the child and repeating these words constantly while making sensory application, such as "shoe" while placing it on the child's foot. Success has been reported with some children who have learned to crawl, to sit, and, in some cases, to stand and to walk.

The educable child is often not discovered to be retarded until he starts school, and is not able to keep up with his class. Special classes can do much to help these children adapt to social living; many achieve quite good adjustment, and may be absorbed into society with little discrimination.

SPECIFIC CONDITIONS OF MENTAL DISABILITY
Mongolism (Down's Syndrome)

Although as many as 200 causes of mental retardation have been identified, it is still difficult to establish a specific etiologic diagnosis for most.[*] One condition that is relatively easy to diagnose from clinical observation, and which has recently been the subject of intense study through cytogenetics, is mongolism.

Mongolism occurs approximately once in 600 births in the Caucasian population.[†] This condition apparently has been known for a long time, but no attempt at a description of its clinical features appears in medical literature, until that of Down in 1866. In 1959, the chromosomal etiology of mongolism was first confirmed and published. Much is still to be explored concerning the intricacies of chromosomal aberrations, but studies have brought interesting knowledge and exciting possibilities for the future. Present knowledge is far too complex for exposition here; the student is referred to the many articles that have been written, some of which are indicated in the suggested readings at the end of the chapter.

A simplified review of human genetics reminds us that, normally, each body cell contains 46 chromosomes which transmit the heredity of the cell from generation to generation. The chromosomes consist of 22 pairs of autosomes and 2 sex chromosomes. Each chromosome carries genes, which are the biologic units of heredity. Normally, the cell division, or

[*] American Medical Association: Mental Retardation, a Handbook for the Primary Physician. P. 1. Chicago, American Medical Association, 1965.

[†] Miller, J., and Dill, F.: The Cytogenetics of Mongolism. New York, The National Foundation—March of Dimes, 1966.

mitosis, which commences immediately following fertilization of the ova, produces cells with a stable number (46) of chromosomes.

Errors in cell division may occur, causing numerical changes in the chromosomal complement, or structural changes of chromosomes, such as translocations and inversions. These chromosomal errors are involved in mongolism, as well as in other types of abnormalities. (Fig. 97)

The most common type of mongolism is caused by a chromosomal trisomy, in which the total number of chromosomes in each cell is 47; a single chromosome appearing three times instead of twice. In the autosomal trisomy of mongolism, the chromosome in the 21 position is affected, and this type of mongolism is called trisomy 21. This condition appears to be maternal-age dependent, appearing more frequently in children of mothers over the age of 35. The cause for this age dependency remains unclear at this time, with several theories suggested but not proved.

A type of chromosomal translocation appears in certain mongoloid

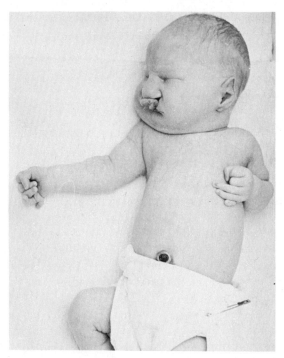

Fig. 97. One type of chromosomal error not associated with mongolism. Autosomal trisomy 13—15 (D₁).

An infant with trisomy 13—15 has multiple anomalies. Characteristics includes cleft lip, extra digits arising next to the fifth finger, cerebral and cardiac defects, and other anomalies.

offspring of younger women. This appears to be an inherited tendency, with one or both parents being carriers. A rare type, called mosaicism, shows a mixture of two cell types, one with 46 and another with 47 chromosomes.

Recurrence risks are low for the group of trisomy 21 with 47 chromosomes. In translocation mongolism, chromosomal studies should be carried out on parents and possibly on other close relatives, if the parents ask for genetic counseling. Mosaicism may also call for genetic studies.

Mongolism is relatively easy to diagnose by the clinical manifestations; therefore, chromosomal studies are not usually indicated except for purposes of genetic counseling and research. Such studies are highly specialized and expensive at present, necessitating taking the child to a medical center at which facilities are present.

Clinical Manifestations of Mongolism

Certain classical symptoms of mongolism are present, but in varying degrees. Some mental retardation occurs, with the majority of mongoloids falling in the moderately or severely retarded group.

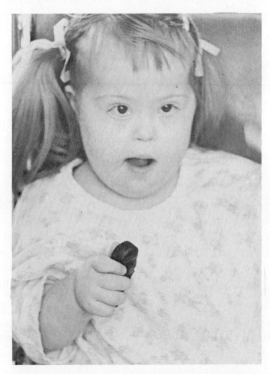

Fig. 98. Mongolism may be a fact of life for this child, but of equal importance is the love and acceptance she receives.

The mongoloid child has a disordered growth of the skull and long bones, resulting in a small skull, a short nose with flat bridge, a small oral cavity, and short extremities. The bony orbits are small and an epicanthal fold is present, giving the child an Asian appearance. The tongue frequently protrudes because of the small oral cavity; tongue sucking is common, causing fissuring and furrowing—the so-called scrotal tongue.

Muscle tone is exceptionally poor in a young mongoloid, allowing him to assume relaxed postures not seen in the normal infant.

The hands are short and broad, with an incurved fifth finger and abnormal palmar lines. There is an abnormally wide space between the first and second toes of the feet.

Not all mongoloid children exhibit all of the symptoms described above, nor do they all have the same degree of mental retardation. Additional abnormalities that appear with some frequency are cardiac defects, and leukemia. (The reason for the high association of acute leukemia with mongolism is not clear at the present time.) (Fig. 98)

As a general rule, these children are good-natured and fairly easily handled, although haphazard discipline is as harmful for them as it is for any child. They deserve the same love, stimulation and acceptance offered to all children, and they respond to the limit of their capability.

Phenylketonuria

Treatment for the Child With Phenylketonuria

The history of phenylketonuria (PKU) is a most interesting one. A mother in Norway had sought help for her two retarded children from many doctors. She was haunted by the idea that these children had a peculiar odor, but no one seemed to be interested. Finally, in the early 1930's, a Norwegian biochemist and physician, Dr. Ashborn Fölling, on examining the children discovered that the musty-smelling urine of both reacted with ferric chloride to give an unusual green color. Further chemical study showed that the reaction was caused by the presence of phenylpyruvic acid, an abnormal urine constituent.

Interest in this discovery was widespread, and simple ferric chloride testing was carried out in institutions for the mentally retarded in many countries. A number of positive reactions were obtained, and using statistics gathered, an estimate of one in 20,000 to 40,000 live births was made. Later testing of newborn infants in the United States suggests that the incidence is more nearly one in 10,000. This does not appear to be a high incidence, but the factor that makes this so interesting is contained in the discovery that the severe mental retardation accompanying the condition can be avoided through diet.

This is an hereditary autosomal recessive disorder. Figuring in reverse from the figure 1:10,000, it can be determined that one in 50 persons in the population is a carrier of PKU. These figures are assumptions only, as the exact incidence of disease and carriers is not yet known.

The basic defect in PKU is a lack of the enzyme phenylalanine hydroxylase, which in normal metabolism changes the essential amino acid phenylalanine to tyrosine. Because of this error, phenylpyruvic acid spills over into the urine.

The affected newborn is protected at birth by his mother's normal metabolism, but as soon as he ingests milk, phenylalanine begins to build up to serum levels about 20 times above normal. The high level of phenylalanine is apparently responsible for the mental retardation. A recent finding has been that some mothers with high phenylalanine levels have given birth to children with normal phenylalanine levels, but who were grossly retarded.

The untreated infant with PKU has a markedly arrested mental development, resulting, in most cases, in a severely retarded child. Some never learn to walk or to talk, and require total care. In addition to the gross mental retardation, they are generally extremely irritable and destructive. The majority have abnormal EEG's, and about 25% have convulsions. Physical growth is usually relatively normal, coloring is generally blond, and eczema is fairly common. The musty, characteristic odor is persistent and pervasive.

The importance of testing all newborn infants was discussed in chapter six. Siblings of a newly diagnosed infant should also be tested, even if no retardation has been noted by the parents. Damage cannot be undone, but the adverse progression may be slowed or even halted.

A case history points up the importance of alertness. A severely damaged child, already institutionalized when urine testing was initiated on a widespread scale, was discovered to have phenylketonuria. On request of the parents, a retarded cousin was also tested and found to be phenylketonuric. Being thus alerted, the birth of another child in the family was awaited with interest. The newborn was repeatedly tested, and when serum phenylalanine rose to abnormal levels during the first week of life, she was immediately placed on a low phenylalanine formula. As she grew, her mother adhered strictly to the low phenylalanine diet prescribed for her, and the child—now at the age of three—falls within normal limits in all respects of development.

How long she will need to follow the strict diet is not yet known with any degree of certainty. Responses differ among affected children, and our knowledge is not yet complete enough to enable us to predict with confidence. Mental deficiency, if caused by high serum phenylalanine levels, is thought to be preventable in those children started on the low phenylalanine diet before significant amounts of milk have been ingested.

Although it is thought that brain damage in untreated children occurs before the age of three, with little deterioration beyond that age, some children untreated until after the age of three have shown notable improvement. Generally speaking, older children, if it has been possible to keep them on the restricted diet, respond with an improvement in behavior, making their care easier. Present day thinking is that the optimum time to start treatment is during the first week of life, and that any affected child has a good possibility of showing some mental improvement if dietary treatment is instituted and adhered to before the age of three. Possibly the patient should continue dietary treatment until adolescence—or perhaps beyond—although this remains to be verified.

Prevention and Control

Successful prevention or control of the mental deficiency of phenylketonuria is dependent on the maintenance of a low phenylalanine diet. Phenylalanine is an essential amino acid necessary for body growth, and thus it cannot be omitted entirely from the daily diet. Normal serum levels are 1 to 3 mg./100 ml.: levels reached as a result of the disease can become as high as 60 mg. Although it is not known to what levels phenylalanine may be allowed to climb without causing damage, the dietary goal is to keep the level between 2 to 6 mg./100 ml.

All normal protein contains phenylalanine in significant amounts; however, the body cannot maintain normal growth and repair without protein. After considerable experimentation, synthetic foods made with modified casein hydrolysate have been perfected, several of which are commercially available. In the United States, the American-made product Lofenalac is generally used. Lofenalac is a powdered formula composed of low phenylalanine casein hydrolysate in which minerals, vitamins, fat and carbohydrate have been incorporated. When reconstituted with water, it has the appearance and consistency of milk. It is taken as a beverage, and is used in place of milk in special recipes. The formula has a nut-like flavor, that is well accepted by most children.

Lofenalac is the principal source of protein in the diet, but it is too low in phenylalanine to meet the entire daily requirement. Low protein vegetables and fruits are added in measured amounts, providing some variation in the diet. The diet may be further varied by using Lofenalac in special low phenylalanine recipes for ice creams, sauces, breads and pastries. The diet remains severely limited, however, and frequently meets with resistance when it is introduced to an older child.

Families need assistance and supervision from the public health nurse, the dietician and from the physician. Long-range guidance is essential for the continuation of a successful program.

Foods that must be omitted from the diet.

breads	cheese	peanut butter
flour (all kinds)	milk	eggs
meat, fish, poultry	nuts	legumes

Example of low phenylalanine menu for one day for a two-year-old.*

Breakfast	Dinner	Mid-afternoon

½ cup dried rice cereal† with 3 oz. formula, sugar

⅓ cup orange sections

6 oz. formula

½ cup cooked carrots

2½ tbsp. mashed potato made with formula and 1 tsp. butter

½ cup applesauce

6 oz. formula

2 animal crackers

6 oz. formula

Supper

3 tbsp. green beans

3 pear halves

6 oz. formula

Formula for this age consists of 26 measures Lofenalac, 1 oz. milk, 20 oz. water. (One measure equals one tablespoon).

Fruits and low-protein vegetables form the basic supplements to the Lofenalac formula, and small servings of cereal, potato, or arrowroot cookies may be added to the daily diet. Special food lists and recipes have been prepared, with "equivalents," so that the menu may be varied within the prescribed amounts of phenylalanine.‡

Dietary management is difficult for any child whose variety of foods is restricted; it becomes particularly difficult if it must be this sharply restricted for many years. Children who have never tasted the forbidden foods usually accept the restrictions more readily than the older child who has become accustomed to a varied diet.

BIBLIOGRAPHY

America's Children and Youth in Institutions—1950–1960–1964. Washington, U. S. Government Printing Office, 1965.

A Proposed Program for National Action to Combat Mental Retardation. A Report of the President's Panel on Mental Retardation. Washington, U. S. Government Printing Office, 1962.

American Medical Association: Mental Retardation, a Handbook for the Primary Physician. Chicago, American Medical Association, 1965.

Centerwall, W., and Centerwall, S.: Phenylketonuria. Washington, U. S. Government Printing Office, 1965.

Dittmann, L.: The Mentally Retarded Child at Home. P. 36. Washington, U. S. Government Printing Office, 1965.

Garell, D.: Metabolic defects associated with mental retardation. Amer. J. Dis. Child. *104*:401, 1962.

Heber, R. I.: Modifications in the manual on terminology and classification in mental retardation. Amer. J. Ment. Defic., *65*:499, 1961.

* After Centerwall, W., and Centerwall, S.: Phenylketonuria. Washington, U. S. Government Printing Office, 1965.

† Do not use "protein fortified" cereals.

‡ Lyman, F., and Lyman, J.: Dietary management of phenylketonuria with Lofenalac. Arch. Pediat., 77:212, 1960.

Holtgrewe, M.: A guide for public health nurses working with mentally retarded children. Washington, U. S. Government Printing Office, 1964.

Lyman, F., and Lyman, J.: Dietary management of phenylketonuria with Lofenalac. Arch. Pediat., 77:212, 1960.

Miller, J., and Dill, F.: The Cytogenetics of Mongolism. New York, The National Foundation—March of Dimes, 1966.

Polani, P.: Cytogenics of Down's syndrome. Pediat. Clin. N. Amer., 10:423, 1963.

Schild, S.: Parents of children with phenylketonuria. Children, 11:92, 1964.

Solnit, A., and Stark, M.: Mourning and the birth of a defective child. Psych. Study of Child, 16:523, 1961.

The American College Dictionary, p. 276. New York, Random House, 1964.

Wolff, I.: Nursing Role in Counseling Parents of Mentally Retarded Children. Washington, U. S. Government Printing Office, 1965.

SUGGESTED READINGS FOR FURTHER STUDY

Bryant, K. N., and Hirschberg, J. C.: Helping the parents of the retarded child. Amer. J. Dis. Child., 102:52, 1961.

Forbes, N. P., *et al.*: Maternal phenylketonuria. Nurs. Outlook, 14:40, (Jan.) 1966.

Hillsman, G.: Now I am a person. Nurs. Outlook, 11:172, (Mar.) 1963.

————: Genetics and the nurse. Nurs. Outlook, 14:34, (Jan.) 1966.

Houglan, M.: The mentally retarded contribute also. Nurs. Outlook, 11:175, (Mar.) 1963.

Jubenville, C.: Day-care centers for severely retarded children. Nurs. Outlook, 8:371, (Jul.) 1960.

Lockwood, D.: The Lizard Eaters. Don Mills, Ontario, Longmans, Green & Co., 1964.

Logan, H.: Me and my shadow. Nurs. Outlook, 14:54, (Jan.) 1966.

————: My child is mentally retarded. Nurs. Outlook, 10:445, (Jul.) 1962.

Murray, M.: Needs of parents of mentally retarded children. Amer. J. Ment. Defic., 63:1078, 1959.

O'Neal, J.: Siblings of the retarded: II individual counseling. Children, 12:226, 1965.

Owens, C.: Parents' reactions to defective babies. Amer. J. Nurs., 64:83, (Nov.) 1964.

Rody, N.: Severely retarded children taught self-feeding in 2–4 months. Hospital Topics, 43:101, (Aug.) 1965.

Schreiber, M., and Feeley, M.: Siblings of the retarded. 1. a Guided group experience. Children, 12:221, 1965.

Shotwell, A. M., and Shipe, D.: Effect of out-of-home care on the intellectual and social development of mongoloid children. Amer. J. Ment. Defic., 68:693, 1964.

Thorndike, R., and Hagen, E.: Measurement and evaluation in psychology and education. 2nd ed. New York, John Wiley & Sons, 1961.

Townes, P.: Genetic counseling. Pediat. Clin. N. Amer., 13:337, 1966.

U. S. Department of Health, Education and Welfare: Feeding Mentally Retarded Children, A Guide for Nurses Working with Families who have Mentally Retarded Children. Washington, U. S. Government Printing Office, 1964.

17

Problems of Every Day Living

THE CHRONICALLY ILL CHILD

We can be justly proud of the considerable progress made in reducing childhood mortality rates. When we look at children who are growing up to be self-respecting, well-integrated individuals, we know that a half-century ago, many of them would not have had this opportunity. Diphtheria and tuberculosis, to name only two conditions, all too often marked the premature end of a promising life. Today these conditions, as well as many others, are rare among the children of the United States, as well as among children in many other parts of the world. Many of the diseases that took such a heavy toll of children's lives now respond to treatment, and we owe much to those whose work has brought about this progress.

There are, however, still children who develop illnesses that respond poorly to treatment, or not at all. Cancer, in the form of leukemia and other neoplasms, is still high on the list of the major causes of childhood death. Cystic fibrosis requires careful nursing, with prognosis still poor. Childhood nephrosis has yielded only slowly to research, although the mortality rate has been lowered to 50 per cent or less. This is a cold comfort to the parents of the child within the 50 per cent: for them, it still adds up to 100 per cent.

Rheumatic carditis is also a crippler of children, bringing a reduced expectancy for living a healthy, normal life. There are many other conditions for which little hope of cure can be expected at present. Research is continually seeking for a break-through, and the future appears hopeful; but in the meantime, we must care for these children with the means at our disposal.

Children with chronic illnesses are generally cared for at home, and are seen in the hospital only for diagnosis and beginning treatment, or for care during exacerbations, or, for many, terminal care.

Understanding the problems faced by these children and their parents helps make the nurse's care more effective as well as furthering her development as a teacher.

When we see a child go home from the hospital with a diagnosis of leukemia or nephrosis, we have a feeling of sadness about the difficult days ahead. Too frequently, however, we do not understand exactly what

325

is involved in his home nursing care. As nurses, we *need* to understand this if we are to fulfill our functions as members of society.

Take a moment to consider what the role of a nurse means. As a student, the nurse may have seen herself as operating within the four walls of a hospital or a school, but she becomes increasingly aware that her influence and her responsibilities reach out much further. In her neighborhood, her community, and in her home, she does not cease to be a nurse. Perhaps as a saleswoman she could shed her identity, but as a professional woman, as a nurse, her role is an integral part of her entire life. Her advice is sought, her opinion is respected, and her influence is great; therefore, it behooves her to have a solid foundation of understanding and information. She must not be rigid, but will find her concepts ever changing as she herself grows; and she will be faithful to her principles if she understands them.

The Chronically Ill Child at Home

Sally, the third child in the family, has been petted and loved by her older brothers—her slow growth confirming her place as the baby of the family. Recently, however, she has become irritable, anorexic, and uninterested in life in general. A physical examination revealed a metabolic disorder and her mother has been obliged to assume the responsibility for a careful diet, prevention of infections, medications, treatments, and allowance for rest that is essential for such a child's care. What does this mean to Sally in terms of daily living? Her older brother is home from school with the sniffles and a slight fever. He sees no reason for staying in bed, hops in and out, and is driving his mother to distraction. Peace is finally secured when his mother finds an activity that occupies both children, with Sally a willing helper to her big brother. He throws off the infection and is back in school in a day or two; but to Sally, who has quickly picked it up, it is a major complication, perhaps sending her back to the hospital: yet it is difficult to keep the children apart.

Perhaps Sally has been invited to a neighborhood birthday party, but her diet does not allow her to eat the party foods without harm. Is Sally to be kept away from all activity? If so, what effect is this going to have on her emotional life?

Sally's diet is monotonous and uninspiring, and she lacks appetite, yet it is essential that she eat the proper foods. It is easy to suggest that the diet be made colorful and interesting, but to a busy mother, this is not quite as simple as it sounds. Suggestions are in order.

Perhaps we can make suggestions that would be helpful for this mother, or for others with home care problems. In this instance, one of the major considerations is to get the uninterested child to eat. If the child is on a restricted diet, there seems little one can do to break the monotony, but the surroundings can be made more pleasant. A mother must discipline herself to make the mealtime pleasant and to avoid nagging or any other unpleasantness. Naturally, she is anxious and concerned about her child's poor appetite, but she is not going to get the child to eat by nagging. Any kind of unpleasantness at the table makes mealtime an unwelcome occasion. She must save any reprimands and discussion of unpleasant subjects for another time and place.

Colorful surroundings help make the mealtime more agreeable. A gaily decorated placemat makes the meal more exciting. The older children can crayon or paint all sorts of gay scenes on an oblong piece of shelf paper, which can easily be discarded as occasion demands. Cheap, embossed napkins lend themselves readily to decoration with crayons or paint and gaily striped drinking straws make variety. Tiny tea sets or doll dishes occasionally add charm and novelty, and do not give the impression that huge amounts of food must be eaten.

Children love flowers, and certainly a cut flower or two on the table adds charm and beauty. Common garden flowers that can be handled and sniffed are most appreciated.

Perhaps the diner would occasionally like to dress up, with a hat, a pair of high heels and a purse, for a society luncheon to which her pet doll or stuffed animal is also invited.

Eating is an aesthetic pleasure as well as a necessity for the maintenance of life. Anything that adds beauty and color to the meal may also stimulate the appetite; the food itself is more tempting if it is bright and colorful. Vegetable food coloring can change some drab-looking foods, and molds or fancy shapes can make foods more exciting.

Neighborhood parties often may be fitted into, or around, the diet of the restricted child, with decorations and prizes heavily played up while foods are kept quite simple. The excitement of partying itself means more than the kind of refreshment, especially to small children.

These seem like simple, perhaps trivial, considerations, but daily living with a chronically ill child is not kept on a high pitch of crisis; it is, largely, monotonous and wearisome.

Daily care. The child who must be kept in bed for weeks presents a most trying problem to himself and to his family. If he is suffering from one of the sequelae of streptococcal infection, such as rheumatic fever, chorea, or glomerular nephritis, he probably feels quite well after the acute phase, and deeply resents the restrictions placed upon him. If he is in a cast for the correction of a congenital anomaly, he is mechanically restrained. The long, enforced inactivity is hard for an eager, active child to accept. We must be able to keep him physically quiet to prevent heart or body damage while at the same time, prevent him from withdrawing his eager interest from living. It is not a simple task.

For the busy mother, the most important consideration is to have the bed in an easily accessible place. If the family lives on one level, this is not too difficult to achieve; if there are stairs to climb, perhaps the nurse can help the parents convert a downstairs room into a temporary sick room. A hospital bed with its added height and raised head rest is a great convenience in the home. Many communities maintain a central supply cupboard from which hospital equipment may be rented or borrowed. The nurse can find out if such is the case in her community. Many city drug stores or supply houses also maintain such a rental service, although this may become too expensive.

Hospital beds, although useful, are not imperative. Blocks can be placed under the regular bed to raise it to the desired height, and back rests can be improvised from inverted straight chairs, or made from packing cases. (Fig. 99)

A most important item is an over-bed table for play or eating. It can be simply supplied by placing a board across the bed, resting the ends on the backs of chairs; or a sturdy carton may be used by turning it upside down and cutting the sides down to make leg room.

A child needs diversion to keep him from complete boredom, and to prevent a loss of interest in activities for his age. This is difficult if he is allowed a minimum of activity and if his callers are restricted. Television is good in limited amounts, but is no good at all for a steady diet. The American Heart Association has source material for children's quiet activities. In the foreword to the booklet *Have Fun—Get Well!** this state-

* Dodds, M.: Have Fun—Get Well! 10th ed. New York, American Heart Association, 1964.

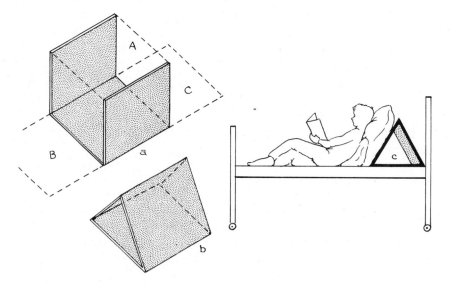

Fig. 99. A homemade back rest. A carton is cut as illustrated to make a triangular support.

ment is made: "Time stretches out like a great desert for the patient who must spend a long convalescence in bed." Many quiet activities can be carried out in the home that would be difficult or impractical in a hospital setting, and the suggestions in Chapter 4—*The Play Program*—for children on bed rest, can of course be used at home as well as in the hospital.

SCHOOLWORK AT HOME. Eventually, as the child progresses toward health, the doctor allows the child to resume his schoolwork at home. The nurse can help by telling the parents how to get in touch with the school authorities to arrange for home teaching or, better still, she can take care of this herself.

Before the child is allowed schoolwork, however, it is of great importance that he does not lose contact with his schoolmates. It is easy for a child to lose interest in life outside his home if he is prevented from participating in its activities, and it is equally difficult for him to step into such activities when he is again allowed to do so. The world does not stand still while he is isolated from his age mates; they will have developed skills in sports, knowledge of the world about them, and understanding of group living and cooperation. It will be difficult indeed for him to catch up, and any help we can give him along the way is essential. One way to help is to encourage his class to write letters to him, and teachers are usually happy to make this a part of their school activities. In this way, projects in which the class is interested can be extended to include the child at home.

EXTRACURRICULAR ACTIVITIES. If the sick child is a member of the scouts or of similar groups, he can participate in many projects, sending and receiving information to and from the group. Perhaps eventually, when the time comes, an occasional meeting can be held in his home.

If the child is encouraged to help plan his own program, it will make more sense to him. At the start of a long convalescence, the most important thing for the nurse and the parents is make certain that the child thoroughly understands his condition, his treatment, and his limitations. Only then can he accept his limitations and cooperate with his treatment.

Children are eager to learn and are curious about their bodies. A child with rheumatic fever can understand a simple diagram showing the heart functions. He may want to draw a diagram himself, or put together one of the plastic circulatory systems found in the toy departments. Children kept in bed for any condition can understand and profit by simple, straightforward explanations and drawings. A normal child sees no fun in illness and is willing enough to help in furthering his recovery if he understands the reasons. Naturally, interest flags at times and cannot be kept at a continuous high level; frequent encouragement may be needed.

RESISTANCE TO INFECTION. Chronically ill children have poor resistance to infection, and need much more careful watching than does the healthy child. Mothers must protect them from becoming overtired, from becoming chilled, and from contact with others whose own sniffles or cough appears trivial, but which could become a serious condition in the child with low resistance. This task includes keeping the other members of the family in the best possible health, rather than making the child a person apart from the family group.

As the child becomes older, mother must then learn to relax and to let him start to take over the management of his own daily living. This is a difficult thing to do because she has protected and worried for so long. She feels that all her careful work may become undone, yet for the sake of the child's future independence and emotional stability, she must do this. It takes both patience and wisdom to help him learn to respect his limitations while keeping a cheerful and optimistic view of possibilities for the future. The child who cannot go on a week-long camping trip with his group, may become expert in some other area that contributes as much or more to his general self-respect and sense of belonging.

PARENTAL ADJUSTMENTS. The adults in the child's life have adjustments to make as well. When a parent feels uncomfortable over a child's deformity or physical lack and tries to hide it or to keep him out of public view, she usually convinces herself that she is protecting him from pity or ridicule. Actually, it is her own pride and self-esteem that she is protecting; unfortunately, she is instilling the idea into the mind of the child that he has something of which to be ashamed. This is clearly brought out in the story of Nancy, as told by her mother. Nancy had a grotesque deformity of her legs and feet that her mother took great pains to hide. Nancy, however, was a friendly child who loved people, and who never for a moment lost faith that she could one day do all the things she wished, and who never worried about how other people saw her. Her mother writes;

"I hadn't known that I was so obviously sensitive about Nancy's body. But underneath, I realized, there was a feeling that I kept hidden and nameless even to myself. It was shame—shame that showed itself in cringing when I took Nancy out in public, in avoiding the questions in people's eyes, in being so quick to cover the deformity. Sometimes I had called it 'embarrassment' and scolded myself for it. Now I knew it was shame and despised myself for it. . . . In the unmasking of it, its power was gone. I'd never be ashamed again. Never as long as I remembered that shame is a festering kind of selfishness."*

Home discipline. Another troublesome problem is that of discipline. Certainly the child is less tempted to break the rules if he knows and understands them, and if he has enough occupation to keep him con-

* Hamilton, M.: Red Shoes for Nancy. P. 76. Philadelphia, J. B. Lippincott, 1955.

tented. For the child who must stay on bed rest, this is at best a long and tedious process against which the best of children rebel occasionally. Firmness, understanding and imagination are necessary, because the child needs strength from the whole family to help him build his own. It is in the child's best interest that he does not become "spoiled" or neurotic; he is happier and more secure if he is treated in the same manner as the others. Rules should be kept simple, but once they are made, they must be enforced, and violations dealt with kindly but firmly. This makes happier relations for the entire family.*

Care of the Child Whose Prognosis is Poor

We have talked about the child who has had his activity restricted, although he feels quite well. What do we do for the child who is miserable, steadily deteriorating physically, and whose interest is difficult to sustain? Children do not give up easily, but eventually even they need some hope for the future, to sustain them. There is nothing to be gained —and much to lose—by telling the child that he will never be well and able to participate in normal living, even though evidence does point in this direction. Children have great faith. They believe that adults are all-powerful, and accept their verdicts as simple truths. It is indeed a serious matter to rob a child of hope. Perhaps—who knows—next year or even next month, the breakthrough may come and research may have found a way to alleviate or even cure those conditions now believed to be incurable. Therefore, it would seem to be only good sense to keep the child in the best condition possible; emotionally, physically, and spiritually.

If an anxious, tired mother can occasionally get away from her constant attendance of her sick child, both she and the child will profit. In some communities, homemaker services can provide a mother substitute for a few hours weekly under such circumstances. It may take some persuading the first time to convince a mother that she should leave, but when she does get away for a short while, she undoubtedly finds the little, everyday vexations are not the overwhelming problems they seemed to be, and everything will tend to go along a bit more smoothly.

THE CHILD WITH A FATAL ILLNESS

When a child is discovered to have a disease for which we have as yet found no cure, we feel extremely helpless. The child may have been unwell and may have failed to progress normally for a period of time, or the onset of symptoms may have been very recent, as is usually the case in childhood leukemia.

---

* The film *Valiant Heart* brings out this aspect of home nursing very well. (American Heart Association).

The shock to the parents, on hearing that their child will not recover, is so deep that they cannot grasp the import of the information they have received. It takes time and a considerable emotional effort before any sort of adjustment can be made. The nurse, whether she is in a hospital situation, in public health, or just acting as a friend, will undoubtedly find herself called upon for support in such cases; and this is a difficult service for her to give.

Nursing Support of the Parents

Most nurses find it extremely difficult to face a child's impending death. It has been said that we all, both doctors and nurses, become too emotionally involved in these situations. We tend to lose perspective, to identify too much with the child, to take it all into ourselves. It becomes exceedingly hard to be the listener or to give comfort to those near to the child. We feel as one with them, and we look for comfort ourselves.

Because of this, and because the nurse cannot work with children for any length of time without being presented with this type of situation, it becomes important that she spend some time preparing herself. It is a poor time to start preparation when confronted with the actual situation.

When young nurses are asked the question "How do you answer the parents when they ask you 'Is my child going to die?' " their answers show both a need to consider this question and a reluctance to do so. The answers frequently are somewhat as follows: "I would say 'You will have to ask your doctor,' or, 'We are all going to die sometime,' or 'No one can be sure of the future.' "

These are evasive answers, and they satisfy no one. When the child asks "Nurse, is this bug I have the kind that kills people?" the nurse may say, "Why, do you think it might be?" or in some other way try to get at his thinking. This is good, but where does she go from there? She knows that he does have a disease from which he is not expected to recover, but does she tell him that, or does she say "Why don't you ask your doctor? I'm not allowed to tell you." Certainly, she does not like either choice, but what does she do?

No one has stereotyped answers for these questions, and no two situations are alike. The point to be made here, however, is that in order to be of any help whatever, the nurse must have considered the problem very carefully before the situation arose and have formulated some ideas and convictions of her own.

After the parents have had their conference with the doctor, they quite possibly will ask you, the nurse, what is wrong with their child; or, is it true that the child has leukemia? You may be quite certain that they are not asking for a detailed explanation of the child's disease, or of the laboratory findings. Perhaps they do not ask in as pointed a manner, but talk instead about the child of a friend or neighbor who had similar symptoms. Or they may ask for your opinion about their doctor. They may want to discuss a newspaper or magazine article about some condition that seems similar to that of their child. Actually, what they are asking for is reassurance; they want you to tell them they are mistaken; that they misunderstood the doctor; or even that perhaps the doctor is mistaken.

Perhaps you can say something like this: "I think Dr. X is an excellent pediatrician. Why don't you tell me, as well as you can remember, what he told you about Michael?" This may open the way for them to recount the doctor's words, and in the process, speak of their own feelings and fears.

Although this is not the time to go into detailed explanations of symptoms or treatment, the nurse does have an opportunity to clear up gross misconceptions if they make the picture darker than it needs to be. She must be careful not to contradict anything the doctor has said, but she can suggest that the parent may have misunderstood. She never suggests that the situation is worse than the parent sees it, even though she suspects that it is not being told exactly as the doctor explained. Perhaps this was as much as the parent could absorb at the time, and it is not the function of the nurse to force her further. A physician has had much experience in dealing with people and generally can understand the parents' reaction. Perhaps he has been aware that these people cannot take the full burden of knowledge at this time, and is giving it to them as they show that they can accept it. Again, nothing is gained by anticipating all the problems and difficulties that must eventually arise. The parents are to discover these soon enough, and need not be burdened with them unnecessarily in advance.

What we are really saying is that the nurse must be willing to listen. She cannot give out false assurance to the parents, nor should she try to impress upon them the gravity of the disease. Her warm, sympathetic manner, her undivided attention, her entire attitude toward the child and the parents are the important factors right now.

Later on, the parents will remember her understanding manner, and may feel that here is a person to whom they can turn. Then suggestions for care, as well as help in finding places and persons from whom they can receive additional help, are welcomed and acted upon.

The young nurse may feel that she is too immature or is too inexperienced to function adequately in such a situation. She is accustomed to see parents as authority figures, and who is she to give advice and comfort? If, however, she has come to understand herself, to accept her position as one of authority as well, she should find that she can handle herself well at these times.

Doctors believe that someone in the child's family must be clearly aware of the child's condition and of its ultimate outcome. If the doctor has been vague or indecisive, the parents may frantically go from place to place, seeking non-existent help. They can exhaust both their financial and emotional resources without having helped their child. They might rather conserve these resources toward making the child as comfortable and happy as possible, for as long a time as he has left. The doctor must not, of course, say that there will never be any help available; but instead present the facts as honestly as he knows how, and ought to assure the parents that should a reliable new treatment be discovered, he will be among the first to use it.

Nursing Support of the Child

The next person to be considered is the child himself. There appears to be no reason to tell a young child that he has a fatal illness. Taking hope away from a child robs him of all incentive, and all effort, to get what he can from life itself. A child has blind faith in his doctor; whatever he is told, he believes. If the doctor tells him that he is going to die from his disease, to the child's understanding the doctor is willing him to die; he could prevent it if he would. If a doctor takes the time to explain a particular treatment to a child, he will cooperate to the best of his ability, but he cannot understand or accept his own death.

Nature is very merciful, and as the disease progresses, the child is gradually weaned away from his strong urge to live, his perception becomes dulled, and he no longer has the acute fear and worry that he may have had earlier.

Perhaps we need to examine what death means to a young child. According to Nagy,* it is thought about mainly in terms of motor function. In a study done on a large group of children, she drew several conclusions. She found that the very young child can recognize death as a physical fact, but cannot separate it from life. Thus dead persons can still move, eat and drink, hear and feel. The only restriction comes from outside sources, such as being buried.

When a person goes out of a child's life, even temporarily, he is considered as dead, so that death means living under changed circumstances. Thus, the only painful thing about death to a small child is the fact of separation itself.

As a child grows older and begins to accept and to understand reality, Nagy concludes "he recognizes the fact of physical death but cannot separate it from life—he considers death as gradual or temporary." Eventually, he comes to accept the definitiveness of death, first as a person who "carries people off," but eventually he begins to understand its personal nature and its universality.

The adolescent, however, lives in such an intense present, according

---

* Nagy, M.: The child's view of death. *In* Feifel, H.: The Meaning of Death. P. 79. New York, McGraw-Hill, 1959.

to Kastenbaum,* that only the "now" seems real to him. Death (his own) is something for the future, thus vague and confusing.

Most normal persons seem to look back on their childhood as the period in which they least feared death, because it seemed most remote. It seems probable that even the seriously ill child does not see death in relation to himself. The older person who is caring for the child may find that he is confusing his own thoughts with the child's more immature ones. When you see a small child seriously ill, do you believe that he sees the illness in the same manner as you perceive it? The only way that you can get a glimpse of his understanding is to remember your own thoughts and emotions when you were his age. Relate to some landmark from the time when you were five or six, or nine or ten, and feel now whatever you felt then. Of course you are not this particular child, and you never were, but you may be able to understand him a little better.

For example, a tiny girl stood with her parents at the graveside of her baby sister. This made such an indelible impression on her that she never forgot it, but no memories of fear or despair were attached. Although it was sufficiently impressive to stay in her mind, it had no connection with herself as a person. Another child of six years, attending her father's funeral (he had been ill for a long time) had no conscious feeling of deprivation. She did think about the fact of death as she saw it, but her only feeling was one of guilt, because she had no impulse to cry as the others did. Her greatest emotions were of curiosity and of fantasy. How could the angels come, as she had been told in Sunday school, and, taking her father by the hand, lead him up the big golden stairs straight to God, when he so obviously was lying right there in full view? This was a fearful child, imagining dreadful calamities which could, and perhaps would, happen to her, but the sight of death did not bring these thoughts back. It just did not seem to concern her.

It would seem that death itself is not fear-provoking to a child, but the thought of separation is. A child is willing to face anything he can imagine if his mother is with him. She is his strength, his shield from harm, his ego. In a very real sense, his ideas of God come to him through his ideas about his parents. Therefore, separation from his parents is the greatest fear during childhood. The child who becomes separated from his mother in a crowd does not think of himself as lost; it is his mother who is lost. Perhaps he thinks that she has deserted him—he can never be entirely sure that he has not deserved this. It is the most panic-provoking situation that a child knows.

What then can the thought of death mean to a child but such a sepa-

* Kastenbaum, R.: Time and death in adolescence. *In* Feifel, H.: The Meaning of Death. P. 99. New York, McGraw-Hill, 1959.

ration? Certainly his parents, the all-powerful, are letting him go, and are deserting him. It seems extremely doubtful that any amount of explanation or assurance could be effective. He is faced with the devastating fact that his parents are leaving him, and that is all that he can really understand.

An older child understands his situation a bit better and may pretty well know the outcome, but he might not ask. Any bright child has undoubtedly heard such conditions as his discussed on television or in the neighborhood. If he has normal curiosity he can readily look up the meaning in a medical book or in some other source. In this day, there is but a small chance that the average child might not have a considerable knowledge of his condition.

If he does not ask, even if you are quite sure that he understands his disease, there seems little point in bringing up the subject. If the young person would prefer not to have his suspicions confirmed, it would seem that his wishes should be respected. With the newer drugs and treatments used today, children live many months with conditions that have no ultimate cure, and during this time, they may have periods of remission during which they feel quite well. It is difficult at such times to believe in one's own death, nor should the child be asked to do so. It seems unnecessarily cruel to destroy anyone's hope.

There is a considerable divergence of opinion about this. Some believe quite strongly that the older child certainly knows that all is not well, and may have confused and disturbing ideas from hearing and reading things that he only half understands, and can better adjust to facts that are, after all, inevitable. This is the belief held at the National Cancer Institute* where children with malignancies are cared for with sympathy and understanding.

Others, who have the same interest in the child's comfort and support, would not follow this line of reasoning. Susan, age 12, knew that her disease was called leukemia and asked, "Am I going to die from it?" The answer given her was "People do die from leukemia, there are several different types. Yours is not the type people die from." Susan lived for three years with long remissions during which she felt quite well, but even when she came into the hospital with severe symptoms and in intense pain, she remained confident, taking medicines and accepting treatments with courage.

In The Story of Gabrielle,† the child and her mother were greatly supportive of each other. Gabrielle never asked about her condition, and although her mother suspected that she knew, she felt that her daughter, a courageous child who believed in frankness, would prefer not to be

---

* Truth sustains leukemic children. Medical World News, 6:62, (Sep. 3) 1965.
† Gabrielson, C.: The Story of Gabrielle. New York, World Books, 1956.

told. Once, when Gabrielle was in great pain, her mother's courage deserted her, whereupon Gabrielle turned to her and said severely, "I expect you to go through all these things without breaking down."

Of course the nurse must find out from the parents, and from the doctor, what they have been telling the child, and how much they wish the child to know. The nurse must respect the parents' wishes and act in accordance with them, even though she may not agree completely. The child belongs to his parents, and this may be the only way that they are able to cope with the situation. If she is greatly disturbed over their attitude, she may be able to guide them to some qualified person who can help them reach something better, but she never tries to force her own beliefs on them.

Although the nurse believes that she may need to be the person to give support to the grieving parents when a child dies, this does not mean that she should appear detached and reserved. It is supportive and comforting for a parent to know that the child was loved by his nurse, and that she, too, is grieving over his death.

BLOOD DYSCRASIAS
Anemias of Childhood

A knowledge of the physiology of the circulatory system, including an understanding of the terms used, is quite necessary for the adequate nursing care of a child with anemia. For a review of the normal circulatory system, refer to the selections at the end of the chapter.

Anemia is a common childhood blood disorder. It may be the result of an inadequate production of red blood cells or of hemoglobin, or from an excessive loss of either red cells or of hemoglobin. The following are examples of the more common types of anemia found in childhood; there are many others.

1. Inadequate production of erythrocytes or of hemoglobin, as in iron deficiency anemia and in anemia of chronic infection.
2. Excessive loss of red cells, as in hemorrhage.
3. Hemolytic anemia associated with congenital abnormalities of erythrocytes or hemoglobin, as in thalassemia or sickle cell disease.
4. Hemolytic anemia associated with acquired abnormalities of erythrocytes or hemoglobin, from drugs, chemicals, or bacterial reaction.

Iron Deficiency Anemia

Iron deficiency is the most common nutritional deficiency among children in the United States, and is most often caused by an inadequate iron intake. Other causes can include an inadequate supply of iron at birth, as in cases of prematurity, and, occasionally, in those of twin births. In normal, full-term pregnancies, a maternal iron deficiency must be quite severe to affect the child, and probably does not occur in the general population. Impaired iron absorption is also found in certain gastrointestinal diseases, but the great majority of children with iron deficiency anemia have a poor intake of iron-producing foods.

Iron deficiency anemia is a hypochromic, microcytic anemia, occurring primarily in children between one-half and two years of age. The healthy, full-term infant has stored up before birth a supply of iron sufficient for the first three to six months of his life, after which he is dependent on an intake of iron-containing foods for the supply necessary to maintain adequate blood formation.

Immediate causes of iron deficiency. In the United States, iron deficiency is more commonly the result of poor feeding practices than of economic stress. Babies with an inordinate fondness for milk, sometimes taking an astonishing amount, have their appetites satisfied, and show little interest in solid foods. Mothers sometimes misunderstand the learning of the infant requires transfer from sucking to chewing and swallowing motions, and think the baby is showing a dislike when he pushes his food out with his tongue. Babies need time to adapt to the new manner of taking food, and a mother needs considerable patience and persistence. A baby undoubtedly is going to register his surprise and his impatience with this attempt to satisfy his hunger, but he learns quickly and will become an enthusiast for the newer method, especially if he can still have his comforting bottle.

Infants and toddlers have come into the hospital with a history of taking two to three quarts of milk daily with no other foods accepted, or at best, only foods with a high carbohydrate content. (Some confusion still exists: the belief that "milk is a perfect food ," so why not let him have all he wants?) Examples are many; the nine-month-old who was entirely bottle-fed, with no vitamin or mineral supplements; the two-year-old who doesn't care for vegetables and fruit, but enjoys pancakes with the family, and so forth.

Clinical Manifestations and Laboratory Findings. The affected children are large, fat and pale. Anorexia and listlessness are common, as is an increased irritability. The pallor becomes accentuated, with a waxy and sheetlike aspect as the disease progresses. Hemoglobin falls to levels as low as 3–9 Gm./100 ml. and the erythrocyte count may be low normal.

Treatment. The treatment·of iron deficiency anemia caused by faulty nutrition is mainly concerned with correcting the diet. This often is quite difficult, and may require the impersonal atmosphere of a hospital. Foods rich in iron are offered to the child, high carbohydrate foods are withheld, and milk is limited to one pint daily. Patience and strict adherence to the rule on everyone's part is necessary, until the child learns to accept the diet. Oral intake of medicinal iron, such as ferrous sulphate (preferably given between meals) supplements the diet. Therapy for six to eight weeks is needed to bring the child back to good health.

A few children have a hemoglobin so low, or their anorexia so acute, that they need additional therapy. An iron dextran mixture for intramuscular use (Imferon) is available, which is markedly efficient in bringing the hemoglobin to normal levels. A special technique for administering this medication, called the Z tract method, is necessary to avoid leakage into the subcutaneous tissues.*

Home Care. The most important aspect of treatment for this condition is education for the parents. They need to understand the importance of iron in their child's diet, and the foods that are best for meeting this need. One mother was quite severely criticized in the pediatric outpatient clinic because of her child's anemic condition. "Mrs. Black," said the pediatrician, "you simply have to give your child more foods that contain iron." Mrs. Black looked at him in bewilderment and exclaimed, "But doctor, after liver—what?"

A nurse has a splendid opportunity to teach good nutritional habits in such a situation—habits that may improve the health of the entire family. She can guide the mother to the green and the yellow vegetables, to the use of egg yolk, and to iron-rich fruits such as peaches; in addition, of course, to liver. Some of the pamphlets published by commercial food companies are excellent for teaching parents, and perhaps can refresh the nurse's memory as well. These give the iron and the vitamin content of foods, and list the requirements for various age levels.†

Prognosis is excellent for restored health in iron deficiency caused by poor iron intake with dietary correction. If untreated, anemia becomes progressive, with possible resultant cardiac failure.

Sickle Cell Disease

Sickle cell disease is an hereditary condition occurring principally in the Negro race. It is inherited as an asymptomatic trait if only one parent has the sickling trait, but if both parents carry the trait, one out of four offspring will have the disease. The sickling trait occurs in 7 to 9% of American Negroes, with the disease itself having an incidence of 0.3 to 1.3%.

Etiology. An abnormal hemoglobin (hemoglobin–S) is responsible for the sickle-like shape of the red cells. Destruction of the abnormal cells results in a hemolytic anemia. The cells are also apt to clump, causing infarcts in the spleen and in other organs, thus bringing on the so-called sickle cell crisis.

Onset and Manifestations. Clinical manifestations rarely appear before the child is six months of age, with the disease itself frequently diagnosed during the preschool period. The sickling trait may be demonstrated fairly early, but there is no way to tell whether this is the trait only, or if it will develop into the disease.

---

* See appendix.

† One such publication is Facts About Foods, H. J. Heinz Co., Pittsburgh, 1961.

Sickle cell trait is asymptomatic and needs no treatment. Sickle cell disease causes a chronic anemia with hemoglobin levels of 6 to 9 Gm./ 100 ml., or lower. Easy fatigability and anorexia are the usual manifestations of any form of anemia. The frequent sickle cell crises, however, make the disease a serious one.

Sickle Cell Crisis may be the first clinical manifestation of the disease, with frequent recurrences during early childhood. This disturbance presents a variety of symptoms. The most common symptom is severe, acute abdominal pain, together with muscle spasm, fever, severe leg pain that may be muscular, osseous, or localized in the joints, which become hot and swollen. The abdomen becomes board-like, with an absence of bowel sounds, making it extremely difficult to distinguish the condition from an abdominal condition requiring surgery. The crisis may have a fatal outcome caused by cerebral, cardiac or hemolytic difficulties.

Treatment. The child should be kept in optimum health between crises. Small blood transfusions help to bring the hemoglobin level near normal, but the increase is only temporary. Treatment for crises is supportive and symptomatic. Bed rest is indicated, with the main treatment consisting in the use of analgesics for the relief of pain, and vigorous oral hydration. Water is preferred, because it is free of electrolytes, but if sufficient water cannot be taken, intravenous glucose in water may be used. Crises tend to become less frequent as the child grows older.

Oral iron intake has no effect on sickle cell disease, and splenectomy has no effect on the disease either, but it may be done if the spleen enlargement causes discomfort.

Prognosis is guarded, and depends on the severity of the disease.

Thalassemia (Mediterranean Anemia)

Thalassemia is a serious hereditary blood disorder appearing principally in persons of Mediterranean origin, such as Greeks, Syrians and Sicilians, or in their descendants elsewhere. In this condition, hemoglobin formation is faulty, and red blood cells are of abnormal size and shape and are rapidly destroyed.

The hypochromic, microcytic anemia resulting from this disorder is not present at birth, but appears after a few months of life. As in sickle cell anemia, it is manifested as a major or a minor trait. Clinical manifestations in a minor trait are minimal, limited to slight pallor and occasionally a slight enlargement of the spleen. These children remain unaffected by the slight anemia, but genetic counseling may be indicated. Should such persons marry individuals carrying the same trait, one in four of their children can be expected to have the major form. Unfortunately, the expectation of one in four offspring developing the hereditary condition is misleading to many persons, who think that if one child is defective, the next three will not be. Too often, it has not been made clear to them that there is no order of succession, and the one-quarter of the offspring who are affected may follow each other.

Thalassemia major produces a severe irreversible anemia requiring frequent transfusions, and shortening the affected person's lifespan. Although life expectancy is somewhat better than has been supposed, a person with this disorder rarely lives beyond the third decade.

Clinical Manifestations. Early in the disease, it may be difficult to distinguish it from other types of anemia, including iron deficiency, or from other hemolytic disorders. The nature of the disorder is confirmed by an examination of the blood of the patients' parents.

Pallor, poor appetite and fever may be early manifestations. Splenomegaly appears early, and may reach disabling proportions. The most striking changes are skeletal, and exceed those of other hemolytic anemias. Changes in the facial bones give a characteristic appearance, and there is a tendency toward protusion of the teeth.

Another characteristic is the muddy, bronze color of the skin, caused by hemosiderosis, after months or years of transfusions. Growth becomes markedly retarded, and cardiac enlargement is common.

Treatment. Transfusions are required at frequent intervals with an effort to maintain hemoglobin at or above 6 Gm./100 ml., with care taken to avoid overloading. In certain cases, splenectomy may be helpful.

Prognosis is very poor. With careful treatment, some children may live to adulthood, but at best, must lead lives of limited activity. The most serious problem presented is the prevention or control of cardiac failure.

LEUKEMIA IN CHILDREN

Leukemia is still a major pediatric problem, with no cure yet in sight. The ability to produce remissions, during which the child feels quite well, has brightened the picture, but the disease is still fatal within a year or two years of the onset.

Leukemia in childhood is usually acute, with the lymphocytic type predominant. A pronounced rise in occurrence has been noted in recent years, particularly in the United States. Active research continues with several theories being tested, but no conclusive evidence has been discovered. A familial incidence has been noted on occasion, and multiple cases have appeared in a community during a certain period. Other possible leads, such as a higher incidence following radiation exposure have been followed, but no constant cause and effect relationship has as yet been isolated. An unexpectedly high incidence of acute leukemia has been found in association with mongolism, but again, the significance is not clear.

Incidence and Appearance of Clinical Manifestations. The highest incidence of leukemia occurs in the age group under five years. Clinical manifestations of the disease appear with surprising abruptness in many affected children, with few, if any, warning signs. Presenting manifestations are frequently lassitude, pallor and loss of appetite. Other early or presenting symptoms are fever, bone and joint pain, sore throat, or hemorrhages into the skin or the mucous membranes.

Nausea and vomiting, headache, diarrhea and abdominal pain, although seldom presenting signs, frequently occur during the course of the disease. Anemia and easy bruising are present, and enlargement of the spleen is common, although less common than in chronic leukemia. Intracranial hemorrhage is the most common immediate cause of death.

Diagnosis. Bone marrow aspiration must always be carried out for a definitive diagnosis of acute anemia. The bone marrow shows an overgrowth of leukopoietic tissue, with few hemopoietic elements.

Treatment. In addition to symptomatic, palliative measures, certain drugs have been found to produce remissions during which time the patient may feel well and show no clinical manifestations. Remissions may be partial or complete, lasting for a period of weeks, and occasionally, for months. The antimetabolite drugs interfere with the metabolism of leukemic cells, but have little adverse effect on normal cells. The effective drugs in this class are the folic acid analogs, Methotrexate and Aminopterin, and the purine antagonist, 6-Mercaptopurine.

The use of steroids, in conjunction with the antimetabolates, produces the most complete and longest remissions. An alkylating agent, Cytoxan, is also used to induce remissions.

Antimetabolite drugs are capable of producing toxic effects, including nausea, vomiting, diarrhea, ulceration of the buccal membrane and interference with hemopoietic activity. Toxic effects of Cytoxan include bone marrow depression, alopecia and, occasionally, cystitis. The well-known side effects of steroids include the retention of fluids, giving a typical cushingoid appearance, nervous system irritation and the formation of gastric ulcers. These effects must be watched for and reported while the patient is being treated with these drugs. Whether they will be discontinued or reduced depends on the severity of the reaction and upon the judgment of the attending physician.

As the disease progresses, the leukemic cells tend to become resistant to the drugs, and remissions no longer occur. Survival without special therapy averages approximately nine weeks. With adequate treatment, average survival is from one to two years.

Home Care for the Leukemic Child

Hospitalization for leukemic children is limited to diagnostic procedure and to the institution of therapeutic measures whenever possible. The child at home is allowed to live a normal life as much as he is able. The family needs to unite to make the home pleasant and cheerful, and should make a particular effort to keep anxiety and discouragement away from the child. Parents may need special encouragement about this, and may appreciate an understanding, sympathetic friend for support.

Over-indulgence and undue permissiveness tend to make the child anxious and confused, however, and is not in his best interest. Short periods of hospitalization for exacerbations quite possibly are going to be necessary, as well as admission for terminal care.

Nursing Care of the Critically III Child

Physical care for a child in the terminal stages of a wasting disease (such as leukemia) is aimed at providing all possible comfort for the patient. Frequent turning is necessary, but painful, and is dreaded by the child. Unhurried movement, a soft, gentle touch, and careful handling, helps minimize the pain. Abrupt movements should be avoided, and necessary analgesics should be used as indicated. Cleansing of bleeding, ulcerated areas in the mouth must be very gentle in order to prevent further trauma.

Emotional support for the child and his parents is of equal importance. Parents, singly or together, are allowed and encouraged, to stay with their child and to perform as much of his cares as they are able. It frequently comforts a mother to know that she is doing something for her child, rather than watching helplessly. Nurses should avoid urging parents to go away "for a little rest" at such a time. Instead, they should understand that most parents need to be with their children, and the nurse should do all she can to add to their comfort at the child's bedside. The nurse should be constantly available and as understanding and receptive to requests as possible. She may think a suggestion to call the doctor, or to perform some nursing act, useless or unnecessary, but if such acts ease things for the parents, she should cheerfully perform them. Nurses are human and may make mistakes, perhaps many; but avoiding disturbing conditions or assuming an indifferent manner should never be among them.

HEMOPHILIA

Hemophilia is one of the oldest hereditary diseases known. A law in the Talmud forbade the circumcision of a boy born into a family in which older sons had bled uncontrollably following circumcision—an indication that the female carrier status was understood.

In modern times, a famous example of a carrier is that of Queen Victoria. One son, three grandsons, and six great-grandsons had the disease, while six of her female descendents were carriers. Thus the condition has occurred in several royal houses of Europe. No records of hemophilia can be found in the ancestors of Queen Victoria, and it is assumed that a mutation took place in her X chromosome. The hereditary line of Queen Elizabeth II, however, has been entirely free from this disorder.

Recent research has demonstrated hemophilia as a syndrome of several distinct inborn errors of metabolism, all resulting in the delayed coagulation of blood. Defects in the synthesis of protein give rise to deficiencies in any of the factors in the blood plasma needed for thromboplastic activity. The principle factors involved are factor viii (AHG), factor ix (PTC), and factor xi (PTA).

Mechanism of Clot Formation

The mechanism of clot formation is complex. In a simplified form, it can best be described as occurring in three stages.

1. Prothrombin is formed through plasma-platelet interaction.
2. Prothrombin is converted to thrombin.
3. Fibrinogen is converted into fibrin by thrombin.

Fibrin forms a mesh that traps red and white cells and platelets into a clot, closing the defect in an injured vessel. A deficiency of one of the thromboplastin precursors may give rise to hemophilia. This progression of events is diagrammed in Fig. 100.

Reference to one of the specialized texts on the circulatory system is necessary for a detailed discussion and for better understanding of the clot-forming mechanism.*

Recognized Types of Hemophilia

Factor VIII deficiency (hemophilia A; AHG deficiency; classic hemophilia). Classic hemophilia is inherited as a sex-linked recessive mendelian trait with transmission to affected males by carrier females. An asymptomatic carrier mother is capable of transmitting the trait to half of her sons, who will have the disease, and to half of her daughters, who

---

* One good source for further study is: Smith, C.: Blood Diseases of Infancy and Childhood. 2nd ed., chapter 26. St. Louis, C. V. Mosby, 1966.

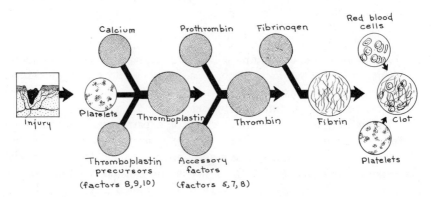

Fig. 100. Formation of a blood clot.

will be carriers. It was formerly believed that the disease appeared in male offspring of carrier mothers only, but it is now known that a union of a carrier female and a hemophilic male may produce a daughter with classic hemophilia. Severe classic hemophilia has occurred in daughters of carrier mothers and non-hemophilic fathers, possibly as a spontaneous mutation.

Hemophilia A (classic hemophilia) is the most commonly found type, and is also the most severe. It is caused by a deficiency of antihemophilic globulin (AHG)—the factor viii necessary for blood clotting.

Factor IX deficiency (hemophilia B; PTA deficiency; Christmas disease). Christmas disease was named after a five-year-old boy who was one of the first patients diagnosed as having a deficiency of factor *ix*.

This deficiency constitutes about 15 per cent of the hemophilias. It is a sex-linked recessive trait appearing in male offspring of carrier females, caused by a deficiency of one of the necessary thromboplastin precursors, factor ix, the plasma thromboplastin component (PTA). In either hemophilia A or hemophilia B, as many as 25 per cent or more of the affected persons can trace no family history of the disease. It is assumed that spontaneous mutations have occurred in some of these cases. Hemophilia B (Christmas disease) is indistinguishable from classic hemophilia in its clinical manifestations, particularly in its severe form. It may also exist in a mild form, probably more frequently than in hemophilia A.

Factor XI deficiency (hemophilia C; PTA deficiency). This exists as an autosomal dominant trait, appearing in both males and females. Sporadic cases may also be observed, as in the other hemophilias. The deficient factor is plasma thromboplastin antecedent (PTA), factor xi. Bleeding is generally milder than in the AHG and the PTC deficiencies, hemorrhage usually being by trauma, and rarely spontaneous.

Von Willebrand's syndrome (vascular hemophilia; pseudohemophilia). Von Willebrand's syndrome is classified with the hemophilias. It is a mendelian dominant trait present in both sexes, and is characterized by prolonged bleeding time.

Clinical Manifestations and Diagnosis

Clinical manifestations in any type of hemophilia are similar, and are treated by transfusions to supply the deficient factor, and by measures to prevent or treat complications. In severe bleeding, the quantities of fresh blood needed may easily overload the circulatory system. It therefore becomes important to know the type of deficiency, in order that concentrated plasma containing the necessary factor may be administered when a transfusion is considered necessary.

Diagnosis of hemophilia is made by a careful examination of family history and of the type of bleeding the patient presents. Abnormal bleeding dating from infancy, in combination with a family history, suggests hemophilia. A markedly prolonged clotting time is characteristic of severe AHG or PTC deficiency, but mild conditions may have only a slightly prolonged clotting time. It must be kept in mind that in a number of instances, no family history may be obtained.

AHG deficiency may be determined by the prothrombin consumption test and by the prothrombin generation test. The prothrombin generation test will identify the PTC defect.

Treatment

Treatment of any of the hemophilias consists primarily in supplying the missing factor. In addition, other measures are concerned with the application of coagulants and local pressure to sites of external bleeding, and prevention or treatment of complications.

The AHG factor is extremely labile, disappearing from blood or from stored plasma within a few hours. When introduced into the circulation, its life-span is correspondingly short, necessitating repeated transfusions until bleeding is controlled. Although PTC and PTA factors are more stable than AHG, stored plasma or blood does not appear to be so effective in controlling bleeding in any of these deficiencies as does fresh frozen plasma.

Type-related Transfusions. 1. In instances of extensive blood loss, fresh whole blood, less than 24 hours old, is usually necessary for the initial treatment.

2. Single donor, fresh frozen plasma is made from freshly collected blood and is stored in individual containers at a temperature under −20° C. The AHG factor, under these conditions, remains potent for varying periods of time, estimated to be as long as a year according to some studies. When it is needed, the plasma is thawed quickly and is used at once. Teamwork between the laboratory and the ward is necessary to prevent any delay between thawing and administration.

3. Lyophilized, freshly collected, pooled plasma may be stored under normal refrigeration (making this a convenient preparation for use while traveling, or in areas where fresh frozen plasma is not readily available). The lyophilized (dried) plasma may be reconstituted with the provided diluent and made ready for use within minutes.*

Clinical Manifestations and Management

Hemophilia is characterized by prolonged bleeding, with frequent hemorrhages into the skin, the joint spaces, the intramuscular tissues and externally. Bleeding from tooth extractions, brain hemorrhages, and crippling deformities are serious complications. Death during infancy or in early childhood is not unusual in severe hemophilia, and results from a great loss of blood, intracranial bleeding, or from respiratory obstruction caused by bleeding into the neck tissues.

---

* Provided by Hyland Laboratories, sold in United States and many other countries.

Excessive bleeding may follow circumcision, contraindicating circumcision if hemophilia is present. A young infant beginning to creep or walk bruises easily, and may often cause serious hemorrhages from minor lacerations. Bleeding frequently occurs from lip biting, or from sharp objects put in the mouth. Tooth eruption seldom causes bleeding, but extractions require specialized handling, and should be avoided by preventive care, if at all possible.

Topical fluoride applications to the teeth are of particular importance to these children. Particular attention should be paid to proper oral hygiene, well-balanced diet and to proper dental treatment. Although parents may be aware of the benefits to the teeth from a well-balanced diet and from the avoidance of in-between snacks without toothbrushing, damage frequently occurs before the patient's first visit to the dentist. Parents should be encouraged to bring their affected children to the dentist very early, in order that they may secure assistance in setting up a well-balanced diet, and in establishing good dietary habits. In this manner, the child also becomes familiar with the dental office before any care is actually needed. Parents may also appreciate any help in the selection and the use of proper equipment such as a toothbrush, tooth paste and dental floss. The parents need to use care in their selection of a dentist who understands the problems presented, and who will set up an appropriate program of preventive dentistry.

Nosebleeds in affected children are frequent, but can usually be controlled with a Gelfoam pack soaked in topical thrombin solutions and maintained by gentle pressure. Bleeding from any source in a hemophiliac, however, indicates the titer of AHG or other deficient factor is below a critical level; therefore, transfusion of whole blood or fresh frozen (or lyophilized) plasma is indicated.

Bleeding, of course, must be controlled by the use of blood or of plasma containing the deficient factor. If a tooth extraction becomes necessary, the patient is hospitalized for the extraction. Plasma is given previous to, and following, the surgery. The tooth socket is packed with Gelfoam, or with Oxycel soaked in concentrated topical thrombin and maintained with pressure. A dental cast may be used in those areas in which pressure can be maintained only with difficulty. If bleeding recurs two or three days after the extraction, the clot should be removed and a fresh pack should be introduced.

Bleeding into the joint cavities. This frequently occurs following some slight injury, and seems nearly unavoidable if the child is to be allowed to lead a normal life. Pain, caused by the pressure of the confined fluid in the narrow joint spaces, is extreme, requiring the use of sedatives or of narcotics. Prompt immobilization of the involved extremity is essential to prevent contractures of soft tissues and the destruction of the bone and joint tissues. Emergency splints are available, and should be kept in every hemophiliac's home. Ice packs should also be available for instant use. Before leaving for the hospital, a splint and cold packs should be applied, and if any great length of time is required for transportation, a transfusion of quick-frozen or Hyland plasma should be given. (Fig. 101)

A bivalve plaster cast may be applied in the hospital for the immobilization of the affected part. Orthopedic surgeons disagree as to whether collected blood in the affected joint should be aspirated.

After bleeding has been stopped, the cast may be removed, and gentle traction may be applied to restore motion and alignment. Passive physiotherapy is used to help prevent the development of joint contractures. A fairly large number of patients who have had repeated hemarthroses have, however, developed functional impairment of their joints despite careful treatment.

Most children with hemophilia have their lives interrupted by frequent hospitalization. Nurses and auxillary personnel should be well informed concerning the necessary care for a hemophilia patient, as well as the care needed by a particular child.

A small child may be placed in a crib with padded sides to protect him from bruises. This, however, isolates him from the rest of the world. Coming at the same time as separation from mother, this isolation is especially hard to bear. His choice of toys is going to be quite severely limited, because anything that could possibly cause injury must be avoided. Even if he is feeling well, he is quite possibly going to be kept in his crib, because no one will have enough time to watch him carefully. His prospects are rather dismal, and they present a strong point in favor of allowing his mother to stay with him.

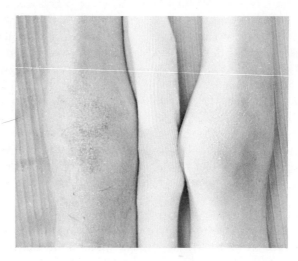

Fig. 101. Bleeding into joints in hemophilia.
The knees are swollen and painful.

Particular attention must be paid to treatments and procedures in order to avoid pain or additional bleeding. Medication should be given orally, if possible, but if injections are ordered, care must be taken to choose and to rotate sites, avoiding bruised areas or hematomas. The medication must be injected slowly, after which manual pressure should be applied for five or more minutes. A pressure dressing and an ice pack may be used instead. Venipunctures should be done by experienced persons.

During daily hygiene, the nails should be trimmed to prevent scratching, and adequate skin care should be given to prevent irritation. Oral hygiene is important, and if a tooth brush is used, it should have very soft bristles.

If internal bleeding is present, vital signs must be watched carefully for signs of shock, and excretions should be examined for the presence of blood. If the bleeding is into the joints, the nurse should take care to avoid additional pain or injury. A bed cradle can keep the weight of the blanket off painful areas. The knee is the most commonly affected joint, and only a slight degree of motion may lead to more bleeding. Careful turning and handling are essential.

Emotional Support in the Hospital

A small child very quickly learns how to get his own way, and if his mother has been understandably apprehensive about her child's condition, he will quite possibly enter the hospital determined to get it. He does not expect any one to cross him too much, because he can always have a temper tantrum.

How, indeed, can a nurse maintain needed discipline for a child who can so easily injure himself? Freddy was an excellent example. He was allowed to play about the ward, and was completely undisciplined. If he was prevented from climbing, snatching toys from others, or from running in the corridor, he promptly responded with a full-blown temper tantrum, throwing himself on the floor and banging his head enthusiastically. The suddenness and the violence of his reactions frequently took the nurses by surprise, and it required nimbleness on their part to pick him up and carry him, kicking and screaming to his crib where he could do minimal damage to himself. Placing him in the safest possible place, and drawing the curtains around his unit seemed to be the best response to his anger. He deeply resented being watched, and could not respond to reasoning or affection when he was emotionally upset.

The nurse may frequently avoid such occasions if she uses a little forethought. If the dispute is not particularly important, as is often the case, flexibility is in order. Failure to make necessary restrictions because a child might react is not in his best interest, nor will it contribute to his emotional welfare.

For an older child, frequent hospitalizations, treatments and school absences are difficult to accept, and he needs considerable help. He can learn to understand his condition, and can learn the need for caution in his life. Occupational activities suitable for his age, and placement in the ward with others of his age and with his interests, are important adjuncts to his emotional well-being.

Home Care

A child with hemophilia is perfectly well between bleeding episodes, but the fact that bleeding may occur as the result of very slight trauma, or often without any known injury, causes considerable anxiety. For an unknown reason, bleeding episodes are more common in the Spring and Fall. There also appears to be some evidence that emotional stress can initiate bleeding episodes.

Parents experience continual anxiety over such questions as how much activity to allow their child, how to keep from overprotecting him, and how to help him achieve a healthy mental attitude and yet protect him from mishaps that may cause serious bleeding episodes. In some way, they must help him toward autonomy and independence within the framework of his limitations. There certainly will be times when the emotional effect of social deprivation and restrained activity must be weighed against possible physical harm.

The financial strain on the family is considerable, as is so frequently the case when a child has a long-term chronic condition. Children who have had several episodes of hemarthrosis may be crippled to the extent of needing crutches and braces, or even use of wheelchairs. Measures toward rehabilitation require hospitalization, with possible surgery, casts, and other orthopedic appliances. Rehabilitative measures have been remarkably successful when in the hands of competent orthopedists, but they take long periods of time and cannot be hurried.

A hemophilic child usually suffers much loss of school time. One college student reported an average attendance of approximately 25 days a year, with only a few weeks of home tutoring during high school. Another hemophilic boy had excessive absences but was assisted with a school-to-home telephone hookup when he was absent.* The child who must frequently interrupt his schooling, for whatever reason, suffers a considerable handicap. Each child should be considered individually, with as normal an environment as possible planned for him.

Both a child and his family must accept his limitations, and yet realize the importance of normal social experiences. School, health, and com-

---

* Proceedings, Institutes on Hemophilia, sponsored by The National Hemophilia Foundation, Columbia University and Tulane University. Copies may be obtained from The National Hemophilia Foundation, 25 West 39th St., New York, New York, 10018.

munity agencies must be prepared to assist the family with counseling and encouragement, and enable them to bring up their affected children in a healthy manner, both emotionally and physically.

Rehabilitation

Extensive crippling resulting from hemophilic arthropathies presents a difficult task for rehabilitation. Prompt and thorough care of any injuries as they arise helps minimize crippling. Many children, however, develop deformities severe enough to limit successful daily living.

Rehabilitation for the correction of flexion deformities requires hospitalization for periods of weeks for treatment with corrective casts. When the best possible correction has been obtained, braces usually are fitted for maintenance of the correction.

Braces are frequently needed for a period of years, during which, they must be kept in perfect repair, adjusted to the patient's growth, and replaced as necessary. Rehabilitation of the severely crippled patient requires a long period under specialized orthopedic care, but the results have been eminently worthwhile.

The nurse should be aware of the resources in her community, both for family counseling and for financial assistance. State chapters of the National Hemophilia Foundation provide information, form parent groups, support the establishment of special clinics, and provide a diversity of other services.

BIBLIOGRAPHY

Burchenal, J. H., *et al:* Chemotherapy of neoplastic diseases in children. Advances Pedia., *12:*189, 1962.

Dodds, M.: Have Fun—Get Well! 10th ed., New York, American Heart Association, 1964.

Feifel, H.: The Meaning of Death. Pp. 79, 99. New York, McGraw-Hill, 1959.

Gabrielson, C.: The Story of Gabrielle. New York, World Publishers, 1956.

Hamilton, M.: Red Shoes for Nancy. P. 76. Philadelphia, J. B. Lippincott, 1955.

H. J. Heinz Company: Facts About Foods. H. J. Heinz Company, Pittsburgh, 1961.

Iverson, T.: Leukemia in infancy and childhood. Acta Paediatrica, Supplement no. 167, 1966.

Rosenthal, M. C.: Management of Hemophilia. New York, The National Hemophilia Foundation.

Smith, C.: Blood Diseases of Infancy and Childhood. 2nd ed. St. Louis, C. V. Mosby, 1966.

The National Hemophilia Foundation: Blood or Blood Products. New York, The National Hemophilia Foundation.

————: Proceedings: Institute on Hemophilia, 1964–1965. New York, The National Hemophilia Foundation, 1965.

The Valiant Heart (film) M.P.O. Productions, distributed by the American Heart Association, 14 mm., sound, 28½ minutes.

Truth Sustains Leukemic Children. Med. World News, *6:*62, 1965.

SUGGESTED READINGS FOR FURTHER STUDY

Carpenter, K., and Stewart, J. M.: Parents take heart at city of hope. Amer. J. Nurs., *62:*82, (Oct.) 1962.

Dargeon, H.: Tumors of Childhood. Chapter 12. New York, Paul V. Hoeber, 1960.

Geis, D.: Mothers' perceptions of care given their dying children. Amer. J. Nurs., *65:*105, (Feb.) 1965.

Glaser, B., and Strauss, A.: Dying on time. Hospital Topics, *43:*28, (Aug.) 1965.

Knudson, A. G., and Natterson, J. M.: Participation of parents in the hospital care of fatally ill children. Pediatrics, *26:*482, 1960.

Leikin, S.: Leukemia: current concepts in therapy. Pediat. Clin. N. Amer., *9:*753, 1962.

Miller, R.: Etiology of childhood leukemia. Pediat. Clin. N. Amer., *13:*267, 1966.

Pappas, A., *et al.:* The problem of unrecognized "mild hemophilia." J.A.M.A., *187:*772, 1964.

Pearson, H.: Newer concepts in the genetics of the thalassemias. Pediat. Clin. N. Amer., *9:*635, 1962.

Scott, R.: Sickle cell anemia. Pediat. Clin. N. Amer., *9:*649, 1962.

Wagner, B.: Teaching students to work with the dying. Amer. J. Nurs., *64:* 128, (Nov.) 1964.

Whissell, D. Y., *et al.:* Hemophilia in a woman. New York, The National Foundation—March of Dimes, 1965.

White, D.: Living with hemophilia. Nurs. Outlook, *12:*36, (Jul.) 1964.

Wolf, A.: Helping your child to understand death. New York, Child Study Association of America, 1958.

Zuelzer, W. W., and Flatz, G.: Acute childhood leukemia: a ten-year study. Amer. J. Dis. Child., *100:*886, 1960.

18

Other Disorders of Childhood

COMMUNICABLE DISEASES OF CHILDHOOD

Many of the common communicable diseases are becoming remarkably *uncommon*—a very satisfying fact. Within very recent memory, widespread epidemics of poliomyelitis were annual occurrences; today, a majority of young nurses have never seen an active case. Many people still living remember losing brothers or sisters from diphtheria, or can recall vividly the stories their parents told of this dreadful disease, which was once so common. In the United States today, it is possible for the diagnosis of an occasional case to be missed, because the attending physician may never have seen one.

Smallpox still occurs throughout the world, but rumors of a suspected case in North America or Western Europe is sufficient reason to send large numbers of people to health stations for revaccination. The most recent disease earmarked for eradication is measles, a disease by no means as simple and innocuous as people have been inclined to believe. The list goes on, including such conditions as whooping cough and typhoid fever.

None of these changes have just "happened." Considerable education has been necessary: at one time, laws for compulsory protection against smallpox were resisted and evaded. Even now, public health surveys show that large numbers of people—children and adults—are inadequately protected against conditions for which there is a safe, effective immunization. It is quite possible that epidemics could occur in any community, triggered by a few sporadic cases. Few people have an immunity to these diseases from frequent exposure to them, or from previous inapparent infection.

Suggested schedules for providing acquired immunity through inoculation change frequently as research continues to isolate causative factors and to devise preventive measures. The approved timetable for inoculation against communicable diseases, as revised in 1966, is given in Chapter 9.

The following outline of communicable diseases contains the conditions still widespread among children, as well as some of those rarely seen in the United States today. It is well for a practicing nurse to be aware of certain signs and symptoms, although she should not *expect* to see these once common diseases. The descriptions are admittedly sketchy. For a comprehensive discussion, a nurse should consult a specialized text.*

Definition of Some Common Terms

Antibody. A protective substance in the body produced in response to the introduction of an antigen. *Antigen.* A foreign protein that stimulates the formation of antibodies. *Antitoxin.* An antibody that unites with and neutralizes a specific toxin. *Carrier.* A person in apparent good health, who harbors in his body the specific organisms of a disease. *Carrier State* is also a feature of the incubation period, the convalescence, and the post-convalescence of some infectious diseases. *Enanthem.* An eruption upon a mucous surface. *Endemic.* Habitual presence of a disease within a given area. *Epidemic.* An outbreak in a community of a group of illnesses of similar nature, in excess of the normal expectancy. *Erythema.* Redness of the skin produced by congestion of the capillaries. *Exanthem.* An eruption appearing upon the skin during an eruptive disease. *Host.* A man, an animal, or a plant that harbors or nourishes another organism. *Immunity.* Passive—acquired immunity by administration of an antibody. Active—immunity acquired by an individual as the result of his own reactions to pathogens. Natural—resistance of the normal animal to infection. *Inapparent Infection.* Infection in a host without recognizable clinical signs. *Incubation Period.* The time interval between the infection and the appearance of the first symptoms of the disease. *Macule.* A discolored skin spot not elevated above the surface. *Pandemic.* A world-wide epidemic. *Papule.* A small, circumscribed, solid elevation of the skin. *Pustule.* A small elevation of the epidermis filled with pus. *Toxin.* A poisonous substance elaborated by certain organisms such as bacteria. *Toxoid.* A toxin that has been treated to destroy its toxicity but that retains its antigenic properties. *Vaccine.* A suspension of attenuated or killed microorganisms administered for the prevention of a specific infection.

Communicable Diseases Common or Once Common Among Children

Diphtheria. INFECTIOUS AGENT. Corynebacterium diphtheriae, the Klebs-Loeffler bacillus.

SOURCE OF INFECTION. Discharges from the mucous membranes of the nose and the throat, the skin, from other lesions, or from infected persons.

* Texts on communicable disease are easily available. For an up-to-date, quick, authoritative reference, The American Public Health Association publishes a handbook, *Control of Communicable Disease in Man,* 10th ed., 1965. (Obtainable from many State Health Departments, some college bookstores, or directly from the Association, 1790 Broadway, New York, New York.

Raw milk, contaminated with infectious material, may be a vehicle. Carriers (meaning certain persons who have had an apparent or an inapparent attack of diphtheria and still harbor the bacillus).

IMMUNIZATION AGENT. Diphtheria toxoid, usually combined with tetanus toxoid and pertussis vaccine (DPT) for small children; adult type (DT) given after the age of 12. Diphtheria antitoxin should be given if the presence of the disease itself is suspected. Antitoxins are developed in horse serum, and can cause a severe anaphylactic reaction in allergic persons; therefore, a skin test for sensitivity should be made first. A sensitivity test is not necessary for the toxoid.

INCUBATION PERIOD. Usually two to five days, may be longer.

SUSCEPTIBILITY. Infants born of immune mothers are relatively immune until about the sixth month of life. One attack does not always produce persisting immunity. Following an attack, a person may become a carrier.

PERIOD OF COMMUNICABILITY. Variable, until 2 negative nose and throat cultures are obtained in succession, and at least 24 hours apart. Usually, communicability ceases about two weeks after the inception of the disease, unless the person becomes a carrier.

CLINICAL MANIFESTATIONS. A sore throat, with the formation of a grayish membrane in the tonsillar region, frequently extending into laryngeal region as disease progresses. A raw, bleeding surface is left if this membrane is peeled off. Generalized toxic symptoms of fever, headache, malaise, and of body aches. Nasal diphtheria (less frequent) has lesions limited to the nose, and produces no constitutional symptoms unless it spreads to the throat. Toxins produced by the bacilli, and circulated in the bloodstream, cause paralysis, involving any muscle or group of muscles, in about 10 to 15 per cent of all cases.

TREATMENT—NURSING CARE. Immediate administration of diphtheria antitoxin if the disease is present or if it is suspected, after testing for sensitivity to horse serum, is necessary. Strict bed rest should be maintained, at least until afebrile, or longer if there is cardiac involvement. Tracheotomy may be a life saver.

COMPLICATIONS. Many. Motor and sensory nerve paralysis, myocarditis, and laryngeal stenosis, are the most common.

TREATMENT OF CARRIERS. Procaine penicillin intramuscularly daily for seven days usually removes the bacilli. Two negative cultures in succession, 24 hours apart, must be obtained.

Infectious Parotitis (mumps). INFECTIOUS AGENT. The virus of mumps.

SOURCE OF INFECTION. Saliva of infected persons.

IMMUNIZATION AGENT. Live and attenuated vaccines are available, but of limited value, give short period of protection. Immunity acquired from infection during childhood preferable, to avoid more serious consequences of attack after adolescence.

INCUBATION PERIOD. 12 to 26 days.

SUSCEPTIBILITY. General, but not so highly communicable as measles or chickenpox, although inapparent attacks may occur.

PERIOD OF COMMUNICABILITY. Possibly six to seven days before, and up to nine days after the swelling appears.

CLINICAL MANIFESTATIONS. Fever, swelling and tenderness of one or both of the parotid glands. The gland becomes painful and tender, and causes difficulty in chewing.

TREATMENT—NURSING CARE. Bed rest if indicated, but it is not mandatory. Diet should be adjusted to patient's ability to chew.

COMPLICATIONS. Meningoencephalitis in children and orchitis in the adolescent and in adult males. Nerve deafness may occur.

Pertussis (whooping cough). INFECTIOUS AGENT. Bordetella pertussis, the pertussis bacillus.

SOURCE OF INFECTION. Discharges from the laryngeal and the bronchial membranes of infected persons.

IMMUNIZATION AGENT. Pertussis vaccine, usually given combined with diphtheria and tetanus toxoids. (DPT)

INCUBATION PERIOD. Commonly a week or two, does not exceed 21 days.

SUSCEPTIBILITY. General. Many inapparent cases. Occasionally, second attacks occur.

CLINICAL MANIFESTATIONS. An acute disease involving the trachea, the bronchi and the bronchioles. The initial stage, with an irritating cough, continues for one or two weeks. The cough gradually becomes paroxysmal, with the second stage lasting from one to two months. There is a characteristic crowing or inspiratory whoop. A paroxysm is frequently followed by vomiting. This is a severe condition in infants, with a high mortality rate.

TREATMENT—NURSING CARE. Careful nursing care is essential, especially for the seriously ill infant, who may need oxygen, and perhaps a tracheotomy. The infant must be fed after vomiting to prevent severe debilitation. Older children should not be allowed to expose others, but profit from being allowed out-of-doors in mild weather.

COMPLICATIONS. Bronchopneumonia is a frequent complication. There can be convulsions, especially in infants, and hemorrhage from severe paroxysms.

Poliomyelitis (infantile paralysis). INFECTIOUS AGENT. Poliovirus types 1, 2, and 3.

SOURCE OF INFECTION. Direct contact with infected persons, feces and with pharyngeal secretions.

IMMUNIZATION AGENT. Sabin oral or Salk vaccine for types 1, 2, and 3.

INCUBATION PERIOD. Range from three days to three weeks.

SUSCEPTIBILITY. General. Probably many inapparent infections among unprotected persons.

PERIOD OF COMMUNICABILITY. Virus isolated from throat secretions as early as 36 hours, and from feces 72 hours after infection. The virus persists in the throat for about a week and in feces for three to six weeks, or longer.

CLINICAL MANIFESTATIONS. Fever, headache, gastrointestinal disturbance, stiffness in the neck and in the back, and paralysis in the paralytic type.

TREATMENT—NURSING CARE. Bed rest, use of a hard mattress and of bed boards. Body hot packs to relax muscles. For the bulbar type, tracheotomy may be required, and a tank-type respirator is needed for respiratory failure.

COMPLICATIONS. If it is the paralytic type, muscular paralysis may be permanent, causing atrophy of the affected muscles.

Rubeola (measles, red measles, regular measles). INFECTIOUS AGENT. Measles virus.

SOURCE OF INFECTION. Person to person, from nose and throat secretions, droplet spread, and from articles freshly contaminated with nose and throat secretions. These may be air-borne.

IMMUNIZING AGENT. Live, attenuated vaccine or inactivated vaccine.

INCUBATION PERIOD. 10 to 14 days.

SUSCEPTIBILITY. Universal. One attack usually confers immunity.

PERIOD OF COMMUNICABILITY. About four days before the rash to five to six days after the rash appears.

CLINICAL MANIFESTATIONS. Coryza, with a dry cough and a moderate fever. Photophobia. There are Koplik spots on the buccal membrane for a few hours, disappearing before the rash appears. A maculopapular rash appears on the third or fourth day, starting behind the ears, around the hair line, and spreads over the entire body.

TREATMENT—NURSING CARE. Symptomatic. Protect the eyes from glare. Tepid baths and soothing lotion relieve itching. Provide a humidified atmosphere for a troublesome, harsh cough. Fluids, diet as desired and bed rest.

COMPLICATIONS. Pneumonia, nephritis, otitis media, and encephalitis.

Rubella (German measles, three day measles). INFECTIOUS AGENT. Virus of rubella.

SOURCE OF INFECTION. Direct contact, droplet, and freshly contaminated articles. It may be air-borne.

IMMUNIZING AGENT. None at present, several are in the process of research.

INCUBATION PERIOD. 14 to 21 days.

SUSCEPTIBILITY. Universal. One attack usually confers immunity. The condition may be confused with other rashes.

PERIOD OF COMMUNICABILITY. About a week before and at least 4 days after the onset of the rash.

CLINICAL MANIFESTATIONS. Mild catarrhal symptoms and mild fever may be present. There may be enlargement of the postauricular, the suboccipital or the postcervical lymph nodes. No Koplik spots. There is a rash resembling measles or scarlet fever. The symptoms may be mild and go unnoticed.

TREATMENT—NURSING CARE. Bed rest if febrile.

COMPLICATIONS. Rare, except in newborns contracting the infection in utero. (See *Congenital Rubella*).

Scarlet Fever (Scarletina). INFECTIOUS AGENT. Group A beta hemolytic streptococcus.

SOURCE OF INFECTION. Discharge from the nose, the throat, from the purulent lesions of infected persons and from contaminated objects.

IMMUNIZATION AGENT. Immunity conferred by an attack of the disease, and probably by unrecognized infections of toxigenic strains of hemolytic streptococci. Antibiotic treatment may give type-specific temporary immunity.

INCUBATION PERIOD. Usually one to three days.

SUSCEPTIBILITY. Scarlet fever is a streptococcal sore throat with a toxic rash. The incidence of scarlet fever has been decreasing in the United States for many years.

PERIOD OF COMMUNICABILITY. During incubation and the clinical illness, about 10 days. Adequate penicillin therapy usually eliminates the carrier state in 24 hours.

CLINICAL MANIFESTATIONS. Acute sore throat, headache, fever, and vomiting, followed within 24 to 72 hours by a diffuse, papular, bright red erythema. Petechiae are present on the soft palate, and the tongue shows raised papillae, giving it the name "strawberry tongue."

TREATMENT—NURSING CARE. Strict bed rest, as in any streptococcal infection. Penicillin, codeine or aspirin should be given as needed, and fluids, as well as treatment for complications.

COMPLICATIONS. Otitis media, laryngitis, cardiac disorders (which may be transient) and meningitis.

Typhoid Fever. INFECTIOUS AGENT. Salmonella typhi, the typhoid bacillus.

SOURCE OF INFECTION. Patients and carriers, through the feces and the urine of infected persons. From direct contact, contaminated water, raw food and vegetables, milk, and milk products. Flies may be sources of infection under certain conditions.

IMMUNIZATION AGENT. Typhoid vaccine. Commonly used in areas of possible exposure. Reinforcement is recommended every 3 years.

INCUBATION PERIOD. Usually one to three weeks.

SUSCEPTIBILITY. General, with some immunity through unrecognized infections.

PERIOD OF COMMUNICABILITY. Usually from the first week through convalescence, until three negative stool and urine cultures are obtained in succession, at least 24 hours apart. The patient may become a carrier.

CLINICAL MANIFESTATIONS. Fever, malaise, ulceration of Peyer's patches in intestines, an enlarged spleen, rose spots on the trunk, emaciation, fatigue, and anemia.

TREATMENT—NURSING CARE. Bed rest, proper nutrition, and maintenance of fluid balance. Tepid sponges for the reduction of fever, and transfusions for anemia. Chloramphenicol is the drug of choice for treatment. The doors and windows of the patient's room should be screened against flies. Stools and urine should be mixed with disinfectant before being discarded. Family contacts should not be employed as food handlers during the period of contact. Carriers must register with health authorities, are not allowed to act as food handlers, and are instructed in personal hygiene. Cholecystectomy is highly effective for ending the carrier state. Carriers must have six consecutive negative cultures taken one month apart before being released from supervision.

COMPLICATIONS. Hemorrhage and bowel perforation is less common in children than in adults. Urinary infections and nervous complications may follow.

Varicella (chickenpox). INFECTIOUS AGENT. The varicella zoster virus.

SOURCE OF INFECTION. Respiratory secretions of infected persons (droplet). Articles soiled by discharges from the mucous membranes and from the skin of infected persons. Air-borne.

IMMUNIZING AGENT. None.

INCUBATION PERIOD. Two to three weeks.

SUSCEPTIBILITY. Universal: one attack confers a long immunity. A second attack may appear years later as herpes zoster. Herpes zoster has been known to be an original manifestation in a few children.

PERIOD OF COMMUNICABILITY. About one day before the rash to six days after first crop of vesicles.

CLINICAL MANIFESTATIONS. Sudden onset of a slight fever, a maculo-papular skin eruption, which then becomes vesicular and leaves a granular scab. The rash appears in crops, with several stages of maturity present at the same time. There is severe itching and generalized lymphadenopathy.

HERPES ZOSTER. This is a localized manifestation of same virus. Vesicles appear along the nerve pathways, and severe pain is usually present. It is rare in children, but it does occur.

TREATMENT—NURSING CARE. Measures to relieve itching and to prevent infection from scratching include starch baths and calamine lotion. Fingernails should be kept short and mittens should be used if scratching not controlled. The disease varies from mild to severe. Bed rest should be ordered, as well as sedation if itching cannot otherwise be relieved.

COMPLICATIONS. Secondary bacterial infection from scratching. Encephalitis and hemorrhagic complications are rare. Fatal chickenpox has occurred in patients receiving corticosteroid therapy. Such persons should be protected from exposure. If they are exposed, dosage should be reduced as rapidly as possible.

Variola (smallpox). INFECTIOUS AGENT. Variola virus.

SOURCE OF INFECTION. Respiratory discharges from infected persons, from lesions of the skin and from the mucous membrane. Separated scabs may remain infectious for years.

IMMUNIZING AGENT. Cowpox virus by vaccination.

INCUBATION PERIOD. From a week to 16 days.

SUSCEPTIBILITY. Universal. Second attacks rare.

PERIOD OF COMMUNICABILITY. From the first symptoms until all of the scabs disappear.

CLINICAL MANIFESTATIONS. Sudden onset of fever, malaise, headache, severe backache, and abdominal pain, with prostration for about three to four days, followed by a rash similar to that of chickenpox. The lesions, however, are deeper.

TREATMENT—NURSING CARE. Symptomatic treatment and adequate nutrition, (may require tube feeding). Sedation should be given as needed.

COMPLICATIONS. Bacterial infections of the skin are not so common since the use of antibiotics. Bronchopneumonia is relatively common.

Vaccination against smallpox. METHOD. Cleanse the site with ether or acetone. The closed tube containing the vaccine is removed from the freezer unit of the refrigerator just before use, the two ends are broken off, and the contents are squeezed onto the skin by means of a small rubber bulb. The accompanying sterile needle is used to prick the skin through the drop of vaccine (six to ten times) care being taken to penetrate only the epidermis. The area should not be made to bleed. The vaccine is rubbed into the site with the needle, and the site is allowed to dry. The site is not to be bandaged.

REACTION. On the third to fifth day, a red papule appears, followed by a vesicle, which in turn becomes covered with a scab. The scab drops off on about the twenty-first day, leaving a pitted pink scar that eventually fades to white.

A mild fever, headache and malaise usually accompanies the local reaction. The vaccinated area becomes hot and tender on about the ninth day, and the regional lymph nodes become enlarged and painful.

A mild reaction indicates that partial immunity was present before vaccination. An area of redness and induration appearing within 8 to 72 hours, which then fades, usually indicates a complete immunity. No reaction to the vaccine generally indicates poor technique or inactivated virus. A lack of response to repeated vaccinations may indicate an immunity. Vaccination should be repeated every three to five years, and whenever there is a possibility of contact with the disease.

CONTRAINDICATIONS TO VACCINATION FOR SMALLPOX. A serious condition, called eczema vaccinatum, results when an infant with eczema is vaccinated. The eczematous skin becomes covered with vesicles resembling the primary one, and the infant becomes seriously ill. The mortality rate is as high as 40 to 50 per cent. This reaction also takes place if the infant's exposure is to the vaccination of another person.

Other conditions that are contraindications to vaccination are leukemia, hypogammaglobulinemia, acute illnesses and corticosteroid therapy.

CARE OF THE CHILD WITH A COMMUNICABLE DISEASE (ISOLATION PRACTICES IN THE HOSPITAL)

Although children are rarely hospitalized for the uncomplicated childhood diseases, there is still a need for the practice of aseptic technique, a routine more commonly known as *isolation*.

Medical centers and large hospitals may have departments exclusively for patients with communicable diseases, but the majority of smaller hospitals set aside only certain rooms in which contagious patients may be kept separate from the rest.

Isolation may be advised for one of two reasons. Either a child with a communicable disease must be prevented from infecting other patients, or the seriously ill, or chronically ill child may need to be separated from the ward for his own protection.

Infectious Conditions Requiring Isolation

One condition that commonly places a child or an infant in isolation is diarrhea. The majority of cases of diarrhea seen in our hospitals are not of infectious origin, except during certain epidemics. Diarrhea may result from a variety of causes. Food allergies and improper feeding (over-feeding or under-feeding) or a poorly balanced diet may be the cause. Certain nutritional diseases such as celiac disease or cystic fibrosis have accompanying diarrhea. Certain drugs or emotional tension are causative factors. None of these, of course, are infectious.

Infectious organisms that produce diarrhea generally produce severe symptoms. Diarrhea may be of staphylococcal origin, or may be the result of infection by Salmonella, Shigella, Escherichia coli, or by certain viruses. The difficulty in differentiating an infectious diarrhea from one of an allergic or of metabolic origin, stems from the impossibility of determining the causative mechanism from a gross examination of the stool. Stool cultures are necessary to determine the presence of an infectious organism, and stool cultures take a period of time to grow. Therefore, a child with diarrhea of unknown origin is usually placed on an isolation routine until negative cultures can be obtained.

Another cause for isolation is a diagnosis of meningitis. Meningitis may also result from a variety of causes, not all of them infectious. The disease may have a viral origin, be the result of a bacterial infection, or may instead be caused by a meningeal irritation. Other causes could be mentioned as well. Because the cause is often in doubt, these patients are carefully isolated until no further question of communicability exists.

Although children are not ordinarily hospitalized for uncomplicated measles, mumps or chickenpox, many children admitted for other reasons reach the end of an incubation period from a previous exposure, and cheerfully infect their fellow patients. When this happens, the child is frequently sent home, if possible, or moved away from the department. Unfortunately, the period of greatest communicability occurs before a diagnosis is made.

Conditions Requiring Separation of the Child for His Own Protection

A child whose resistance to infection is low, may be placed in *protective technique.* Such children cannot afford to have any infectious condition superimposed on their present one. Children with chronic, debilitating diseases such as nephrosis or leukemia, are readily susceptible to infection and must be guarded. The burned child, particularly, must be diligently protected.

The major difference between aseptic technique and protective technique is simply that an article coming out of a contaminated room must be freed from infection, in some manner, whereas only articles free from infectious material may be taken into the room of the protected child. Rules for either procedure are outlined in the appendix. They may be modified to fit the needs of a particular hospital, but in any case, they are both cumbersome and time-consuming. To the uninitiated, it seems like an endless amount of taking off and putting on, until someone asks "Where is the time to take care of the patient?" It is a good question. One would suppose that a patient whose condition required as much specialized procedure as this must be a patient who needed lengthy and skilled nursing care. No doubt this is usually the case, yet one sees many of these children alone and unattended for long periods of time. If the child cries too much, someone goes to the corridor window (if there is a window) and tries to cheer him from the outside. His play things are limited. "You can't take that in the room, he's isolated," we say. No one has the time to put on a gown and a mask, and scrub for three minutes, just to go into the room to play or to hold him for a while. "He will only cry when I put him back; besides, I have other patients who need my attention. He will probably wet my gown or vomit on my shoulder, and then my uniform will be contaminated." Therefore, unless a child is seriously ill, he is likely to go through a traumatic experience of frustration and loneliness, with little sympathy extended to him.

It is quite possible that a serious study might reveal newer and better methods for the protection of patients from cross infection without the amount of precious time spent in routine preparation. Too often it is just that—routine. One is led to wonder if some nurses believe germs only land on the front of a gown, inasmuch as the backs of their uniforms remain completely uncovered. Again, the nurses appear to believe that germs go to sleep at night, and are active only when someone is around to see that a technique is not broken, Ultimately, aseptic technique is only relative, particularly with so many people going in and out of an isolated room.

This is not meant to be a plea for discarding necessary precautions, not by any means. We must simply ask if we believe these precautions are necessary; we should be conscientious about observing them. If we think of them as just another routine, they should be evaluated or changed, or observed as indicated. This is exactly a nurse's own field, and is an important area of study. If these routines *are* necessary, and they may well be, then we must discover some other way to meet the emotional needs of an isolated child.

CONVULSIVE DISORDERS

Convulsive disorders are not uncommon in children; they are estimated to occur in about five per cent of children under the age of five years. Convulsive seizures may occur from a variety of causes. The most common form of seizure is the febrile convulsion that occurs in association with fevers and acute infections.

Febrile Convulsions

These are usually in the form of a generalized seizure, occurring early in the course of a fever. Although usually associated with high fever (102° to 106°), some children appear to have a low seizure threshold and convulse when a fever of 100° to 102° is present. Febrile convulsions appear most commonly in children under the age of four years.

An isolated convulsion may cause no harm, but repeated convulsions may result in brain damage. Evidence indicates that in some children a febrile convulsion may initiate such a process. Acute pharyngitis, tonsillitis, otitis media and pneumonia are the most common systemic conditions associated with febrile seizures.

A child who has one convulsion should be studied thoroughly. The child's history concerning all phases of his health and of his level of development; documentation of the attack; a complete physical and neurological examination are all called for.

Prevention and treatment for febrile convulsions. Prompt report of elevated temperatures is essential for all hospitalized children. Some pediatricians write orders for treatment if the child's temperature rises above a fixed point. Aspirin and tepid sponges are often ordered for reduction of fever.

Management of convulsions. The child is placed in a horizontal position, with his head turned to one side to prevent aspiration. A padded tongue blade placed between his teeth prevents him from biting his tongue, and will keep his tongue from falling back into his mouth and obstructing his airway. Mouth suctioning is helpful in control of saliva. Whether a course of daily anticonvulsive medication is initiated after a single seizure associated with fever is a matter of divided opinion.

Epileptic Seizures

Epileptic seizures may be caused by injuries or by infections of the meninges and the brain, or may be the result of certain organic or degenerative changes. In many instances, no cause can be determined, and the condition is then labeled idiopathic epilepsy. Onset of seizures of unknown cause is usually between the ages of four and ten years.

The most frequent types of epileptic seizure occurring in children are grand mal and petit mal. Other types of less frequent incidence are minor motor seizures occurring almost entirely in the infant age, and focal seizures involving one part of the body.

Grand mal seizures may be preceded by an aura, although children may have difficulty describing it. The attack consists of a sudden loss of consciousness, with generalized tonic and clonic movements. The initial tonic rigidity changes rapidly to generalized jerking movements of the muscles (clonic phase). The child may bite his tongue or lose control of his urine and his bowel functions. The jerking movements gradually diminish, then disappear, and the patient relaxes. The seizure may be brief, lasting less than a minute, or it may last thirty minutes or longer. Following the attack, some children return rapidly to an alert state, while others go into a prolonged period of stupor.

Petit mal seizures last for only a few seconds, rarely longer than 20. The child loses consciousness and stares straight ahead, but does not fall. He becomes immediately alert following the seizure and continues conversation, but does not know what was said or done during the attack. Petit mal attacks have a high frequency of recurrence, which may be as high as 50 to 100 in a single day. Petit mal seizures usually decrease or stop entirely at adolescence, but they may be succeeded by grand mal attacks that may persist into adult life.

Treatment

Complete control of seizures is the main goal, and this is achieved through the use of anticonvulsant therapy. A number of anticonvulsant drugs are available and are used according to their effectiveness in controlling seizures, and their least degree of toxicity. Phenobarbital, Mebaral and Dilantin given singly, or in combination, have a relatively low toxicity. Mysoline may offer control if these have been unsatisfactory.

Approximately sixty per cent of patients gain complete control of grand mal and focal seizures with the use of these medications.*

Phenobarbital or Milontin, or the two in combination, may control petit mal seizures. (Other drugs of choice are Celontin, Tridione and Paradione.) Phenobarbital is the least toxic of any of these; it may, however, be the least effective.

Many of these drugs have an adverse effect on the hemopoietic, hepatic or genitourinary systems. Periodic tests and examinations are made when these drugs are used, with the drug in question immediately discontinued and replaced by another at the first sign of reaction.

Long-Term Management

Although no accurate figures are available, epilepsy is a common disease. Because of the stigma attached to the condition, some victims make great efforts to conceal their condition. It is probably wiser not to use the term "epilepsy" when explaining the diagnosis to young children. Livingston recounts the instance of a very young child who told his playmates he had epilepsy.† The playmates told their parents, who in turn forbade their children to play with the child, saying that epileptics were "crazy" and "insane."

Epileptic children should be given the same opportunity to receive an education as that provided for other children. Schools, in the past, have often been reluctant to accept these children, either providing no opportunity for education, or by placing them on home instruction. With better understanding, attitudes have changed, and most epileptic children now attend regular classes. Problems still exist, however, mainly because of the lack of understanding of the condition by the general public, and because of the notion, still prevalent among many parents, that epilepsy is shameful; as well as a belief that nothing can be done.

The following narration of the experiences of two epileptic persons illustrates the difficulties experienced by many. Attitudes are slowly changing, but much education concerning the nature and treatment of this disorder is still needed.

A Child Who Desperately Needed Help

Helen S., a senior student nurse receiving her public health experience in a small suburban town, had the responsibility for visiting the elementary school in her area. While she was still getting acquainted, the school principal asked her to stop in his office for a conference.

"We have a little girl in the second grade whom we are probably going to ask to leave school," he said. "She so disrupts the entire grade that the teacher can't handle the situation any longer. Part of the time she is sweet

---

* Farmer, T., (ed.): Pediatric Neurology. New York, Harper and Row, 1964.
† Livingston, S.: Living With Epileptic Seizures. P. 202. Springfield, Illinois, Charles C Thomas, 1963.

and loving—too loving in fact. She rushes up to her teacher, regardless of what is going on, kisses and hugs her fiercely, and upsets order and discipline completely. At other times, she is sullen and uncooperative, refusing to take part in the schedule. She hits the other children and has even hit the teacher —for no reason at all. She is an epileptic and has had several seizures in school, frightening the rest of the children. Parents are starting to object, and the teacher says she must go."

The principal said that he had talked with Susie's mother, who said that her daughter was getting medicine and that nothing more could be done for her. He was reluctant to accept such a defeatist attitude and wondered if the student nurse could help in any way.

Helen made a visit to Susie's home, where she met the child's mother, a pleasant woman who seemed to have accepted the situation as something the family had to live with. The other children went their own way, ignoring Susie as much as she would let them. The child was definitely resented in the neighborhood, and the tale of her misdemeanors was long.

Susie's mother admitted that she "was so wild she climbed the wall," and that she had no control over the child. Susie frequently had "staring" episodes during the day as well as frequent generalized convulsions. Questioning revealed that she had been examined two years before at a seizure center, and had been started on medication, although her mother did not know the name of the medicine—"two kinds of pills," she said. Shortly afterward, the family had moved to another state. Susie had not been examined in the meantime. Her mother continued to give Susie the original pills, but she said they did her no good. She had taken Susie to a doctor once, but nothing came of it, and after the pills were used up, she did nothing more.

Helen discussed the situation with her, strongly urging that Susie be taken to the seizure center in the city for an evaluation. Mrs. S. felt, however, that her husband earned too much for them to be eligible for this kind of service, and yet with a household of children, they could not afford to pay a specialist. She seemed to feel that because Susie did have epilepsy and because the examination two years ago had done nothing more than confirm this, that there was nothing more to be done. She was willing, however, to let Helen make inquiries at the center in the city as to whether they would work with Susie.

Helen did visit the seizure center, which had been opened a short time previously, and after describing the situation, she was able to arrange for Susie's acceptance. Susie was given a complete physical and neurological examination, including an electroencephalogram and psychological testing, and started on a combination of Dilantin and phenobarbital.

Back at school again she became quite manageable, and no more seizures were noted. She was, however, thought to be drowsy and rather slow to respond, and medications were adjusted in an effort to meet her needs. Her parents now began to realize that this was not a hopeless situation, and they were now much more inclined to continue the treatment. Susie's mother was no longer afraid to discipline her and risk another attack. A better understanding of her daughter's condition made her realize that Susie's unacceptable behavior was not the result of her physical condition, as she had supposed. It was rather an expression of her child's deep-seated resentment of the rejection she had received, and of bewilderment over the complete lack of discipline and restraint despite the fact that the other children in the family had to behave. The entire atmosphere was improving, and it seemed likely that this little girl could eventually be helped to achieve a more normal and satisfying life.

Mary T. was a young woman with a somewhat different background. She was an attractive teenager, and worked in the housekeeping department of a hospital. Her sympathetic, cooperative manner made her well liked by both patients and nurses, although they wondered why an intelligent young person was content to spend her days dusting and cleaning. Mary explained this by saying that she had dropped out of high school and had an insufficient education or training for any other sort of employment.

One day, however, the entire unit on which Mary worked was shocked when she had a severe generalized convulsion. The housekeeping supervisor was angry that Mary had concealed her epileptic condition, and thus her dismissal was imminent. Mary tearfully confided to her nursing friends that her life had been miserable. She had not been accepted at school, and had found high school so traumatic she had dropped out. Her seizures, although infrequent, were completely uncontrolled, and she dared not accept dates, or participate in any social life. She had neither close friends, nor any family to help her.

Mary also believed that her condition was hopeless, and she was close to complete despair. Now that she had been forced by this most recent seizure to acknowledge her difficulty, the interested nursing personnel were able to persuade her to seek medical help, and the housekeeping department agreed to keep her on as an employee if she would accept the treatment.

The physician who examined her assured her that she could be helped. His confident, optimistic attitude gave her the first hope she had ever known. Drugs were found to control her seizures completely. After two years without a seizure, Mary had adjusted to the normal social life of any young person, and shortly thereafter was married. She became a well-adjusted member of society, with just a little more sympathy and understanding of the problems of young people than an average person.

The Epileptic in the Community

Parents and older children are entitled to receive complete and accurate information concerning their disorder. The advances in medical understanding, and the ability to control seizures with newer medications take away the hopelessness of the situation and provide the possibility of a normal, well-adjusted life for a majority of affected persons. They also need to understand that epilepsy does not inevitably lead to mental retardation. Studies indicate that continued and uncontrolled seizures increase the possibility of mental retardation, and that the longer the epilepsy is uncontrolled, the greater the possibility of mental retardation.* The data point up the importance of the early discovery and control of seizures.

Although the general outlook is optimistic, there is no point in concealing the nature of the restrictions with which the epileptic is presented. The likelihood is that an epileptic will be forbidden by law to drive a

* Wallace, H.: Health Services for Mothers and Children. P. 370–371. Philadelphia, W. B. Saunders, 1962.

motor vehicle in many, but not all, states. Most states lift the restriction for a person whose seizures are completely controlled, but some do not.

A person whose seizures are under control should be able to obtain employment and perform the work normally expected of any employee, but he may find that he is not accepted. There are also some occupations from which he will find himself excluded by state law or by social custom.

Marriage for an epileptic is still forbidden in certain states, some of whom designate marriage by an epileptic, granting a license to marry, or performing the marriage of an epileptic, as a crime.* These laws should be considered archaic, because there seems no reason for an epileptic to forego marriage, provided he and his partner understand the nature of his disorder, and accept it.

Whether an epileptic should have children is difficult to answer until a genetic mode of transmission is established. The general opinion is that this decision must be an individual matter, with the consideration that the risks of transmission do not appear, at this time, to be much greater than in the normal population.

ACUTE GLOMERULONEPHRITIS

Acute glomerulonephritis is a condition that appears to be an allergic reaction to a specific infection, most often a group A beta hemolytic streptococcal infection, as in rheumatic fever. Not all strains are nephritogenic; one type (12) appears to be the most common of nephritogenic strains, but several others have been identified.

Acute glomerulonephritis occurs most frequently in children between the ages of three and seven years. As a rule, the child is not very ill, and it is often difficult to impress on parents the seriousness of this condition.

Pathology. The kidneys are slightly enlarged and pale, with changes in the glomerular capillaries, which permit the passage of blood cells and protein into the glomerular filtrate. In a majority of cases, these changes are reversible, but there is no way to predict which cases will show complete recovery or will instead develop into chronic nephritis.

Clinical manifestations. Presenting symptoms appear one to three weeks after the streptococcal infection. Most frequently, the presenting symptom is grossly bloody urine; periorbital edema may accompany or precede the hematuria. Fever may be as high as 103° or 104° at the onset but falls in a few days to about 100°. Slight headache and malaise are usual, and there may be vomiting. A transient hypertension appears in 60 to 70 per cent of patients during the first four or five days, returning to normal in about a week.

Oliguria is usually present, and the urine is of a high specific gravity

---

* Livingston, S.: Living With Epileptic Seizures. P. 227. Springfield, Illinois, Charles C Thomas, 1963.

and contains albumin, red and white blood cells and casts. The blood urea nitrogen level is elevated, and the serum albumin is usually low.

Complications. Cerebral symptoms occur in connection with hypertension in a small percentage of cases, consisting mainly in headache, drowsiness, convulsions and vomiting. When the blood pressure is reduced, these symptoms disappear. Cardiovascular disturbance is present in many patients, but has few clinical manifestations in the majority, and is apparent only in electrocardiographic tracings. In most children, this condition is transient, but in some, it goes on into cardiac failure.

Treatment. Although the child usually feels quite well in a few days, it is important that he be kept in bed until clinical manifestations subside. This generally occurs two to four weeks after the onset. Penicillin during the acute stage is given to eradicate any existing infection. A fluid diet is offered for the first few days, followed by a soft to full diet as acute symptoms subside. Low salt or low protein diets are not prescribed except in the presence of edema or renal failure. The treatment for complications is symptomatic.

Nursing care. Bed rest must be enforced until acute symptoms and gross hematuria have disappeared. The child should be protected from being chilled, and from contact with persons with infections. When he is allowed out of bed, he should be prevented from becoming fatigued.

Urinary output must be carefully recorded. Fluids may be restricted, particularly if oliguria is present. If fluids are limited, the day nurse has the responsibility of making sure that an allowance is made for both evening and night fluid intake. Because intake is greatest during the daytime, an allowed intake of 800 cc. might be apportioned approximately in a ratio of 500 cc. for daytime to 200 cc. in evening, and 100 cc. for nighttime, or in some similar pattern.

Blood pressure readings must be accurate. Considerable deviation of pressure readings is possible if the wrong size cuff is used. For accurate readings, a cuff should cover one-third of the distance between the child's elbow and his shoulder. If it is possible, the same cuff should be used each time. Children's blood pressure is not always easy to read correctly, and the child's tendency to resist or to move about does nothing to help. Any doubt as to the accuracy, or any marked deviation from the previous readings automatically calls for a check by another nurse.

Specific gravity of the voided urine, as well as tests for any urinary protein are also part of nursing procedure. Tests such as the Addis count or urine concentration require preparation.*

Continuing care. Traces of protein in the urine may persist for months after the acute symptoms disappear, and an elevated Addis count, indicating urinary red cells, persists as well. Parents are taught

---

* See the Table in the Appendix.

to test for urinary protein routinely, and to collect the urine for an Addis count about every three months, until all evidence of kidney damage disappears. If the urinary signs persist for more than a year, the disease has probably assumed a chronic form.

Prognosis for recovery. In spite of such grave implications, a recovery rate of 82 per cent or higher is reported. In an additional, small number of children, the condition progresses into chronic nephritis. Mortality rate figures for the acute condition are about 2 per cent.

CHILDHOOD NEPHROSIS (LIPOID NEPHROSIS; NEPHROTIC SYNDROME)

Childhood nephrosis is a condition whose main clinical manifestation is a generalized edema that becomes so great that the child may double his true weight. It has a course of remissions and exacerbations, lasting for months, or more commonly, for years. Although the mortality rate remains high, present-day management has allowed many more children to survive until the disease disappears spontaneously, than had previously been the case. Previously, before the availability of effective antibacterial agents and corticosteroid therapy, recovery rates were estimated as low as 30 per cent. Some present-day estimates place the recovery rate at as high as 75 per cent with the use of intensive steroid therapy. In view of the long intervals between recurrences, which commonly occur, final evaluation of present-day data must be deferred until later. The peak incidence of the onset is between one and five years.

Etiology. The etiology of childhood nephrosis is not known. It appears to occur independently of other conditions. In some instances, however, a relationship to glomerulonephritis has been found, and many specialists believe chronic glomerulonephritis may be a progression from childhood nephrosis.

Clinical manifestations. Progressive edema, commencing insidiously and becoming marked, is the outstanding clinical symptom. Extreme ascites is common in untreated cases, and may cause severe respiratory embarrassment. Anorexia, irritability, and loss of appetite develop. Malnutrition may become severe. The generalized edema masks the loss of body tissue, causing the child to present a chubby appearance, but after diuresis, the malnutrition becomes apparent. These children are unusually susceptible to infection, and repeated acute respiratory conditions are the usual pattern.

Laboratory findings include marked proteinuria, with large numbers of hyaline and granular casts in the urine. Hematuria is not usually present. Blood serum protein is reduced, and the total serum globulin level is normal or increased, with a reversed serum-globulin ratio.

Treatment. Steroid therapy has proved to be the most effective method for inducing diuresis, most successful if it is started early in the course of the disease. Clinical improvements from the use of steroids can be anticipated in those patients who do not have irreversible kidney damage. Prednisone has proved to be a satisfactory drug, although cortisone is also used. The drug is given daily in divided doses for ten days to two weeks, until after diuresis has been established. Thereafter, an intermittent course of steroid therapy is maintained, with a program of a certain number of days on therapy, followed by the same number of days off, and then repeated. Such a course is followed for about one year, with adjustments made in the dosage.

Diet is general, high in carbohydrate and without additional salt, but it is otherwise not restricted.

Long-Term Care

Affected children are usually hospitalized for diagnosis, a thorough evaluation of his status in regard to his general health and specific condition, and for the institution of therapy. A course of penicillin is given to clear up any concurrent infection, and unless unforeseen complications develop, the child is discharged with complete instructions for management.

A written plan is most useful to help parents follow the program successfully. They must keep a careful record of home treatment, and bring it to the clinic or to the physician's office at regular intervals.

This home record includes the daily weight, taken at the same time each day, a daily record of urinary proteins, and a daily record of medications as to the kind, the amount, and time given.

The parents must be taught the reactions that may occur with the use of steroids, and also be made to understand the adverse effects of abrupt discontinuance of these drugs. If these things are well understood, the incidence of forgetting to give the medication, or of neglecting to refill the prescription, should be reduced or eliminated entirely. Parents also need to feel free to report promptly any symptoms that they consider caused by the medication.

Special care to keep the child in optimum health is important, and intercurrent infections must be reported promptly. Exacerbations are common, and parents need to understand that these will probably occur, and to report rapidly increasing weight, increased proteinuria or signs of infections for a possible alteration of the therapeutic regimen and the specific antibiotic agents as indicated.

An Addis count is obtained at intervals of two to three months; the parents need to know the necessary procedure to follow when making the urine collection for this test.

Caring for the child at home follows the same pattern as that for any chronically ill child. Bed rest is not indicated except in the event of an intercurrent illness. Activity is restricted only by the edema, which may slow the child down considerably, but otherwise his normal activity is beneficial. Sufficient food intake may be a problem, as it is in other types of chronic illness. Fortunately, there are usually no food restrictions, and the appetite can be tempted by attractive, appealing foods.

Complications from kidney damage necessarily alter the course of treatment. Failure to achieve satisfactory diuresis, or the necessity of discontinuing the use of steroids because of adverse reactions, will call for a reevaluation of treatment. The presence of gross hematuria suggests renal damage. Any persistence of abnormal urinary findings following diuresis presents a less hopeful outlook.

The outcome of the disease cannot be predicted, however, and a length of time with a number of exacerbations does not appear to indicate an unfavorable outcome. Mortality rates are still high, but the prospects for recovery, with no residual damage, are much brighter than before the present course of treatment was instituted.

BIBLIOGRAPHY

American Public Health Association: Control of Communicable Disease in Man. 10th ed. New York, American Public Health Association, 1965.
Cooper, L. Z., and Krugman, S.: Diagnosis and management: congenital rubella. Pediatrics, 37:335, 1966.
Farmer, T,. (ed.): Pediatric Neurology. New York, Harper and Row, 1964.
Gellis, S., and Kagen, B. (ed.): Glomerulonephritis, p. 361, and The nephrotic syndrome, p. 364, In Current Pediatric Therapy. Philadelphia, W. B. Saunders, 1964.
Hammil, J., and Carter, S.: Current concepts: febrile convulsions. New Eng. J. Med., 274:563, 1966.
Heggie, A.: Rubella: current concepts in epidemiology and teratology. Pediat. Clin. N. Amer., 13:251, 1966.
Livingston, S.: Living With Epileptic Seizures. Springfield, Illinois, Charles C Thomas, 1963.
————: What hope for the child with epilepsy? Children, 12:9, 1965.
McGrory, W. W., and Shibuya, M.: Poststreptococcal glomerulonephritis in children. Ped. Clin. N. Amer., 11:633, 1964.
Pickering, D., and Kerr, G.: The management of childhood nephrosis. G.P., 23:111, (Mar.) 1961.
Wallace, H.: Health Services for Mothers and Children. Philadelphia, W. B. Saunders, 1962.

SUGGESTED READINGS FOR FURTHER STUDY

American Academy of Pediatrics: Report of the Committee on the Control of Infectious Diseases. Red book, 15th ed. Evanston, Ill., American Academy of Pediatrics, 1966.
Eisner, V., et al: Epilepsy in the families of epileptics. J. Pediat., 56:347, 1960.
Harlin, V. K.: An obligation to epileptic children. J. Amer. Med. Wom. Ass., 20: 535, 1965.
Korsch, B., and Barnett, H.: The physician, the family and the child with nephrosis. J. Pediat., 58:707, 1961.
Lennox, W. G.: Epilepsy and Related Disorders. Boston, Little, Brown & Co., 1960.
Nelson, W. (ed.): Textbook of Pediatrics. 8th ed. Philadelphia, W. B. Saunders, 1964.

UNIT 6

THE SCHOOL AGE CHILD

19

Normal Growth and Development

A child, as he enters the larger world of the schoolroom, is becoming a self-directed, independent person. Physically, he has attained two-thirds of his adult height, as well as two-thirds of his adult weight. He should be gaining one or two inches a year in height, and three to five pounds a year in weight. His growth and development are affected by his play, his rest, his sleep, his nutritional state, as well as by his heredity. Occasionally, a clinic worker may be puzzled by the small size of a healthy appearing boy until she sees his parents. Then she understands that he is only following an hereditary pattern. A large child does not necessarily mean a healthy child.

At about the age of six, he starts to lose his baby, or deciduous teeth. The first to come out are usually the incisors. At about the same time, his first permanent teeth, the six year molars, appear directly behind the deciduous molars. (Fig. 102)

These six year molars are of the utmost importance and merit some discussion. Because they appear in the spaces behind the deciduous teeth, they are often mistaken for deciduous teeth. This is unfortunate because they are the key or pivot teeth which help to shape the jaw and affect the alignment of the permanent teeth. If they are allowed to decay to the point where they must be removed, the child suffers a handicap that may give him trouble later. Education for the care of the teeth, with particular attention to the six year molars, is important. It is disturbing to inspect young children's teeth and see such a large number with decaying six year molars.

Dental hygiene for children includes a routine inspection, with cleaning and application of a fluoride at least twice a year, and conscientious brushing after meals. A well balanced diet is important for healthy teeth. Sweets should be limited to mealtimes.

THE HEALTH OF A SCHOOL AGE CHILD

In general, this is a healthy age for most children. With the notable exception of rheumatic fever, very few major diseases have their onset during these years. Minor respiratory diseases spread among children in the close proximity of the schoolroom, although the incidence tends to decrease after the age of five or six.

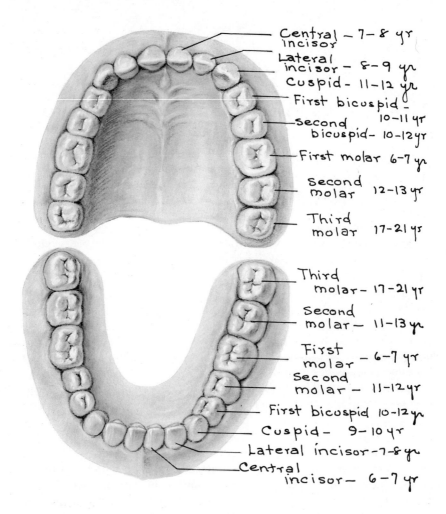

Fig. 102. Eruption of permanent teeth (approximate ages).

Children with head colds, or coughs or sore throats should be kept home from school, kept indoors during cold weather and encouraged to rest as much as possible. With adequate care, a healthy child can throw off these infections easily enough. Unfortunately, the younger brother or sister whom he infects may not come off so lightly, but may instead become seriously ill.

Communicable diseases also make the rounds of the schoolroom among those children who were not immunized during their earlier years, either by inoculation or by the disease itself. Most children, with proper care, recover promptly, but encephalitis and pneumonia may cause severe after-effects.

Skin diseases, such as ringworm or scabies, as well as pinworm infestations, are also easily spread, although present day school health supervision and teaching has reduced their incidence.

Schoolchildren need their full amount of sleep, even though they consider it a waste of time—the day is already too short for their activities. Ten or eleven hours of sleep is still necessary. Rest periods may be needed during the day for the six-, and perhaps even the seven-year-olds.

Nutritional Considerations

The child's appetite should start to improve at five or six years of age. Certainly an adequate diet is important, but other factors, including a pleasant mealtime atmosphere are also important.

Mealtime should never be used for nagging, fault finding, or for correcting a child's manners. A child lives in a child's world, not an adult world. He can learn to accept more readily the adult valuation of manners, soft voices, and all the customs associated with gracious living, if he sees them carried out, consistently, at home.

Indeed he does learn by example. Jimmy's father does not like string beans; everyone knows this, but tonight, Jimmy's mother has served string beans. The father says "Now Bess, you know I don't like string beans. Here Jimmy, have some, they're good for you." Naturally, Jimmy does not like string beans either, and passes them on.

Children frequently go on food "jags," wishing the same food day after day. This soon passes and is unimportant if the child generally gets the necessary nutrients. It does not matter greatly if a child dislikes or refuses a certain food; he is apt to learn to like it later if too much emphasis is not placed on his dislikes. He would have a greater inclination to eat most foods, however, if everyone else accepted them in a matter-of-fact way.

Children like simple, plain foods, are good judges of their own needs if their appetites have not been perverted by coaxing, nagging, bribes or rewards. Even in sickness, an average child knows enough not to eat more than is good for him. A long, debilitating disease may affect him so that he loses his appetite, and strong emotions may cause him to lose interest in food, but force helps little and may have harmful effects.

A child may easily fall into the habit of running into the house frequently and grabbing a handful of cookies or crackers, and then showing a conspicuous lack of appetite at mealtime. Strict curtailment of such snacks may be needed, with only a mid-morning or after-school snack allowed, with perhaps a possible something at bedtime.

A healthy child, full of energy, and generally properly nourished, undoubtedly eats as much as he needs, even though his weight may remain stationary for a time, or show only a very slight gain. Preschool children have sometimes fallen into the habit of dawdling, or of interrupting their meals with play—to mention a few shortcomings—so the school entrance age may be a good time to start afresh. A small child does not have a clear concept of time and may dawdle, until it is too late to eat a good breakfast if he has to clean his teeth, use the bathroom, and get to school on time. He needs a clearly planned schedule, and no doubt plenty of help to keep it.

The health teaching in school reinforces a mother's teaching, sometimes more than she expects, or even likes. Children, at least in the early grades, are greatly impressed by what their teacher has to say. One small boy accused his mother of not serving as many vegetables daily as he thought his teacher had said were necessary; for days, he counted them suspiciously to make sure that he got the right number.*

As a child grows and becomes absorbed in his own private life, he needs direction and discipline in both standards of hygiene and in acceptable table manners—all administered in a cheerful, matter-of-fact way. If he comes to the table with dirt-encrusted hands, he has to be sent back to wash, and may even need to go back a second time to spread the clean area a little further. He expects this, even if he feels it his duty to mumble and to grumble. When the day comes that an average, active boy comes to the table voluntarily with a clean face and with clean hands, a clean shirt, perhaps even a tie, his mother will know that his boyhood days are nearly over.

CHARACTERISTICS OF A SIX- TO SEVEN-YEAR-OLD

His temporary teeth are now beginning to loosen, and he looks forward to the time when one comes out—nor is he above helping this event along by wriggling the loose tooth with his tongue or his fingers. He is quite willing to believe that the dime he finds under his pillow, instead of the tooth he left, was really left by a good fairy.

His belief in magic is real. Usually he still believes in Santa Claus, although this may be from choice rather than conviction. Because his imagination is still keen, he has fears, especially at night, concerning remote, fanciful or imaginary events.

He may lie to escape punishment, or to make himself important, because his ability to distinguish reality from imagination has usually not yet developed fully.

He enjoys group play, but his groups frequently break down into smaller ones of only two or three children. He loves parties, but to him "party manners" are of little importance. His delight in learning is real, and his interest in everything he encounters is intense. Sometimes, to the dismay of his parents, he still shows a lack of discretion. Name calling,

---

* Your Child from six to twelve. P. 113. U. S. Department of Health, Education and Welfare. Children's Bureau, publication no. 324, 1964.

and the use of vulgar words is common. He can rapidly alternate between good and bad behavior.

Physically, this is an age of great activity. He cannot sit still for long. Running, jumping and tumbling are enjoyed for their own sake. He is able to ride a bicycle, and can hop, skip, and gallop at about the sixth or seventh year, and he can keep time to music.

CHARACTERISTICS OF A SEVEN- TO TEN-YEAR-OLD

The six-year-old is moving into a new world, because now a well-adjusted school age child has developed sufficiently to move easily from the small confines of his home into the larger community. He frequently seems to use his home simply as a place of departure. Nevertheless, it is still very much his source of security and strength.

After the age of seven or eight, he tends to shake off his acceptance of parental standards as the ultimate authority in all matters, and is somewhat more impressed by the behavior of his peers.

Physically, his permanent teeth continue to erupt, requiring the same care needed by his temporary teeth. A child has so many absorbing interests at this point, however, that he needs frequent reminders to brush his teeth or to tend to other hygienic matters such as washing his hands, bathing and changing his clothes.

His interest in group play increases, with acceptance into the group or the gang of great importance. These become either boy groups or girl groups. Formed at first mainly for their own sake, they become increasingly project-oriented. Interest in organizations, such as the Scouts and athletic groups, is usually high.

Secret codes and secret language are popular. Individual friendships are formed as well, and they are apt to become quite intense.

Table games, and arts and crafts requiring skill and dexterity are popular, as well as more active pursuits.

Although acceptance by his peers is extremely important, a child will have incorporated into his own personality the normal standards of his parents. He may, under stress, cheat, lie or steal, but he suffers considerable guilt if he has learned that these are unacceptable values. With understanding guidance at home, a let-up of pressures if necessary, and acceptance of him as a person, he should not wander too far from acceptable behavior.

SCHOOL DAYS

A six-year-old is moving into a new world, that of the schoolroom. Perhaps he has attended nursery school or kindergarten and may feel himself to be an "old pro," but he knows that this was not "real" school.

Six-year-old Ruthie dressed up in her new and prettiest school dress and started off with confidence for her first day in the first grade. At noon, an important young lady called home. "Mother, will you pick me up at school and take me to the store? I must buy some school supplies right away. No; I had better not come home first. The supplies might be all gone." So her mother picked up Ruthie in the car and took her to the ten cent store where she carefully selected some crayons, a ruler, an eraser and a pencil. "We have started to study jography," she said. "The teacher asked us where we had spent our vacations, and I told her Pennsylvania. Then I found Pennsylvania on the globe." Ruthie seemed to be off to a good start.

Most children appear eager to start school and go willingly enough. If they have maturational readiness for this experience, are physically healthy and emotionally secure, this eagerness should help them get off to a good start and keep them interested as time goes on.

A child is entitled to an adequate physical examination before entering school, either by a private pediatrician, a child clinic, or by a school physician. Hearing and sight should be checked, defects should be corrected whenever possible, teeth examined, and the general health should be checked. His immunizations should be brought up to date, and he should be re-vaccinated against smallpox and given a booster DPT, unless the child had received these before entering kindergarten. (See immunization schedule in Chapter 9.

Readiness for school is more than physical, however. He should understand certain safety rules, and practice them until they are routine. He should know his full name, his father's name, his street address and his telephone number. It would be extremely helpful if he has met and has become acquainted with policemen, so that he understands one of their duties is to help small children, not to punish them.

He should have learned the function of traffic lights and, hopefully, has watched his family obeying them as a matter of course.

Readiness also includes being able to go to the toilet alone, and to be able to manage his own clothing, with perhaps a little help with the really hard parts of his outdoor wear.

If a child has already attended nursery school or kindergarten, entering the first grade should be pleasing, exciting, and not unduly disturbing. If he has not had that privilege, any preparation should include one, or perhaps several visits to school, a proven ability to accept separation from his home and his mother during the day, and some experience in getting along with other children. He must be able to sit still for short periods of time, and learn to take his turn. Some children who have not matured sufficiently for this experience will do poorly and will dislike school.

EMOTIONAL SUPPORT FOR THE CHILD

An adult can never fully enter into the world of a child. When we say "What makes him act this way?" or when we try to put ourselves in his place, we can do so only to a degree. We know something about how and why a child, under certain circumstances, reacts as he does, because we have studied child reaction and child behavior and because we can also remember our own childhood. We can not know all of the particular factors that influence any particular child's behavior. Neither does the child. He is not good or bad because of any innate goodness or badness, but rather because of the impact of his heredity, his environment, his understanding, and, to a surprising extent, his physical condition.

A child is born with a need to be loved and accepted. When his parents are entirely satisfied with him as he is, he can take his place as a rightful member of the family, with all of the rights and privileges (as well as the restrictions suitable to his age) that such a place provides.

As he grows, his home should be a place where he is accepted for himself. He is expected to make mistakes; if he makes no mistakes, he cannot be learning to be self-reliant. He must be able to turn to his parents when mistakes do occur, and expect to receive direction and advice.

His parents should also make him feel that they think he is the finest child in the world. Not that he can do no wrong; they should recognize that he has to grow and develop. Therefore, they should praise him for his efforts, but should not shame him for his failures, or compare him to others to his own detriment. They should help him to build confidence in himself. A child thrives on praise, and will work to make himself worthy of still more praise.

DEVELOPMENTAL TASKS

In 1950, the White House Conference on Children and Youth presented a scheme of personality development that has been widely used. Building on the sense of trust and autonomy that the well adjusted child should have acquired in infancy and in early childhood, he now turns to the task of finding out what he can do.

The sense of duty and accomplishment, which quite logically grows out of the preceding levels, occupies the period of six to twelve years. This is the period of industry, during which the child is interested in engaging in "real" tasks, and is capable of seeing them through to completion. His developmental learning includes how to cooperate, to lead, to follow, and to observe the rudiments of fair play. He must, however, have his accomplishments noted and rewarded, if he is to develop a sense of achievement and to be able to evaluate himself realistically. If he continually encounters defeat or disparagement—"Bobby does that much better"—he will eventually give up and no longer try.

A good example was Joe, the middle child in the family between a gifted older brother and an equally gifted younger sister, but who was himself rather slow to learn, and appeared to have a rather limited capacity. He was a pathetic, bewildered child who could not do his schoolwork, and whose parents were unable to admit this fact. Never in his life had he been praised for any achievement, nor had he been able to excel in any endeavor. Being thoroughly convinced that he was inferior, he acted that way, and had no incentive to try to reach his own capacity. Granted that he showed a slower rate of learning, he still desperately needed to know that he was good for something.

PROVIDING SEX EDUCATION

Beginning sex education should not, of course, be postponed until school age. The small child who inquires about the difference between himself and his baby sister needs an explanation geared to his understanding.

In today's world, so much emphasis is placed on the importance of truthful explanations that mothers at times become over-anxious. It is obvious that the best teaching can be done by parents who are relaxed and natural, and who fit their teaching into a context of daily living. This is not always easy, however, and many parents feel quite at a loss as to how to work this out.

Intellectually, a mother can accept quite wholeheartedly the concept that she answer the child's questions frankly and simply. Matters become rather more complicated, however, when Sonny chooses the Sunday mother has guests for dinner to ask, "Mommy, where do babies come from?"

For parents who are rather insecure about this, there are excellent booklets that serve as guides for helping children from the preschool age up through young adulthood.

As school age children near the age of puberty, they should be told about the physical changes they should expect, well in advance. A girl who has her first menstrual period at ten or eleven stands a chance of receiving a considerable shock if she has not been prepared. No doubt she has heard various tales from her schoolmates, which admittedly leave much to be desired as a source of information.

In general, girls accept sex teaching best from their mothers, and boys from their fathers. Unfortunately, there are many homes in which either the mother or the father is absent. When a single parent feels inadequate to this task, the various printed aids offer a valuable source of support. These aids are recommended as support for the parents, and provide them with a clearer understanding, allowing them to assume a relaxed attitude. They should not be a substitute for parental guidance. They are valuable, however, as a supplement to parental counselling.*

---

* One excellent series is published by the American Medical Association. Lerrigo, M., and Southard, H.: A Story About You, Facts Aren't Enough, Finding Yourself, Parents' Responsibility, Approaching Adulthood. American Medical Association, 535 North Dearborn, Chicago, Illinois, 1961.

THE DEPRIVED CHILD

Discussions of normal growth and development assume that the child comes from a secure, well-adjusted home, in which there is an ample opportunity for cultural enrichment. Unfortunately, that assumption ignores a sizeable portion of the population which, for a number of reasons, does not have such a background.

Society seems to be awakening to its responsibilities to such children, if only in terms of its own preservation. Enriched nursery school and kindergarten experiences are important ways of preparing for a satisfactory school adjustment for those children whose home life cannot do this for them.

Children who have not been able to achieve a sense of security and trust, because of placement in foster homes, inadequate parents, or because of broken homes, need special understanding, warm acceptance from someone, and intelligent guidance, in order to grow into self-accepting individuals.

THE CHILD IN THE HOSPITAL ENVIRONMENT

Our present hospital policy of early ambulation and of letting the child out of bed whenever this does not interfere with his health or recovery appears to make the child's hospital stay more pleasant, bolsters his morale and is generally desirable. Still, it does call for more thoughtful planning on the part of the nurse in order to take full advantage of the helpful effects, while at the same time, keeping the child from overdoing.

At this age, an average child is quick and alert. He is very much concerned with demonstrating his own competence, and gives himself wholeheartedly to his job. This aspect of development can be of tremendous value to the nurse, if she uses it, in her effort to develop relationships with the children under her care. First of all, however, she must be secure herself before she can relate properly to a child.

Martha had been receiving a rather complicated daily dressing over a long period of time, and had come to learn every step of the procedure by rote. The ritual had eventually banished her fear, but now, a new nurse was to do the dressing, and much of her anxiety returned. The nurse, Miss Brown, recognized Martha's uncertainty and suggested that she needed the little girl's help, because she had not done this treatment for Martha before. From then on, everything went along very well. Sitting on the treatment table, Martha directed the procedure. She told Miss Brown where to find the dressings and how to set up the tray. She told her the order in which to proceed, when to put on her gloves and all the rest. Miss Brown was secure enough to recognize the child's need, and also to take advantage of the child's knowledge and ability.

A few days later, another nurse, who had not done this treatment on Martha before, had to do it. Martha now felt so much a part of the team that she confidently started to play the role that she believed to be hers. The nurse did not have enough security in herself, however, to allow Martha to participate. The first time that Martha said, "We remove that first, then we do this," the nurse said firmly, "I know how to do this, you just sit still." Then she proceeded to do the treatment in her own way. Immediately Martha's anxiety returned, and the entire procedure became a battle between the nurse and her patient. The nurse went away convinced that Martha was a most uncooperative child and reported that she would need help to hold the patient still tomorrow if she was going to be able to maintain any sort of aseptic technique. This seems quite a high price to pay in order to reinforce the nurse's desire to show her authority.

Naturally one does not let the child dictate his own care, but children of this age can understand the reasons behind the various treatments, and if explanations are made, members of the team will usually become enthusiastic, meticulous performers. Then let the nurse beware if she breaks technique!

Helen was a ten-year-old diabetic child who came from a home where affection was present, but where understanding was at a rather low level. She was obliged to take over the management of her own diabetic control if she was to remain in a state of health.

Helen had been admitted twice before for instruction and for control, but this had not been during the pediatric rotation of the student nurse who was now to care for her and give her instruction. Miss Brown was asked to do this and was told that no one was sure how competent the child was, or how much of her previous instruction she had retained. Miss Brown had the task of discovering how much she knew and of proceeding from there.

Helen was a reserved, shy girl, who did not relate easily to new personnel. She indicated, however, that she knew how to draw up the insulin into the syringe, and how to give it. Miss Brown brought a tray containing the insulin syringe, regular and long lasting insulin, and skin antiseptic to Helen's room. Miss Brown said, "Show me how you would prepare the insulin in the syringe." Helen picked up the bottles, carefully shook them, and after deciding which one to put in the syringe first, drew them up correctly. She cleaned the site on her thigh and inserted the needle. She placed the needle in a position which was too horizontal, however, so that it went into the tissue intradermally, instead of subcutaneously. Miss Brown, who had been giving unqualified approval, now suggested that she remove the needle and try again, explaining why. Helen did so, but again placed the needle in the wrong position. Using the greatest possible tact, the nurse removed the needle and demonstrated to the little girl the correct angle for the needle and finished the procedure herself. In spite of the praise for her excellent procedure, Helen's eyes filled with tears, and she appeared distressed that her performance had not been entirely accepted. Miss Brown was distressed over Helen's reaction. She suggested that they both practice later in the day, and use an orange to get the correct angle. This they did, and Helen soon corrected her error. Miss Brown felt that there was more involved here, however, than a mere mechanical error, and spent some time studying the situation.

Helen was a girl with extremely plain features, whose home was in a community in which she did not fit. She had received much rejection in her short life from her peers as well as from others outside her family. Miss Brown

made an effort to establish a genuine friendship with this child and succeeded to the extent that Helen came out of her reserve enough to talk, and
even to begin a show of interest in participating in some activities. Helen's
roommate was a blonde, blue-eyed child who was both the pet of her family
and of the hospital department. Her family and her friends poured in to
visit, walking past Helen without even acknowledging her presence. Personnel waved and smiled to her but seldom noticed Helen. Helen seldom
responded to any overtures anyway, and so she was easily ignored.

One morning, Miss Brown came into the room to find that Helen had
resumed all her defences and failed to respond to any of her overtures. Miss
Brown discovered that the roommate's family had brought several gifts to
her the evening before, had put a pretty bathrobe on her and a dainty cap.

Miss Brown went into action. She spent a long time giving Helen her
bath, lavishly massaging her with a fragrant bathing lotion. She brushed the
child's hair until it shone, and then tied it with a bright ribbon that presented
suitable competition to the other child's cap. The nurse's hope was that the
obvious affection she showed, as well as the extra attention, would help the
child accept her own worth. A conference with staff members was planned
to help them realize that this child needed attention before she could
respond to them. Helen went home before much else could be done, but
Miss Brown became so interested that she planned to see her when she
returned to the diabetic clinic, in order to show her very real interest and
affection for the child.

A healthy child, in mid-childhood, is at a peak of curiosity, enthusiasm
and responsiveness. If we could only take advantage of these qualities,
we would be so much better able to show success in our nursing care.
Nearly every child will enthusiastically participate in his own care if he
understands the reasons.

Preparation for Procedures

A school age child entering the hospital for the first time is interested
in learning about the world around him. If the nurse would take advantage of this interest, she should have little difficulty. For example, a child
who enters for the repair of a heart defect wants to know what is going
to happen to him. Take one of the small plastic hearts that the Heart
Association provides and explain the anatomy, the action and the physiology of a normal heart. Point out the location of his defect, and explain
how it affects the function of his own heart. Show him how it will be
fixed. From there on, it should be easy to explain the reasons behind the
various nursing procedures, and his cooperation can be assured. Of
course he will try to cough, to turn, to accept the unpleasantness of the
chest tubes, the oxygen tent and intravenous fluids—he knows all about
them. Besides the plastic heart, diagrams appeal especially to this age
group, and there are now on the market teaching models of the circulatory
system and of other physiological processes which are fun to put in functioning order and to understand. The child nearly always is admitted
early enough before surgery for the very purpose of getting him accustomed to hospital environment.

There is a distinct advantage present in working with this age group. The nurse should make the most of it. The infant or the preschooler cannot understand, but this child is eager to learn and to know. Knowing gives him an excellent reason for using his own wit and imagination in participating in his own care.

Problems of Discipline

The entire problem of discipline in the hospital deserves careful study. It becomes one of the most frustrating and difficult problems that the nurse meets in the pediatric department.

The dictionary gives several definitions of discipline. Among them are the following.
1. Training to act in accordance with rules,
2. instructions and exercises designed to train to proper conduct or action,
3. punishment inflicted by way of correction and training,
4. the training effect of experience, adversity, etc.

Ruth Strang says that discipline refers to "the teaching of desirable behavior—the guiding of the learning process. The goal of all discipline is self-discipline." She says that discipline should "accentuate the positive."*

It is quite true that the nurse can win if she fights this battle of wills. She has everything on her side; authority, strength, size and reinforcement. What, however, is she likely to end up with after she has secured submission from the child? Surely not a child who has learned to respect authority?

There comes a time in the child's development when he both needs and desires restrictions as a help toward achieving self-control. Of course, when the nurse meets a child in the hospital she finds a person with his personality and character already deeply affected by his home environment. She meets children from widely different home backgrounds, which, of course, does not make her task any easier. A child in the hospital does present many disciplinary problems.

Take that four-bed ward down the hall for example, where four mischievous boys live. Billy has been told by the doctor that he must stay in bed, and he has had the reason for this bed rest carefully explained to him. But Billy feels well enough and sees no great harm in jumping out of bed to adjust the television or to borrow a comic book, or just to sit at the window watching traffic. The nurse comes in and says "Billy, you know that you are supposed to stay in bed." Billy looks around the ward, sees the admiring looks in the eyes of the other boys, and decides. After all, what can the nurse do? It is certainly more fun to be a hero in the eyes of the other boys by defying the nurse than to stay tamely in bed. What to do?

Six-year-old Tommy has learned some very interesting words, and the hospital seems like a good place to try them out. Now, what to do?

* Strang, R.: Introduction to Child Study. P. 216, 344. New York, Macmillan, 1959.

Joey is a boy with many strikes against him. He is shy and withdrawn, and his capacity for understanding does not meet normal expectations. But he loves the company of people, and he especially likes to tag around with the other boys. They don't like this, insult him, tell him to go away, and generally reject him. The nurse sees his stricken face and feels pity for him. What can she do?

This book is not written for the purpose of delving into psychological backgrounds in child illness or child behavior. It is designed to take the child where the nurse finds him, complete with his heredity and background, and try to discover means for making the hospital stay as therapeutic as possible—to the end of sending a child home healthier in all areas than he was on admission.

For present concern, this is a large enough task in itself. Naturally, a child's background is of immense importance in our handling of him, and, indeed, in the objectives we set up for his care. We are not trying at this level, however, to probe into the *whys* as much as the *hows*.

Take Billy's case. Here was a boy who felt that the prescription of bed rest could be observed or ignored according to his whim of the moment. Billy was an intelligent boy of 11 who had a severe dermatitis, with edema of the legs that was increased by walking or standing. The doctor explained to him that bed rest would be beneficial to him while the treatments were being carried out. Billy had been uncomfortable enough before admission to keep him well in line, but now, after he had received permission to use the wheelchair (with his legs elevated) for short periods, he seemed to feel that compliance with these orders was no longer necessary. The other boys were excited by Billy's frequent excursions about the room and also by his attitude of "What are you going to do about it?"

But how to get Billy to stay in bed? Perhaps one way that might help would be to find an occupation absorbing enough to occupy his mind as well as his hands. Assembling a model car or an airplane? A jigsaw puzzle? Surely you can find some interest for this intelligent boy that would lessen his need to defy rules.

It was suggested, in this case, that Billy should be told that the nurse would report these infractions to the doctor with the recommendation that his wheelchair privileges be taken away. This may be necessary. Billy understood the "why" of the restriction, but he chose to ignore it, so here he is—accepting the consequences. Life is not going to be easy with him, making allowances and softening the consequences of his acts. While enforcing necessary limits, we must also be very sure that we are providing an environment within the restricted area that meet his needs—to the very best of our ability.

Restrictions—Are They Necessary?

Naturally, a definite set of rules cannot be written to fit all occasions, or to fit all children. Rules, of course, are as necessary in the children's ward as they are elsewhere, but they should be written primarily for the child's welfare and comfort rather than for the convenience of the ward (although that certainly must be considered as well).

Restrictions against children playing with wheelchairs, especially racing up and down corridors in them, are valid safety measures. If Johnny finds wheelchairs new and fascinating, perhaps someone can find time to push him around in one, even if he does not especially need this form of locomotion.

There may be rules or restrictions that do not seem to make very good sense and may be a carry-over from the past. Children should be allowed, and encouraged, to visit in other wards, to eat together, and to form friendships. A sign on the boy's ward that says in big letters—"NO GIRLS ALLOWED—THIS MEANS YOU," will call for an answer from the girls, "BOYS KEEP OUT." There may be "Nurses may come in except to give shots," or even, "No doctors allowed." This provides for considerable giggling, but no one would be more surprised and hurt than the boys and girls themselves, if the signs were heeded. This certainly is a harmless way to brighten life in the hospital.

BIBLIOGRAPHY

American Dental Association: The Care of Children's Teeth: Questions and Answers. Chicago, American Dental Association, 1956.
———: Your Child's Teeth. Chicago, American Dental Association, 1962.
Blake, F. G.: The Child, His Parents and The Nurse. Philadelphia, J. B. Lippincott, 1954.
Breckenridge, M. E., and Murphy, M. N.: Growth and Development of the Young Child. 7th ed. Philadelphia, W. B. Saunders, 1963.
Child Study Association of America: What to Tell Your Child about Sex. New York, Perma-Books, 1959.
Gesell, A., *et al:* The Child from Five to Ten. New York, Harper & Brothers, 1946.
Lerrigo, M., and Southard, H.: Approaching Adulthood. Chicago, American Medical Association, 1961.
———: A Story About You. Chicago, American Medical Association, 1961.
———: Facts Aren't Enough. Chicago, American Medical Association, 1961.
———: Finding Yourself. Chicago, American Medical Association, 1961.
———: Parents' Responsibility. Chicago, American Medical Association, 1961.
Neisser, E., and Ridenour, N.: Your Children and Their Gangs. Washington, United States Government Printing Office, 1960.
Strang, R.: Introduction to Child Study. New York, Macmillan, 1959.
Watson, E. H., and Lowrey, G. H.: Growth and Development of Children. 4th ed., Chicago, Year Book Publishers, 1962.
Your Child from 6 to 12. United States Department of Health, Education and Welfare: Washington, Government Printing Office, 1964.

SUGGESTED READINGS FOR FURTHER STUDY

Erickson, F.: When 6- to 12-year-olds are ill. Nurs. Outlook, *13*:48, (Jul.) 1965.
Erikson, E.: Childhood and Society. 2nd ed. New York, W. W. Norton, 1964.
Hayes, W., and Gazaway, R.: Human Relations in Nursing. 3rd ed. Philadelphia, W. B. Saunders, 1964.
National Dairy Council: How We Take Care of Our Teeth. Chicago, National Dairy Council, 1965.
Strang, R.: Introduction to Child Study. P. 216, 344. New York, Macmillan, 1959.

20

The Child With Diabetes Mellitus

THE CLASSIFICATION OF DIABETES

An average student nurse has spent considerable class and study time learning about diabetes mellitus and its effect on adults. Perhaps she has done some patient teaching about this. Thus it sometimes happens that she feels this is one area that she knows well enough so that she can spend her pediatric classtime more profitably in other ways.

This train of thought is unfortunate, because the study of diabetes mellitus in children needs a fresh approach. The condition is somewhat the same, but its manifestations are greatly modified by certain factors peculiar to children.

Diabetes mellitus appearing before the age of 15 years is termed *juvenile diabetes* to distinguish it from the type of diabetes mellitus that has its onset in later life. The condition called *diabetes insipidus* is a disease of the pituitary or the hypothalamus gland, and has no relationship to *diabetes mellitus*. Diabetes insipidus is a relatively rare condition, however, and is designated by the entire name. Diabetes mellitus, therefore, is usually simply called diabetes, or juvenile diabetes if the onset occurs during childhood.

INCIDENCE AND ETIOLOGY

An estimated 300,000 children in the United States have diabetes mellitus.* This in itself is of sufficient importance to justify spending additional time learning about its manifestations and its treatment.

Diabetes is now known to be an hereditary disease, probably of a recessive gene character. The wide-spread variability in the manifestation of diabetes mellitus (that is, in its clinical severity and wide range of age at onset) complicates the study of the genetic pattern. In childhood, the presence of an acute infection may, it is believed, be the trigger mechanism activating a latent diabetes.

True diabetes is very rare in the newborn. A transient type of diabetes may be found that clears up shortly after birth, and probably does not recur. True diabetes may occur, however, as early as six months of age,

---

* Juvenile diabetes: *In* Diabetes in the News. Vol. 5, 1966. Published by Ames Co., Division of Miles Laboratories, Elkhart, Indiana.

although the onset is most frequently found between the ages of four and twelve years.

PRESENTING SYMPTOMS

A child is much more prone to a rapid and violent onset than is an adult, who is more apt to have signs and symptoms for varying lengths of time before seeking medical attention. A child is more likely to be losing weight rather than showing a tendency, usually found in the adult, to gain weight. In fact, it may be this failure to gain weight, along with the general impression that he is not up to par, that prompts his parents to bring the child in for a medical checkup, at which time, sugar is found in the urine.

More frequently, however, a child is brought to the physician in a state of acidosis, frequently in a semicomatose state, and sometimes actually in coma. It is, of course, possible that this condition has not appeared so suddenly as it would seem. This is another area in which the nurse in the community has an important role to play. A mother may comment that her baby never seems to be dry, and appears to need diaper changes more frequently than he did formerly. Another mother may find it extremely difficult to toilet-train her toddler; he just won't stay dry long enough. She may also notice, as one mother did, that the child always seems thirsty and wanting a drink. Other children who have been toilet-trained may go back to bedwetting. An increased appetite may also be a symptom, but this often is not so noticeable in the child as it is in an adult.

Symptoms of Diabetic Acidosis

A child developing diabetic acidosis presents the classical symptoms: drowsiness, a dry skin, flushed cheeks and cherry-red lips, acetone breath with a fruity smell, and hyperpnia. There may be nausea and vomiting. If untreated, a child lapses into coma, and exhibits the characteristic Kussmaul breathing, rapid pulse, and subnormal temperature and blood pressure.

Children, as a rule, do not have the residual ability to produce insulin that an adult diabetic may have, and thus they tend to become "complete" diabetics very quickly.

The Nurse's Role in Detection

Whenever a nurse has knowledge of a family history of diabetes, she has an obligation to all members of that family. She needs to be alert to suggestive symptoms in any member, regardless of age. The public in general is not sufficiently aware of the high incidence of diabetes in children, so that the parents may not connect the difficulty in toilet training, or the child's unusual thirst, with any physical abnormality.

The nurse's obligation extends beyond her ability to recognize potential danger signals, however. In her role as an educator, she should make the parents aware of their own obligations. All relatives of diabetics should be considered a suspect group, and should have periodic testing for diabetes.

A nurse need not be an alarmist, but should present the facts in an orderly manner. She should explain the hereditary aspect of the disease, its incidence of onset during childhood among the diabetic population, and the importance of regularly scheduled screening tests.

Recent developments in screening techniques make this a more acceptable idea to the general public. There is now available a filter paper that is to be dipped in urine, dried, and sent to the laboratory to be tested for the presence of sugar. This type of screening has been widely used in statewide campaigns. Persons whose filter-paper reaction indicates the presence of urine sugar are invited to come to a designated center for blood sugar determinations, or to check with their own physicians.

DEFINITIVE DIAGNOSIS

The presence of urine sugar in itself is not indicative of diabetes, inasmuch as it may be the result of overeating, or it may possibly indicate some other condition. A postprandial blood sugar level elevated beyond normal limits, in a child with a history of diabetic symptoms, is strongly suggestive. Most physicians, however, prefer a glucose tolerance test for a definitive diagnosis.

TREATMENT AND FAMILY TEACHING

After it has been determined that a child is diabetic, he is usually hospitalized for a period of time, to stabilize his condition under supervision. The nurse must remember that this is a trying time for the parents as well as for the child, especially if he is old enough to understand its significance. The parent sees his child as someone who "Will always be different," and who will need to take special care of himself all his life. The idea of giving insulin injections is in itself appalling. How easily did you, as a nurse, learn to handle a syringe and a needle? The combination of giving insulin, checking daily urine and calculating diets must appear overwhelming, especially to parents with other children.

Insulin was discovered as recently as 1922. Before that time it was a rare diabetic child who lived to grow up. The parents of a present-day diabetic child almost certainly have heard terrifying stories from friends and from relatives about childhood diabetes. Many of these parents may remember some member of the family, alive at that time, who suffered from all the frequent complications before the advent of insulin.

A child enters the hospital not only for the treatment of his illness and for the regulation of his diet and insulin. He and his parents are there to *learn*. The teaching program in a hospital is concerned primarily with a sound, basic concept of the disease itself. A child can assimilate facts and concepts only as much as his maturational level permits him to. As time goes on, his parents must be his principal teachers; therefore, they must have a satisfactory understanding of the condition. The success of any subsequent teaching about diet, insulin, and exercise and control depends largely on the degree in which the parents grasp the entire picture, as well as the older child mature enough to take the responsibility for some of his own management.

If the hospital does not have a regular instruction program outlined for the patient and for his parents, the nurse should be able to find a number of books and articles to assist her in her teaching, and that would also be valuable for the family to read.

Principles of Diet

Understanding the principles of a diabetic diet is an important aspect of the teaching program. The dietician should be principally responsible for this, but the nurse is the person who ultimately is going to have the task of reinforcing this information, as well as the possibility of having to interpret it.

The present tendency with respect to diet is to put the child on a diet best suited to his nutritional needs for his weight and for his age. Weighed diets are not used so frequently as they were in the past, because many physicians prefer a measured diet, or even a free diet. The measured diet provides a nutritionally adequate diet with the emphasis on protein and vitamin-rich foods. Exchange food lists are used with this diet, and the standard measuring cups and spoons can usually be used. A child on a free diet, should have his nutritional needs carefully considered. The only restriction on the types of food taken is to limit his intake of excessive carbohydrates, such as candy, pastries and cake.

Whether the diet is a measured one with food exchanges, or a so-called "free diet," it is especially important that it be nutritionally well-balanced. It is necessary to find out how much the family understands about basic nutrition and to fill in the gaps when necessary.

A diabetic child needs a liberal amount of protein in his diet, as well as vitamin-rich foods—more than any other child. All this the family must learn and understand.

There are demonstration food trays on the market that are excellent for helping the child learn the basic principles of his diet. These trays are of heavy cardboard with slots cut into the tray for the various cardboard food dishes. All the basic dishes are available in cut-out form, with the nutritional value of the food given on the back of each item. It is as much fun as any game to set up various well-balanced meals on this tray.*

* Food models and display piece obtainable from the National Dairy Council, 111 N. Canal, Chicago, 60606. A catalog of educational materials is available on request.

Urine Reductions

The parents, as well as the child, need instruction in urine reduction. A child of five or six years in not too young to learn, under supervision, the mechanics of urine testing. The parents must be reminded that the tablets, if they are used, are corrosive and harmful, if by chance they are swallowed. The color may be attractive to the child who might want to investigate further. Perhaps the parents should feel the test tube while the tablet is dissolving to discover how hot the solution actually becomes. Any reagent, of whatever type, should be stored away when it is not in use, in order to keep it out of the hands of small children.

A young child in the hospital can watch the nurse while she does the test, and he can help count the drops of urine as they are added. He will be proud of his ability to count, and fascinated over the change of color. Soon he should be able to do it himself under the watchful eye of his mother and should be able to keep his own chart by coloring-in the correct color change.

A child of three or four very quickly learns that there is a relationship between voiding and urine testing, and accepts this as a way of life.

Juvenile diabetes is extremely labile, making it important that urine be tested before each meal, at least until control is established. A second specimen, voided 20 or 30 minutes after the first, will be more accurate and should be obtained, if at all possible. It does present a problem to little tots who have only recently been toilet-trained. When asked to "go potty" they are apt to protest, "But I did go potty," and to feel quite injured that they are not considered to have performed satisfactorily. Usually, it is best to test a toddler's urine every time he voids, because it is entirely unpredictable as to whether he will go at the designated times.

After the child leaves the hospital, urine reductions are usually continued three or four times daily. Clinitest tablets are preferable to the use of Clinistix for routine testing.

Many physicians prefer to regulate the insulin so that a small amount of sugar will appear in the urine, (one plus or trace). They consider the slight spill-over of sugar in the urine to have a less dangerous potential than the possibility of frequent insulin reactions from lowered blood sugar. The physicians who treat in this manner ask to have repeated reductions showing negative results reported for a possible decrease in insulin. Tests for acetone, using acetest tablets, are made at the same time as a blood sugar monitoring device. Any appearance of acetone in the urine should be reported immediately.

A school-age child may have difficulty, or may experience embarrassment over noon-time urine reductions. If he does not go home at noon, the physician may allow him to skip the noon test, or a child may go to the school nurse's office to do the test. One girl collected urine in a tightly corked test tube, carried it in her purse and tested it at home after school.

A child should be taught to keep a record of urine reductions, making a color chart or using one of the prepared charts. Some supervision from the parents is necessary, particularly if the chart is repeatedly negative. Children frequently get bored or angry over the whole thing, and the testing of tap water in place of urine is not unheard of. Charts have even been made up neatly for a week in advance. Parents need to understand the child's emotions, however. Probably some scheme of a routine check —perhaps a weekly test—would be more acceptable than a check based on doubt or suspicion.

Insulin: Type and Method of Injection

Because diabetic children have no residual ability to produce insulin, it is probable (according to our present knowledge) that he will always need to take insulin. Oral medications are frequently useful in maintaining a satisfactory blood sugar level for an adult who has developed diabetes late in life. The child, however, must have insulin supplied to him, although some of the oral medications, when given in conjunction with insulin, assist in its utilization and provides better control. The family should understand, however, that insulin is required, and that the child's requirement is going to increase gradually as he grows.

The type of insulin ordered is determined by the child's needs. Children are usually treated at the start of the disease by doses of regular insulin, given according to color changes in the urine. As soon as possible, the child should be placed on a probable daily dose of long-acting insulin, usually with supplements of regular insulin before meals, given according to color changes in the urine. NPH insulin, intermediate between regular and protomine zinc (PZI) insulin in its length of effect and the rapidity of action, is frequently chosen.

It is important that all children receiving long-acting insulin in the morning have a bedtime snack in the evening, in order to avoid an insulin reaction during the night.

Frequently, children on long-lasting insulin go into shock during the early morning hours. The night nurse must observe the child at least every two hours, note the tossed bedding that would indicate restlessness, note any excessive perspiration, and if necessary, try to arouse him. As the child becomes regulated and observes a careful diet at home, his parents need not watch him so closely, but they should have a thorough understanding of all aspects of the disease.

An example of the sort of thing that can happen in a hospital concerns a six-year-old boy, who, after being put to bed at 9 PM, slept soundly all night. His night nurse became suspicious of a possible reaction at about 4 AM when she found him quite wet with perspiration and discovered his bedding tossed about. She was able to awaken him enough to get a urine specimen, which upon testing showed a strong positive reaction for sugar. Not satisfied, however, she asked advice, but the decision was made that the high sugar ruled out insulin shock, so nothing was done. At 7 AM the child could not be roused. A blood sugar determination revealed hypoglycemia, and intravenous glucose had to be administered to bring the child out of coma. Why did he show glycosuria at 4 AM? The answer is simple; he had last urinated at 9 PM, and sugar-containing urine had been collecting in his bladder all night.

Insulin reactions. Because diabetes in children is extremely labile, the child is subject to insulin reactions. A nurse should take note that a child may not recognize an impending reaction, particularly if he is young. She should also recognize that both she and the parents may have some difficulty recognizing reactions.

An example occurred when two-year-old Donald was hospitalized for the regulation of his diabetic condition. He had entered the hospital in deep coma and now, two weeks later, he was still having some difficulty in adjusting satisfactorily to his diet and his insulin dosage. One day at naptime, he went to sleep in his usual manner, and it did not occur to his nurse that anything was wrong, yet he went into insulin shock during his sleep. When a nurse found him perspiring deeply, and had great difficulty in arousing him from his nap, she realized that these children present somewhat different problems from those of the diabetic adult.

Some of the symptoms of impending insulin shock in children are— any type of odd, unusual or antisocial behavior; headache and malaise; blurred vision and faintness, and undue fatigue or hunger. One small child complained of hunger just before evening tray time, and before the nurse could bring her supper tray, she went into a convulsion. After two such episodes, the nurse learned to have orange juice readily available for the child whenever she complained of hunger. One older child, however, worked a system for obtaining a little extra juice. Every afternoon, he regularly complained of faintness and was convincing enough to get his juice. After a few such episodes, blood sugar determination revealed that his blood level was at the highest at this time of day. He was an intelligent child, and after the tests and their significance were explained to him, he cooperated, and his afternoon reactions ceased.

Most newly diagnosed diabetic children show a decreased need for insulin during the first weeks or months after control is established. This is a natural reaction, and it should be explained to avoid the false hope that the diabetic is "getting better." As the child grows, his need for insulin increases and continues to do so until he reaches full growth. Again, this needs to be explained; the child's condition is not "getting worse."

Another matter that merits discussion is the use of insulin during illness or an infection in a diabetic child. When an ill child is unable to eat his prescribed diet, his mother rather naturally assumes that his insulin dose should be reduced. This is not the case, however; his insulin may actually need to be increased during this period.

In actual fact, this all points up the importance of close supervision by the physician. Parents need to understand this, and should have no hesitancy about reporting any change in the child's health, any recurring insulin reactions, the presistence of more than a small amount of urine sugar, and, in particular, any positive urine acetone reaction.

Methods of giving insulin. The child will not be able to take over the management of his insulin dose as early as he learned to test his urine, but he can watch the preparation of the syringe, and learn the technique for drawing up the dosage. If he can watch until it becomes routine, it might be helpful. By the time he is eight or nine, he should be thinking out his dose and getting the feel of the syringe. He should be drawing up his own dosage and preparing for the time when he will be caring for himself. Just when that comes cannot be stated arbitrarily. No two children mature at the same rate; some may be able to do this quite early. For others, this may be an act of love on the mother's part, showing her

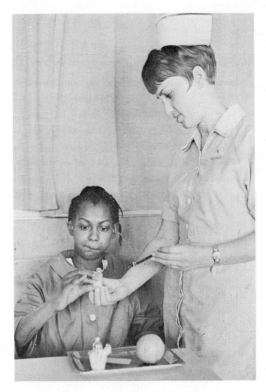

Fig. 103. Learning to prepare insulin.

concern and care for him. A child should be encouraged, however, to take over the management of his therapy as soon as he is ready. *He can learn the importance of the routine and accept the restrictions his disease imposes if he has helped to make the decisions.* (Fig. 103)

Manner of injection. The child and his parents should be taught the correct way to give insulin, and supervised until it is certain that they are injecting the insulin subcutaneously rather than intradermally.

Rotating injection sites is also a matter of considerable importance. If insulin is given frequently in the same location, the area is apt to become indurated and is eventually fibrosed, hindering proper insulin absorption. The atrophic hollows in the skin, or the lumps of hypertrophied tissue, are unsightly as well. Some people, however, appear to have a greater skin sensitivity than others.

Definite instruction should be given concerning the importance of rotating sites. Areas on both the upper arms and the upper thighs can be used, allowing several weeks between the use of the same site, if a plan is carefully mapped out. Starting from the inner, upper corner of the area, each injection is given one-half inch below the preceding one, going down in a vertical line, with the next series starting one-half inch outward at the upper level. The lower abdomen may also be used if necessary. If there is any sign of induration, the local site should be carefully avoided for a period of weeks after all signs of irritation have disappeared.

Occasionally, some people have allergic reactions to the protamine in NPH or protamine zinc insulin (PZI), and have to change to Lente insulin.

Exercise in the Hospital

It would be unrealistic to attempt to regulate a child's diet and insulin dosage if we insist in keeping him unduly quiet in the hospital. We want him to be a normal, active child at home, and thus we teach him that he can resume all normal activities. He needs an opportunity to be active, at the same time learning how to handle his condition. If possible, a child should be allowed to play outside. If conditions do not permit this, he should be able to obtain activity within the hospital, with an opportunity for active exercise, such as bicycle riding, in the physical therapy department and in the playroom.

Continuing Home Care

A diabetic child should carry some form of sugar with him at all times. Candy is useful, although perhaps it presents more temptation to the child than does pure sugar. In cases of doubtful insulin reactions, it is undoubtedly better to give sugar than to withhold it, but frequent reactions indicate a need for a physician's attention.

It is extremely important that a child wear an identification medal or a bracelet, with information about his diabetic status. Identification cards, such as those carried by many adult diabetics, are seldom practical for a child diabetic.

Some of the difficulty encountered in regulating blood sugar stability stems from the variations in an average child's activity. His school day contains many hours of sitting still, interspersed with sports or gymnastics, whereas on weekends and vacation periods, he may be much more active. Theoretically, his greatest periods of activity should come at the time of day when his blood sugar is highest; in practice, this is not always possible for a school child. Many physicians advocate a slight reduction in insulin or a diet increase for those days when the child is more active physically. This calls for good judgement and understanding on the part of the child's parents.

A diabetic child should participate in normal activities for his age, and should consider himself a normal child. He should, however, make his diabetic condition known to at least one friend, and should not go swimming or hiking without a responsible individual nearby, who knows what to look for and who knows what to do if the child should have a reaction.

Some older children are quite sensitive about their condition, and fear that they seem "different" from their friends. Even with the best of instruction and preparation they may feel this way, and wish to keep their condition secret. They must understand that a teacher or some other adult in their environment should be acquainted with their condition. Classroom teachers should know which of their students have such a condition, and should understand the signs of an impending reaction. Any unexplained inattention, blurring of vision, or other unusual behavior, should alert the teacher to this possibility.

Diabetic children under good control need not be kept from such activities as camp-outs, overnight trips with the school band, or other, similar activities away from home. Of course, a child must be capable of measuring his insulin and giving his own injections. Some young people report that a desire to participate in such an activity was the factor that overcame their reluctance to take over this responsibility.

The disposable insulin syringes and needles now on the market simplify traveling for the diabetic. They come several to a package, and are relatively inexpensive. A diabetic must keep in mind, however, that a number of states sell insulin syringes and needles only on prescription— a fact that a young person might not realize if his syringes have been bought in one drug store. When he travels, he should take a prescription with him for presentation if, for any reason, he needs to buy equipment. He must also make sure that a responsible person on the trip knows that he has diabetes, has a knowledge of the symptoms of insulin reaction and diabetic acidosis, and knows what to do. The family with whom he stays on week ends must also have this information.

The Treatment of Insulin Shock

Any indication of an insulin reaction should be treated immediately by allowing the child to take sugar, candy, or orange juice, even if the parents suspect the child of faking. Any normal child breaks the rules once in a while. Repeated reactions, or impending reactions, either real or fancied, call for a checkup by a physician.

Because reactions are apt to progress rapidly, every adult responsible for a diabetic child should clearly understand the procedure to be followed if the child is unable to take any form of sugar orally. Glucagon is a substance that can be administered subcutaneously, brings about a prompt rise in blood sugar, and is invaluable for use as an emergency measure. All parents, school teachers or nurses, and other adults, even temporarily in charge of diabetic children, should have access to this drug and should understand its use.

Glucagon is a hormone produced by the pancreatic islets that also produce insulin. Whereas an elevation of blood glucose results in an insulin release (in a normal person) a fall in blood sugar stimulates glucagon release. The released glucagon in the blood stream acts on the liver to promote glycogen breakdown and glucose release.*

Glucagon is now available as a pharmaceutical product, packaged as a powder in individual dose units. A person preparing the dosage need only add the diluent, which comes with the powdered drug, by the use of a sterile syringe and needle, draw up the solution, and administer it in the same manner as insulin.

Glucagon acts within minutes to restore a child to consciousness, after which he can take candy or sugar. This treatment prevents the long delay occasioned by waiting for a doctor to come and administer glucose intravenously, or waiting for an ambulance trip to the hospital emergency department. It is, however, a form of emergency treatment, and not a substitute for proper medical supervision.

ADOLESCENCE

Adolescence is an extremely trying period for many diabetics, as it is for other young people. Because a normal child has to work through from dependence to independence, so does the diabetic child. Even when a child has accepted much of his own care, he may rebel against the control that this condition places on him. Frequently he becomes impatient, and seems to convince himself that he really does not care about his future health. He may skip meals or drop controls over his diet, or he

* Jacob, S., and Francone, C.: Structure and Function in Man. P. 448. Philadelphia, W. B. Saunders, 1965.

may neglect urine reductions. It can be a difficult time for both the parents and their child. The parents naturally become concerned, and are apt to give the child more controls to rebel against. Special care should be taken by the family, the teachers, the nurses and the doctors to see that these young people find enough maturing satisfaction in other areas, and do not need to rebel in this vital area.

If a child completely understands all aspects of his condition (especially if he has been allowed to assume control of his treatment previously) he should be allowed to continue. Should he run into difficulty, this is a time when an adolescent clinic can be of great value. Here he can discuss his own problems with understanding people, who treat him with dignity and listen to him.

FUTURE HEALTH

According to present knowledge, a person who develops diabetes during childhood will always have diabetes. No way has been found to stimulate the non-functioning Isles of Langerhans in the pancreas to the production of insulin. Since the discovery of a chemical method of producing insulin, however, the lack can be overcome, and a young person can look forward to a life of normal activity.

Present day studies indicate, however, that we have been over-optimistic in our assumption that these persons necessarily escape the serious degenerative diseases common among diabetics in later life. The complications appearing with relative frequency in young adults who have had diabetes for 10 to 20 years, include arteriosclerosis with hypertension and degenerative eye and kidney conditions. Whether such conditions are manifestations of a phase of diabetes not affected by available therapy, or whether they are in large measure the result of insufficient clinical control is not entirely clear at the present time.*

BABIES OF DIABETIC MOTHERS

Babies born to diabetic mothers are among the "high-risk" babies, with a high percentage of stillbirths or early death. These babies tend to be large and plump, with a puffiness resembling a "cushingoid" appearance. They frequently are hypoglycemic and hypocalcemic, and the respiratory distress syndrome appears more commonly than in other full-term infants.

A diabetic prospective mother who places herself early under adequate medical supervision and who adheres conscientiously to her diabetic regime, affords herself and the infant the best chance for a healthy life.

* Nelson, W., (ed.): Textbook of Pediatrics. 8th ed., p. 1324. Philadelphia, W. B. Saunders, 1964.

BIBLIOGRAPHY

Ames Company: Juvenile Diabetes: Diabetes in the News. Vol. 5. Elkhart, Indiana, the Ames Company., 1966.

Bain, H. W., and Chute, A. L.: Diabetes in school children. Pediat. Clin. N. Amer., *12*:919, 1965.

Jacob, S., and Francone C.: Structure and Function in Man. P. 448. Philadelphia, W. B. Saunders, 1965.

National Dairy Council: Food Models and Display Piece. Chicago, National Dairy Council.

Nelson, W., (ed.): Textbook of Pediatrics. 8th ed., P. 1321. Philadelphia, W. B. Saunders, 1964.

Traisman, H. S., and Newcomb, A.: Management of Juvenile Diabetes. St. Louis, C. V. Mosby, 1965.

SUGGESTED READINGS FOR FURTHER STUDY

Greathouse, R. F.: The diabetic child after stabilization. Pediat. Clin. N. Amer., *8*:179, 1961.

Lowrey, G. H.: Management of the Young Diabetic Patient. pt. 1. J. Mich. Med. Soc., *61*:1097, 1962. ibid., pt. 2, *61*:1230, 1962.

Thosteson, G. C.: Observations on the young diabetic child. J. Mich. Med. Soc., *61*:1205, 1962.

21

The Child With
Congenital Heart Disease

It is a great shock to parents when the discovery is made that their child has a heart abnormality. The heart is *the* vital organ; one can live without a number of other organs and appendages, but life itself depends on the heart. To know that an infant is starting life with an imperfect heart is a matter of great concern. Naturally, the question is, "How serious is it?" People have heard about "innocent" heart murmurs. Is there a chance that he can outgrow the condition?—and finally, can it be fixed?

It is a difficult task for a doctor or a nurse to try to answer questions about a child's heart condition. In the first place, a definite answer may not be known. Second, how do you answer encouraging optimism and hope, without giving false assurances and without encouraging unfounded hopes? For example; a mother who mourned and who upset the ward because her child was on his way to heart catheterization. She was sure he would not survive this procedure, and was not helped at all by the assurance that "Children don't die from heart catheterization." Her child *did* die during the procedure. The mother was understandably bitter, and the nurse learned an unforgettable lesson.

The newborn with a severe abnormality, such as a transposition of the great vessels, is blue from the start of his life, and requires oxygen and special treatment from the beginning. A less seriously affected child, whose heart is able to compensate to some degree for the impaired circulation, may not have symptoms severe enough to call attention to his difficulty until he starts to walk. Others may live a fairly normal life and not be aware of any heart trouble until a murmur or an enlarged heart is discovered on physical examination in later childhood. Some abnormalities are slight, and allow the person to lead a normal life without correction. Some may cause little apparent difficulty but need correction to improve the chance for a longer life and for optimum health during the adult years. Some severe anomalies are incompatible with life for more than a very short time, and others may be helped but not cured by surgery. For still others there may be no treatment as yet.

402

EARLY INDICATIONS OF CARDIAC DIFFICULTY

A cardiac murmur discovered early in life is an indication for frequent physical examinations. This may be a functional, "innocent" murmur that may disappear as the child grows older, or it may be the chief manifestation of an abnormal heart or an abnormal circulatory system. The most frequent parental complaint is of feeding difficulties. Infants with cardiac anomalies severe enough to cause circulatory difficulties have a history of being poor eaters, tiring easily from the effort to suck, and fail to grow or to thrive normally.

Manifestations of congestive heart failure may appear the first year of life in infants with such conditions as transposition of the great vessels, large ventricular septal defects, and with other serious defects. One indication of congestive heart failure in infancy is easy fatigability, manifested by feeding problems. The baby tires, breathes hard, refuses a bottle after one or two ounces but soon becomes hungry again. He has greater difficulty lying flat, and appears to be more comfortable if held upright over an adult's shoulder.

Other signs are failure to gain weight, a pale, mottled or cyanotic color, a hoarse or weak cry, and tachycardia. Rapid respiration (with an expiratory grunt), flaring of the alae nasi, and the use of accessory respiratory muscles with retractions at the diaphramatic and the suprasternal level are other clinical manifestations of congestive heart failure. Edema is a factor, and the heart generally shows enlargement. Anoxic attacks (fainting spells) are common.

Treatment for congestive failure includes digitalization, diuretics to reduce any edema, oxygen, and the use of morphine for relaxation. The infant should be placed in a slanting position with the head elevated. An example illustrates the care and treatment of infants in failure.

Baby C, at the age of 28 days, had a history of atelectasis at birth with continuing respiratory difficulties for several days. He was moderately dusky, becoming increasingly cyanotic with feeding, and had been in an isolette with oxygen since birth. A loud, systolic murmur was present. At four weeks of age, he showed no undue respiratory distress, but he had experienced two anoxic spells. He held his breath, became stiff and rolled his eyes. His color became deep red. Cardiac catheterization showed a transposition of the great vessels, with a large patent ductus and an atrial septal defect. He was given a course of digoxin intramuscularly, followed by a maintenance dosage. Mercuhydrin was given for diuresis, and morphine was given for anoxic episodes. Improvement was noted. His color was less dusky, even when he was out of oxygen, and his feeding pattern improved. Because of the patent ductus and the atrial septal defect allowing the mixture of saturated and unsaturated blood, maintenance on medical treatment may be possible for the present.

Because surgery carries less danger for an older child than for an infant, whenever possible affected children should be maintained on medical treatment until the optimal time for surgical procedure.

SURGICAL CORRECTION

The Child at Home Before Surgery

A child with congenital heart disease may show easy fatigability and retarded growth. If he has a cyanotic type of heart disease with clubbing of his fingers or toes, periods of cyanosis and reduced exercise tolerance are evident. This young child assumes a squatting position when he is tired from play. Specific manifestations in several heart conditions are given in the section describing the various types.

Such a child should be allowed to lead as normal as possible a life. Parents are naturally apprehensive and find it difficult not to over-protect the child. They frequently increase their child's anxiety and make him fearful about participating in normal activities. Children are rather sensible about finding their own limitations, and will usually limit their activities to their capacity if they are not made unduly apprehensive.

Some parents are able to adjust well and provide guidance and security for their sick child. Others may become confused and frightened, and show hostility, disinterest or neglect, and stand in great need of guidance and counseling for themselves. Some children have had several periods of hospitalization for respiratory infections, cardiac difficulties or for other reasons.

Routine visits to a clinic or to a doctor's office become a way of life, and the child may come to see himself set apart from others. Doctors and nurses have a responsibility to both the parents and the child to give clear explanations of the defect, using readily understandable terms and illustrating their explanations with appropriate diagrams, pictures or models. A child can accept much and can continue with the business of living if he understands what it is all about.

Hospital Preparation for Surgery

When a child enters the hospital for cardiac surgery, it seldom is his first admission. Generally, it has been preceded by cardiac catheterization or perhaps by other hospitalizations. Admission is scheduled to precede surgery by a few days, in order to give time for adequate preparation. Parents should understand that blood may be drawn for typing and cross-matching and for other determinations as ordered. Possibly additional X-rays may be made, and the child may be photographed.

Apparatus to be used after surgery should be described with drawings and pictures. If possible, the parents and their child should be taken to a cardiac recovery room and should be shown chest tubes, an oxygen tent, and the general appearance of the unit. Judgment should be shown about the timing and the extent of such preparation, because nothing is gained by arousing additional anxiety with premature or excessively graphic descriptions. A young child can become familiar with the surgical dress worn by personnel, with the oxygen tent, and perhaps listen to his heart beat. He should practice coughing, and should understand that he will be asked to cough after surgery, even though it will hurt a little. The preparation described in the nursing care study at the end of the section clearly illustrates what can be done for a young child in order to minimize the strangeness and fearfulness of this type of surgery.

Physical preparation will undoubtedly include pHisoHex baths and shampoos, a Fleet's enema (or Dulcolax suppository) to empty the intestines; careful recordings of vital signs, including blood pressure, weight (preferably taken on the same scales to be used after surgery) and the administration of antibiotics. An anesthesiologist will visit the child the day before surgery, as well as the cardiac surgeon.

Cardiac Surgery

Open heart surgery, using the heart-lung machine, has made extensive heart correction possible for many children who would have been otherwise hopelessly doomed to invalidism and a short life span not many years ago. Machines are now available for infants and small children, although the mortality rate among infants undergoing open heart surgery is still high. If a choice is possible, surgery should be postponed until later childhood.

Hypothermia is a useful technique for providing a bloodless field for the surgeon. The preferred method for inducing hypothermia at present is to cool the blood by the use of cooling agents in the by-pass machine, rather than by packing the child's body in ice.

At the end of surgery, thoracotomy tubes are left in the pleural space so that any collections of fluid or air may be removed by suction, and the blood loss is replaced. The child is taken to the cardiac recovery room to be skillfully nursed by specially trained personnel for 72 hours, or longer if necessary. Children who have had closed chest surgery need the same careful nursing.

Postoperative Care

On admission to the recovery room, the chest tubes are attached to the closed suction bottles, and the child is placed in a croupette or in an oxygen tent. Attachment of a cardioscope to the patient enables the nurse to monitor the heart rate constantly, as well as the rhythm, and the electrocardiogram. (Fig. 104)

Nursing care for a patient following open heart surgery is highly specialized, and requires specially trained personnel. Intravenous blood and fluids are monitored, because great care must be taken not to overload the heart. Chest drainage should be observed for its color and its amount, and recorded. The patient should be turned every hour and helped to cough. Daily chest X-rays should be taken, and the urine output should be recorded. The patient is carefully observed for any signs of hemor-

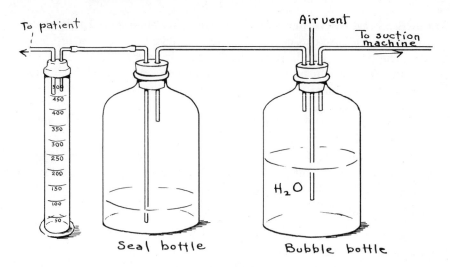

Fig. 104. Water seal chest drainage apparatus.

rhage, shock, infection or cardiac arrest. With all this, the patient must be kept as relaxed and as free from apprehension as possible. Sedation is sometimes ordered for this purpose. Because of the specialized training necessary to care for a child immediately following open heart surgery, no attempt is made here to detail the care given in the recovery or in the intensive care units.

By the time the child returns to the ward, his chest drainage tubes have been removed, he has started taking oral fluids and is ready to sit up in bed or up in a chair. He probably feels rather weak and helpless after his experience, and needs encouragement and reassurance. As he recovers, however, a child is usually quite ready for activity. His improved health provides the incentive. Mothers usually need to reorient themselves and to accept their child's new status—an attitude that is not easy to acquire after years of anxious watching.

The surgeon and his staff evaluate the results of the surgery and make any necessary recommendations regarding the resumption of the child's activities. Plans should be made for both follow-up and supervision, as well as for counseling and guidance, as the parents need it.

The American Heart Association has established standards for centers caring for patients with congenital heart disease, together with recommendations for their use. In general, the facilities needed for this type of cardiac surgery are not readily available outside of medical centers. Crippled children's centers include diagnosis, surgery and follow-up care in their programs. In addition, regional centers for the diagnosis and treatment of children's congenital heart conditions have been established in certain areas with the help of a special grant from the Children's Bureau of the Federal Government.

Open heart surgery requires complicated, highly specialized apparatus that is fantastically expensive. In addition, many hours of service by a large number of professionally trained persons are required. It is with help provided by such programs that an average family is able to take advantage of these professional services.

DIAGNOSTIC TESTS

Electrocardiography

Electrocardiography is of relatively less importance in the diagnosis of congenital heart anomalies than it is in acquired heart disease. Nevertheless, it is still a useful, convenient tool in pediatric cardiology, especially if it is used together with data obtained from clinical and X-ray examination.

Cardiac Catheterization

Cardiac catheterization assists greatly in the evaluation of difficult cases of congenital heart defects. It should be used in conjunction with all of the other diagnostic procedures, such as physical examinations, an assessment of the clinical evidence, roentgenographic examinations and electrocardiographic studies.

Cardiac catheterization has been employed as a diagnostic device for a number of years. It is not entirely benign, a fact that must be kept in mind when giving assurance to anxious parents. The mortality rate, however, is very low. An extremely ill child is at risk regardless of any procedure—or even at rest in his crib. A nurse may feel that the mother is unduly disturbed and may be tempted to give her false assurance, an act that she may deeply regret if the child does not survive.

The patient must be relaxed and without apprehension, but care must be taken to avoid medications that depress respiration. General anesthesia may be employed for very small children, but generally sedation is sufficient.

Right Heart Catheterization

The cardiac catheter is inserted into an exposed vein, frequently the saphenous vein in infants and small children, or perhaps the median basilic vein in older children. The catheter is advanced through the median basilic, the axillary, the subclavian, and the innominate veins, into the superior vena cava, the right atrium, the right ventricle, the pulmonary artery, and from there, usually out into one of the smaller pulmonary branches.

This procedure takes place under intermittent fluoroscopy, with spot films or cine strips taken at particular locations. Blood pressure is recorded and blood samples are taken while the catheter is in the various arteries and heart chambers.

Left Heart Catheterization

If a more complete study is necessary, left heart catheterization is performed. In small children, it is frequently possible to enter the left atrium and the left ventricle by passing the catheter from the right atrium across the foramen ovale. When it is not possible to enter the left ventricle by this route, or, when disease of the aortic valve is suspected, a catheter is passed retrograde from the femoral artery to the aortic arch and the left ventricle.

When left heart catheterization is performed on children over nine or ten years of age, a trans-septal needle may be used to puncture the atrial septum, and the catheter may then be passed through into the left chambers. Some centers use the trans-septal needle on small children as well.

Angiocardiography and cinefluorography are used as necessary during catheterization.

Angiocardiography

Angiocardiography is the term used to describe roentgenography of the heart and the great vessels following the injection of an opaque material. In venous angiocardiography, a radiopaque catheter is inserted (under fluoroscopy) into a peripheral vein, contrast material is injected, and then films are taken.

Although venous angiocardiography has been largely superseded by selective angiocardiography, it is still useful for the diagnosis of certain anomalies of the systemic veins, and in certain very sick infants who can stand little trauma.

Selective angiocardiography has proved to be a more satisfactory method of diagnosing specific heart lesions. The radiopaque catheter is introduced into the heart cavities and the contrast material is injected. Modern equipment permits roentgenograms to be taken rapidly, reproducing quite faithfully the structural changes in the heart.

Cinefluorography

This term describes the taking of motion picture records of successive images appearing on a fluoroscopic screen. This has some advantages over serial angiocardiography. There is less radiation, and it provides a demonstration of pathophysiology, as well as being a useful monitoring system. Cinefluorography and serial angiocardiography compliment each other in the diagnosis of particular conditions.

AN OUTLINE OF THE COMMON TYPES OF CONGENITAL HEART DISEASE

In order to be able to give a child entering the hospital for cardiac surgery intelligent care, the nurse should understand the nature of the defect involved. The more common types of congenital heart disease are briefly outlined here. Several excellent texts are available for more precise and detailed information.

Congenital heart defects are commonly described as cyanotic or acyanotic conditions. Cyanotic heart disease implies an oxygen saturation of the peripheral arterial blood of 85 per cent or less. This condition occurs when a heart defect allows any appreciable amount of oxygen-poor blood in the right side of the heart to mix with the oxygenated blood in the left side of the heart. Defects that permit right-to-left shunting can occur at the atrial, the ventricular or at the aortic level.

Many defects occur in combination, giving rise to complex situations. Many of the complex defects, and most of the rare, isolated defects may never be seen by the average nurse. The only conditions discussed here are common enough to obligate the pediatric nurse to be familiar with their diagnosis and treatment.

Conditions that Ordinarily do not Cause Cyanosis

Ventricular Septal Defect

This is the most common intracardiac defect. It consists of an abnormal opening in the septum between the two ventricles, allowing blood to pass directly from the left to the right ventricle. There is no leakage of unoxygenated blood into the left ventricle, and thus no cyanosis. (Fig. 105)

Small, isolated defects are usually without symptoms, and are fre-

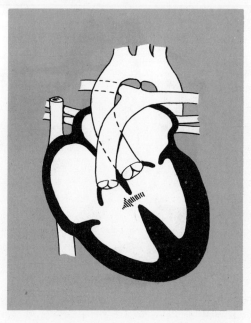

Fig. 105. Ventricular septal defect.

quently discovered during a routine physical examination. A characteristic loud, harsh murmur, associated with a systolic thrill, is occasionally heard on examination. There may be a history of frequent respiratory infections during infancy, but growth and development are not affected. The child leads a normal life.

This type of defect, known as *maladie de Roger,* appears to be compatible with a normal life span. It is usually treated conservatively under medical supervision, but without curtailment of ordinary activity.

In the presence of a large defect, overloading of the left side of the heart, an increased work load for both ventricles, and pulmonary engorgement appear. Congestive heart failure during infancy frequently occurs. Dyspnea, easy fatigability, failure to thrive, and frequent respiratory infections are common. The shunt may eventually be converted into a bi-directional or a right-to-left shunt, as in the Eisenmenger's Complex, making this a cyanotic condition.

Treatment of ventricular septal defects. Surgery is indicated for the repair of large ventricular septal defects with left-to-right shunts. When a shunt reversal has been caused by pulmonary hypertension, surgery is not recommended because the surgical mortality rate is prohibitive.

Corrective surgery should be postponed, if at all possible, until the age of three years, when the surgical risk is less than that for infants.

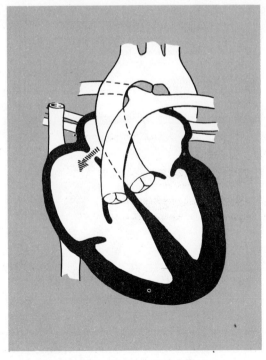

Fig. 106. Atrial septal defect.

A very ill infant may be cared for medically with the use of digitalis, diuretics and antibiotics. A banding procedure has frequently brought about a marked improvement in those infants with large ventricular septal defects who have a large pulmonary blood flow and heart failure. This is accomplished by the application of a nylon cloth band around the root of the pulmonary arterial trunk, causing a reduction in the pulmonary flow and a drop in pulmonary artery pressure. At subsequent corrective surgery, the band is removed.

Corrective surgery of ventricular septal defects is carried out in a dry field, using a bypass machine. The defect is closed by direct suturing, or, if necessary, with a nylon patch.

Atrial Septal Defects

In general, left-to-right shunting occurs in all true atrial septal defects. A patent foramen ovale, which is situated in the atrial septum, however, is present in a large number of healthy persons, and normally causes no problems. This is because the valve of the foramen ovale is anatomically structured to withstand left chamber pressure, and makes the patent foramen ovale functionally closed. (Fig. 106)

True atrial septal defects are common heart anomalies and may occur as isolated defects or in combination with other heart anomalies.

ATRIAL SEPTAL DEFECT—SECUNDUM TYPE. Early in embryonic life, septal structures form to partition the single chambered atrium into both right and left chambers. The ostium primum rises to form a partial partition, followed by the ostium secundum, which completes the atrial partitioning. The secundum defect is in the nature of a hole high in the atrial septum. The child with such a defect is usually symptom-free. Cardiac enlargement and hypertension may appear in later life, however, and bring on the possibility of congestive heart failure. Without surgical repair, the expected life span may be significantly reduced.

ATRIAL SEPTAL DEFECT—PRIMUM TYPE. The ostium primum atrial septal defect is a serious, but fortunately less common, anomaly. The defect is in the lower portion of the atrial septum, and is frequently associated with a deformity of the mitral or the tricuspid valve, or both. It is often found in persons with Down's syndrome.

Treatment of atrial septal defects. The ostium secundum defect is amenable to surgery, with a low surgical mortality risk. Since the advent of the heart-lung bypass machine, this repair can be performed in a dry field, replacing the older "blind" technique. The opening is either sutured or is closed with a nylon patch. The optimum age for surgery is between five and ten years, before irreparable damage has been caused by prolonged pulmonary hypertension.

The repair of the ostium primum defect is feasible, but, at present, surgery carries too high an operative mortality rate to be generally used.

Patent Ductus Arteriosus

The ductus arteriosus is a vascular channel between the left main pulmonary artery and the descending aorta. In fetal life, this allows blood to bypass the non-functioning lungs and go directly into the systemic circuit. After birth, the duct normally closes, eventually becoming obliterated and forming the ligamentum arteriosum. If, however, the ductus remains patent, blood continues to be shunted from the aorta into the pulmonary artery. This results in an overflooding of the lungs and in an overloading of the left heart chambers.

Normally the ductus arteriosus is non-patent after the first or second week of life, and should be obliterated by the fourth month. Why it fails to close is not known at the present time. Patent ductus arteriosus is common in infants who exhibit the rubella syndrome, but most of the infants with this anomaly give no history of exposure to rubella during fetal life.

Clinical manifestations. Symptoms are frequently absent during childhood. Growth and development may be retarded in some children, with an easy fatigability and dyspnea on exertion.

Diagnosis. This can be based on a characteristic, machinery-like murmur over the pulmonary area, a wide pulse pressure, and a bounding pulse. Cardiac catheterization is diagnostic but is not required in the presence of classical clinical features.

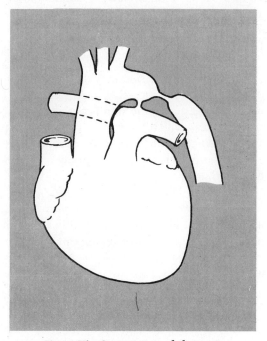

Fig. 107. Coarctation of the aorta.

Treatment. Surgery is indicated in all diagnosed cases, even if they are asymptomatic. Some persons may possibly live a normal life span without correction, but the risks involved far outweigh the surgical ones.

The most serious complication to be considered in patent ductus arteriosus is pulmonary hypertension, resulting from the excessive pulmonary blood flow (and which may lead to cardiac failure). Other complications may include subacute bacterial endoarteritis and pulmonary or systemic emboli. Uncorrected patent ductus arteriosus is believed to be responsible for a sharp reduction in the life expectancy of an average affected person.

Surgical procedures. Surgical correction consists of closure of the defect by ligation or by division of the ductus. Division is the method of choice if the child's condition permits, because the ductus occasionally reopens after ligation. Optimal age for surgery is between two and five years, with earlier surgery for severely affected infants. Prognosis is excellent following a successful repair.

Coarctation of the Aorta

This is a congenital cardiovascular anomaly consisting of a constriction or narrowing of the aortic arch, or of the descending aorta, usually adjacent to the ligamentum arteriosum. (Figs. 107 and 108)

A majority of children with this condition are asymptomatic until later childhood or young adulthood. A few infants have severe symptoms in

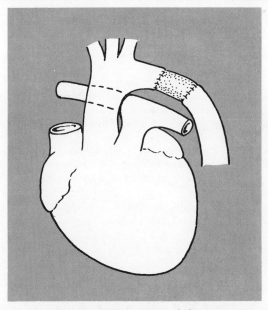

Fig. 108. Coarctation of the aorta
—resected and graft applied.

their first year of life showing dyspnea, tachycardia and cyanosis, these are signs of developing congestive heart failure.

The condition is easily diagnosed from hypertension present in the upper extremities, and from hypotension in the lower extremities. The radial pulse is readily palpable but the femoral pulses are weak or even impalpable. Blood pressure is normal or elevated in the arms and is low or undetectable in the legs. A high-pitched systolic murmur is usually present, heard over the base of the heart and over the interscapular area of the back.

Obstruction to blood flow caused by the constricted portion of the aorta does not cause early difficulty in an average child because the blood bypasses the obstruction by way of the collateral circulation. The bypass is chiefly from the branches of the subclavian and the carotid arteries which arise from the arch of the aorta. Eventually, the enlarged collateral arteries erode the rib margins, and the rib notching can be visualized by roentgen examination.

The uncorrected coarctation may cause hypertension and cardiac failure later in life. The optimal age for surgery is probably between the ages of five to ten or twelve years. Early surgery may be necessary for a gravely ill infant if medical measures fail, but the mortality rate is high.

Surgery consists of resection of the coarcted area with an end-to-end anastomosis of the proximal and the distal ends of the aorta. Occasionally a long defect may necessitate an end-to-end graft, using tubes of dacron or similar material.

Prognosis is excellent for the restoration of normal functions after surgery.

A Boy with Coarctation of the Aorta[*]

Melvin G. was born prematurely and weighed five pounds at birth. His mother gave a history of exposure to rubella during the first trimester of her pregnancy, but a careful examination of the newborn infant revealed no abnormalities. He was discharged on a Similac formula.

When he was two months of age, his mother reported that he was a poor eater and had gained weight slowly. A chest roentgenogram revealed cardiomegaly, but no murmur or other evidence of an abnormal heart condition was noted on physical examination. He was sent home with instructions to visit a pediatric clinic.

At the age of nine months, Melvin was hospitalized for an acute upper respiratory infection. Palor and difficult breathing were noted, and a soft midsystolic murmur could be heard. Chest films revealed both right and left ventricular enlargement and engorged pulmonary vascular markings. He was judged to be in congestive heart failure, with possible pneumonitis.

Treatment included digitalization, oxygen with mist, and antibiotic therapy

---

[*] Condensed from an original study made by Janice O'Sullivan, junior student nurse at University of Oregon School of Nursing. Patient's real name has not been used.

for the respiratory infection. Further investigation of his cardiac status revealed hypertension in the upper extremities—a blood pressure reading in the right arm of 110/60, and a systolic reading in the right leg of 50. Tentative diagnosis was coarctation of the aorta, possibly infantile, with patent ductus arteriosus. In view of his good response to treatment, however, it was decided to treat him medically, and to send him to a cardiac clinic. He was discharged on a daily maintenance dose of Lanoxin.

Melvin continued to eat poorly, remaining in the 10th to the 25th percentile in weight. His height was average, and his developmental progress was within normal limits. His appearance was described as that of an active, but chronically ill infant.

Examination at 18 months revealed a long systolic murmur over the left sternal border and a longer systolic murmur at the apex, but no third sound. Electrocardiography indicated moderate left ventricular hypertrophy. Radial pulses were bounding, and femoral pulses were barely palpible. He appeared to compensate adequately for the cardiac defect on a regimen of low sodium diet and digoxin (Lanoxin).

At the age of two and a half years, an electrocardiogram was essentially within normal limits. Pulses and blood pressure continued in the pervious pattern; a systolic murmur could be heard over the precordium, and a venous hum was heard on the right side, but no diastolic murmur could be heard. Recommendations were to continue with the Lanoxin and with the low sodium diet. A prophylactic course of penicillin was suggested in connection with a proposed tooth extraction.

During his fourth year, Melvin's mother reported that he had leg pains at night severe enough to waken him. Shortly after his fifth birthday, he was admitted to the hospital for cardiac catheterization. Cineangiocardiography revealed a short segment coarctation of the aorta, adult type, but no patent ductus arteriosus. A decision was made to correct the defect surgically, and he was scheduled for surgery one month later.

On his admission for cardiac surgery, he was chosen for the subject of a nursing care study by one of the student nurses. She found him to be a likable, well mannered boy, apparently well adjusted and showing no signs of undisciplined or overprotected behavior. Excellent rapport was established. Melvin was cooperative and calm, accepting the impending surgery with a casual "I had surgery before"; meaning the cardiac catheterization.

On the afternoon before the day of surgery, Janice, his nurse, read him stories, played games with him, and casually discussed the sequence of events for the next day. They talked about Mommy coming early, and the fact that he would not have breakfast. Melvin asked if he would "get a shot"; Janice said he would, and that his mother could hold him afterward until he became sleepy. They talked about the elevator ride, and about the queer operating room garb, which he remembered from the cardiac catheterization. Janice assured him that she would be with him all of the time, which pleased him greatly.

Because he appeared to show no anxiety about surgery itself, Janice talked about what he would see in the cardiac recovery room. She told him about the oxygen tent, and drew a picture of the chest drainage tubes, which interested him. He was quite intrigued with the idea of a little machine that would go "beep" every time his heart beat, and listened to his own heart through a stethoscope, saying "beep" with each beat. He was also interested to know that he would get "food" through a tube in one of his veins. Janice thought that he might be disturbed over his incision, so she drew a picture, explaining to him that it would heal just like a cut finger. Melvin appeared interested and talked freely, but he exhibited no real anxiety.

The physical preparation for surgery included a pHisoHex bath and shampoo, blood determinations and crossmatching, and urinalysis. He received staphcillin, penicillin and streptomycin on the evening and the morning preceding surgery. Preoperative sedation consisted of intramuscular injections of Demerol 30 mgm., atropine 0.2 mgm. and Nembutal 60 mgm. Melvin relaxed and was asleep on admission to surgery.

In the operating room Melvin was positioned in a lateral position with his left side up, was given general endotracheal anesthesia, and had skin preparation with Virac and alcohol. The fifth intercostal space was entered, and a short, narrow coarctation of the aorta found directly proximal to the ligamentum arteriosum. The coarctation was excised, and the aortic ends anastamosed without difficulty. A blood loss of 300 cc. was replaced, chest tubes were inserted, and the incision was closed.

In the cardiac recovery room, the chest tubes were connected to closed suction bottles, and Melvin was placed in a croupette with mist. His heart action was monitored, his vital signs carefully watched and intravenous blood and fluids were given as indicated. Antibiotics and digoxin were continued by intramuscular injection, and morphine was given in sufficient quantity to keep him sedated as ordered. His parents visited him, content to be able to hold his hand through the tent opening.

His vital signs remained stable, his skin was warm to the touch, and his recovery was uneventful. Chest films were taken daily. Melvin was turned and made to cough. On the third day, he was allowed to sit up in bed. Oral fluids were started, the chest tubes were removed, and the oxygen tent was no longer required. On the fourth day, he was returned to the pediatric ward.

Melvin was pleased to be back on the ward, showed Janice his new toys and displayed his incision which was healing "just like a cut." He gradually returned to full activity, and, on the tenth postoperative day, he was discharged. He was to continue with a low sodium diet and with daily Lanoxin, until his return to the clinic in four weeks.

On his return to the clinic, his parents reported that he had been quite active and was feeling well. His weight was still in the 10th to the 25th percentile, but his appetite was improving. A systolic ejection murmur was still audible in the aortic area, but no ventricular overactivity was evident. His blood pressure was 130/80 in the upper extremities, with a systolic reading of 110 in the lower extremities. He was considered to be making good progress. The salt restriction was removed, and digoxin was discontinued. He was to return to the cardiac clinic in six months for further evaluation.

Cyanotic Congenital Heart Defects

Eisenmenger's Syndrome

This term is used to denote a condition in which pulmonary hypertension is present in combination with a ventricular septal defect. The shunting of blood through the defect is reversed, causing a right-to-left flow.

It is believed that the pulmonary hypertension may be a physiological abnormality by itself. The normal newborn has a high pulmonary vascular resistance that falls to adult levels within a few months. In Eisenmenger's syndrome, the pulmonary resistance remains high, and this resistance has probably been present from birth.

Clinical manifestations. These infants show signs of severe heart disease early in life. Feeding difficulties, failure to thrive, recurrent respiratory infections and dyspnea are all associated with this condition. Cyanosis, which increases as the child grows older, is associated with clubbing of the fingers and the toes and with polycythemia. The child may assume a squatting position to relieve fatigue.

Cardiac catheterization and selective angiocardiography are useful for locating the site of the shunt.

Treatment. Attempts to correct this anomaly have been unsuccessful to date. Medical treatment to make the child as comfortable as possible, and perhaps to prolong his life, constitutes the only treatment at the present time.

Tetralogy of Fallot

Tetralogy of Fallot is a fairly common congenital heart defect, involving 50 to 70 per cent of all cyanotic congenital heart diseases. It consists of a grouping of heart defects, the term "tetralogy" denoting four abnormal conditions. These are *pulmonary stenosis, ventricular septal defect, overriding aorta,* and *right ventricular hypertrophy.*

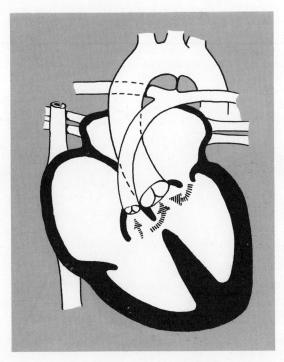

Fig. 109. Tetralogy of Fallot.

The pulmonary stenosis is usually of the infundibular type, in which there is a narrowing of the upper portion of the right ventricle. It may include, however, stenosis of the valve cusps. Pulmonary stenosis results, in turn, in right ventricular hypertrophy.

The aorta appears to straddle the ventricular septum, overriding the ventricular septal defect. This defect allows a shunt of unsaturated blood from the right ventricle into the aorta, or into the left ventricle. (Fig. 109)

Clinical manifestations. The child may be precyanotic in early infancy with the cyanotic phase starting at from four to six months. Some severely affected infants, however, may show cyanosis earlier. It is believed that as long as the ductus arteriosus remains open, enough blood passes through the lungs to prevent cyanosis.

The infant presents feeding difficulties and poor weight gain with retarded growth and development. Dyspnea and easy fatigability become evident, especially when the child begins to walk. Cyanosis becomes grossly severe after the first year, even when the child is at rest.

Exercise tolerance depends somewhat on the severity of the disease, some children becoming fatigued after very little exertion. As the child experiences fatigue, breathlessness and increased cyanosis, he usually assumes a squatting posture for relief. Squatting apparently increases the systemic oxygen saturation.

Attacks of paroxysmal dyspnea are common during infancy and early childhood. An anoxic spell is heralded by sudden restlessness, gasping

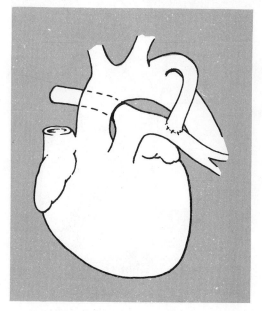

Fig. 110. Blalock—Taussig operation.

respiration, and increased cyanosis, leading into a loss of consciousness and possibly into convulsions. These attacks last from a few minutes in length to several hours and appear to be unpredictable, although stress does seem to trigger some episodes.

Iron-deficiency anemia is a common complication caused by the poor food intake. Polycythemia is usually also present.

Diagnosis. Diagnosis is made by utilizing all available techniques. Roentgen examination reveals a boot-shaped heart contour and a concave pulmonary conus. Cardiac catheterization, using angiocardiography and cine recording helps present a clear picture of the anomalies involved.

Treatment. Treatment is aimed at medical management until the child can tolerate surgery. The constant aim, of course, is to keep the child in the best possible physical condition.

An infant suffering an anoxic spell should be placed in a knee-chest position for the greatest possible relief. Oxygen is administered, and morphine is given to relax any child suffering an anoxic episode. Intravenous sodium bicarbonate has also been proved useful in severe spells. As the child grows older, however, he learns his physical limitations, and the anoxic episodes become fewer.

Anemia, if present, is treated with iron therapy. Surgery on the nose, the throat or on the ears carries the danger of subacute bacterial endocarditis. Therefore, antibiotic therapy is utilized if such surgery is neces-

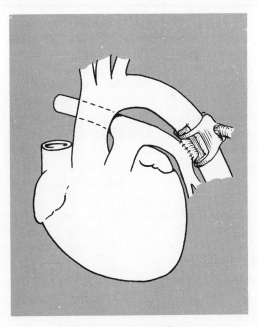

Fig. 111. Potts procedure.

sary. Fevers, vomiting and diarrhea diminish the fluid component of the blood, aggravating the existing polycythemia.

Surgical relief is imperative for these children as early as possible. The average age span for uncorrected cases is not over ten years. Heart surgery does carry a risk, and thus it is necessary for the child to be in the best possible physical condition.

Surgical procedures. Palliative surgery has been in use for several years. Dr. Taussig observed that the infant with tetralogy of Fallot thrived much better as long as the ductus arteriosus remained open. Together with Dr. Blalock, she devised an operation creating an artificial shunt between the pulmonary and the aortic systems. Later, Dr. Potts and his associates devised a similar shunt.

1. BLALOCK-TAUSSIG PROCEDURE. This is an end-to-end anastomosis of a vessel arising from the aorta, usually the subclavian, to the corresponding right or left pulmonary artery. (Fig. 110)

2. POTTS PROCEDURE. This is a side-to-side anastomosis between the aorta and the left pulmonary artery. (Fig. 111)

These procedures do nothing to correct the anatomical defects, but they do relieve the cyanosis and the dyspnea by increasing the flow of blood to the lungs. As the child grows, these shunts tend to become ineffective, but they are useful for carrying the child along in relatively good health until he is a candidate for total correction.

Total surgical correction. This procedure can only be carried out in a dry field, necessitating the use of a cardiopulmonary bypass machine. The heart is opened, and extensive resection is done. The septal defect is closed by use of an Ivalon patch and the valvular stenosis and infundibular chamber are resected.

Total correction is delayed, if possible, until after the age of three to five years. Palliative surgery carries the young child along and does not interfere with later correction. Because of the high surgical risk involved if correction is attempted in infancy, most surgeons prefer the sequence of palliative surgery at an early age, followed by total correction. Some surgeons have attempted total correction on selected infants with reported good results, but the risk for an average infant is still too high.

Successful total correction transforms a grossly abnormal heart into a functionally normal one, as far as we can tell from present knowledge. Most of these children are left without a pulmonary valve, however. Whether this will prove harmful with age we cannot tell as yet.

Transposition of the Great Vessels

In this condition the aorta arises from the right ventricle, and the pulmonary artery arises from the left ventricle, forming two independent, closed circuits. Thus the aortic circuit carries unoxygenated blood to the systemic system, while the pulmonary circuit carries oxygenated blood back to the lungs. This condition is only compatible with life if an associated defect allowing mixing of blood is present, such as an atrial or a ventricular septal defect, or a patent ductus arteriosus.

Clinical manifestations. Extreme cyanosis and dyspnea are present at birth or shortly following. Progressive congestive heart failure appears in most cases, with survival beyond six months uncommon except in instances when there is a good mixture of saturated and unsaturated blood. Growth retardation, with marked clubbing of the fingers and the toes together with severe cyanosis, is the rule for those who survive.

Diagnosis. Laboratory findings include polycythemia and an elevated hematocrit. Definitive diagnosis is made by cardiac catheterization, with the use of angiocardiography and cineangiograms.

Treatment. A number of surgical procedures have been devised, some of which are palliative, and some of which attempt reconstruction of the veins or of the atrial septum.

1. BANDING OF THE PULMONARY ARTERY. This is done when pulmonary blood flow is increased. Some infants appear to get considerable relief from their symptoms as a result of banding.

2. HANLON-BLALOCK PROCEDURE. This involves the creation of an artificial defect in the atrial septum, allowing the mixture of saturated and unsaturated blood.

3. BAFFES PROCEDURE.
   a. Transposition of right pulmonary veins to the right atrium.
   b. Transposition of the inferior vena cava to the left atrium. This procedure has been successful in several patients whose condition allowed this type of surgery.

4. SENNING PROCEDURE. This involves the reconstruction of the atrial septum to divert the flow of blood into proper channels, and has met with some success.

5. MUSTARD PROCEDURE.
   a. Removal of the atrial septum as in the Hanlon-Blalock procedure.
   b. Use of the pericardium to channel blood from the pulmonary veins into the right ventricle.

Palliative surgery presently has a mortality rate of 15 to 35 per cent. The rate in corrective surgery is higher. A method of total correction, designed to connect the aorta and the pulmonary trunk to their proper ventricles·is in the process of research. Success has not been reported yet, but the outlook appears promising.

BIBLIOGRAPHY

Cohlen, S.: Teratogenic agents and congenital malformations. J. Pediat., *63:* 650, 1963.

Gasul, B., Arcilla, R., and Lev, M.: Heart Disease in Children. Philadelphia, J. B. Lippincott, 1966.

Morgan, B., *et al:* Operable congenital heart disease. Pediat. Clin. N. Amer. *13:*105, 1966.

Nelson, W., (ed.): Textbook of Pediatrics. Pp. 901–955. Philadelphia, W. B. Saunders, 1964.

Richman, H.: Casework with a child following heart surgery. Children, *11:*183, 1964.

Roose, J.: Interpretation of rest. Interpretation of bed rest by doctors and nurses. Nurs. Res., *12:*111, 1963.

Pediatric Clinics of North America: Symposium on Cardiovascular Therapy. Pediat. Clin. N. Amer. *11:*, 1964.

Thompson, R.: The cardiac child at home. Nurs. Outlook, *9:*77, (Feb.) 1961.

Wallace, H.: Health services for mothers and children. Philadelphia, W. B. Saunders, 1962.

SUGGESTED READINGS FOR FURTHER STUDY

Blake, F.: Open Heart Surgery in Children: a Study in Nursing Care. Washington, U. S. Government Printing Office, 1964.

Caylor, G. G., *et al:* Pulmonary artery banding in infants with cardiac anomalies other than ventricular septal defects: including an evaluation of a new technique for determining a critical degree of banding. Dis. Chest., *47:*88, 1965.

Nadas, A. S.: Pediatric Cardiology. 2nd ed. Philadelphia, W. B. Saunders, 1963.

Robinson, S., Abrams, H., and Kaplan, H.: Congenital Heart Disease. 2nd ed. New York, McGraw-Hill, 1965.

Rudolph, A.: The infant with heart disease. Pediatrics, *33:*990, 1964.

22

Rheumatic Fever and Rheumatic Carditis

Rheumatic fever is a chronic disease of childhood, occurring as one of the sequelae of Group A beta hemolytic streptococcal infections. It occurs throughout the world, particularly in the temperate zones, but recent studies show it to be more prevalent in the tropics than had previously been reported. For approximately the past 20 years, its incidence has shown a marked decline in the United States, but it is still an important cause of death or disability there as it is elsewhere, among children between the ages of six and twelve years.

CLINICAL ASPECTS

Etiology

Rheumatic fever appears to be a sensitivity reaction precipitated by streptococci. The initial streptococcal infection may be inapparent or unrecognized, and the resultant rheumatic fever manifestation may be the first indication of trouble. An elevation of antistreptoccocal antibodies, indicative of recent streptococcal infection, however, can be demonstrated in about 95 per cent of the rheumatic fever patients tested within the first two months of onset.

Clinical Manifestations

Following the initial infection, a latent period of one to three weeks ensues; in certain cases, the period may be longer. The onset is frequently insidious. The child may be listless, anorexic, pale, and may lose weight. He may complain of vague muscle and joint, or of abdominal pains. Frequently a low grade, late afternoon fever may be the noticeable symptom. None of these are diagnostic in themselves, but if such signs persist, the child merits a medical examination.

Major manifestations of rheumatic fever are polyarthritis, chorea, and carditis. The onset may be acute rather than insidious, with severe carditis or arthritis as the presenting symptom. Chorea, if it is present, generally has an insidious onset.

Polyarthritis. This is an arthritis of the migratory type, moving from one major joint to another; to the ankles, the knees, the hips, the wrists, to the elbows and to the shoulders. The joint becomes hot, swollen, and painful to either touch or movement. Body temperature is moderately elevated, sedimentation rate is increased. Although extremely painful, this type of arthritis does not lead to the crippling deformities that occur in rheumatoid arthritis.

Chorea (Sydenham's chorea). In this manifestation, the affected portion of the body is the central nervous system. Emotional instability, purposeless movements and muscular weakness are characteristic. The onset is gradual, with increasing incoordination, facial grimaces and repetitive involuntary movements. Movements may be mild and remain so, or they may become increasingly violent. Active arthritis is rarely present when chorea is the major manifestation. Carditis occurs, although less frequently than when polyarthritis is the major condition. Attacks tend to be recurrent and prolonged, but they become rare after puberty. It is seldom possible to demonstrate an antistreptococcal antibody rise, because of the generally prolonged latency period, and because of the length of time after the onset before the condition may be recognized.

Carditis. Carditis is a serious manifestation because it is the major cause of death or of permanent disability among children with rheumatic fever. Carditis may occur singly, or it may occur as a complication of either arthritis or chorea. Presenting symptoms may be vague enough to be missed. A child may have a poor appetite or pallor, perhaps have a low grade fever, appear listless and show a moderate degree of anemia. If observed carefully, a slight dyspnea on exertion may be noted. Physical examination reveals a soft systolic murmur over the apex of the heart. Unfortunately, such a child may have been under par physically for some time before the murmur is discovered.

ACUTE CARDITIS. This may, however, be the presenting symptom, particularly in young children. An abrupt onset of high fever, perhaps as high as 104°, tachycardia, pallor, poor pulse quality, and a rapid fall in hemoglobin are characteristic. Weakness, prostration, cyanosis and intense precordial pain are frequently present. Cardiac dilatation usually occurs. The pericardium, the myocardium, or the endocardium may be affected.

Other rheumatic fever manifestations. Epistaxis is common, and may be severe. *Subcutaneous nodules* are shot-like, hard bodies felt on the extensor surface of certain joints, particularly on the elbows, the knees and the wrists. They are painless and do not occur in every case, but if they are noted, they provide one criterion for diagnosis. *Erythema marginatum* is another useful diagnostic aid, when it is present. It consists of a recurrent, pink, characteristic rash, which appears on the trunk or on the extremities, and migrates from place to place. It never appears on the face.

TABLE 22–1. JONES CRITERIA (MODIFIED) FOR GUIDANCE
IN THE DIAGNOSIS OF RHEUMATIC FEVER

Major Criteria	Minor Criteria
Carditis	Fever
Polyarthritis	Arthralgia
Chorea	Prolonged P–R interval in the ECG
Subcutaneous nodules	Increased ESR, WBC, or presence of
Erythema Marginatum	C–reactive protein
	Preceding beta hemolytic streptococcal infection
	Previous rheumatic fever or inactive heart disease

Diagnostic Criteria

Rheumatic fever is difficult to diagnose, and it is sometimes impossible to differentiate it from other diseases. The possible serious effect of the disease demands early and conscientious medical treatment. It is unfortunate, however, to cause apprehension and disrupt the patient's life if the condition proves to be something less serious. The nurse should naturally not attempt a diagnosis, but she should understand the criteria on which a presumptive diagnosis is based.

The Jones criteria (modified), a guide based on criteria formulated in 1944, is generally accepted as a useful rule for guidance when making a decision as to whether to treat the patient for rheumatic fever. The list is divided into major and minor categories.*

The presence of two major, or one major and two minor criteria, is accepted as an indication of a high probability of rheumatic fever if supported by evidence of a preceding streptococcal infection. It is not infallible, because no one criterion is specific for the disease, and other additional manifestations are helpful aids toward a substantiation of the diagnosis.

Laboratory Tests

The chief concern while caring for a patient with rheumatic fever is the prevention of residual heart disease. As long as the rheumatic process is active, progressive heart damage is possible. Bed rest, therefore, is essential in order to reduce the work load of the heart. How long the period of bed rest should last cannot be arbitrarily stated. It is generally agreed that a child should be kept in bed until both laboratory and clinical evidence of the disease have disappeared.

Laboratory appraisal tests, although they are nonspecific, are useful for an evaluation of the activity of the disease. Two commonly used indicators are the *erythrocyte sedimentation rate,* and the presence of

---

* The American Heart Association has issued the Jones Criteria (revised) 1965. It retains the diagnostic criteria and lists other manifestations that may support the diagnosis.

C-reactive protein. The erythrocyte sedimentation rate (ESR) is elevated in the presence of an inflammatory process, and is nearly always raised in the polyarthritis or in the carditis manifestations of rheumatic fever. It remains elevated until after any clinical manifestations have ceased, and after any subclinical activity has subsided. It seldom rises in uncomplicated chorea. Therefore, ESR elevation in a choreic patient may point toward cardiac involvement.

C-reactive protein. This is not normally present in the blood of healthy persons, but it does appear in the serum of acutely ill persons, including those ill with rheumatic fever. As the patient improves, C-reactive protein disappears.

Leukocytosis. This also is an indication of an inflammatory process. Until the leukocyte count returns to a normal level, the disease probably is still active.

Medical Treatment

Medications used in the treatment of rheumatic fever include salicylates and corticosteroids. Salicylates are given in the form of acetylsalicylic acid (aspirin) to children, with the daily dosage calculated according to the child's weight. Remarkable relief from polyarthritis is afforded by the use of this drug. The continued administration of a relatively large dosage may cause toxic effects, because individual tolerance differs greatly. The child's nurse must assume the responsibility for noting any signs of toxicity and must report them promptly. Tinnitus, nausea, vomiting, and headache are all signals of toxicity. Salicylates tend to interfere with the synthesis of prothrombin. Purpura, ecchymotic skin manifestations or frank hemorrhage may be the result. Of particular importance is the toxic reaction of hyperpnea, which may lead to respiratory alkalosis and to metabolic acidosis.

In the presence of mild or severe carditis, corticosteroids appear to be the drug of choice because of their prompt, dramatic action. Neither drug is expected to alter the course of the disease, but the control of the toxic manifestations of this disease contribute to the patient's comfort and to his sense of well-being, and help to reduce the burden on his heart. This is of particular importance in acute carditis with congestive failure. Because a premature withdrawal of a steroid drug is likely to cause a relapse, its use is continued until any evidence of activity has subsided. It is then gradually discontinued. Toxic reactions are naturally to be watched for and reported as well.

Because the presence of group A streptococci prolongs the rheumatic activity, a course of penicillin should be given to eliminate these organisms from the child's body.

Corticosteroids and salicylates are of little value in the treatment of uncomplicated chorea. Sedation with phenobarbital for relaxation, or the use of a tranquilizer such as chlorpromazine (Thorazine) helps to relax the child. Strict bed rest is necessary, and with protection such as padding the bed sides if the movements are severe. When the chorea is complicated by a heart condition, the treatment should include therapy for that condition too.

Bed rest. Prolonged strict bed rest is no longer considered necessary for every patient with rheumatic fever. The psychological trauma that so many children suffered from such a program brought about a careful study of the effects of controlled activity. It was concluded that many children were being needlessly restricted.

The prevailing manner of treatment, in the absence of carditis, advises bed rest until the acute manifestations of polyarthritis, chorea or fever have abated. Following the cessation of clinical symptoms, sedentary activities may be permitted until all rheumatic activity has subsided and the drug therapy has ended. If no relapse has occurred after one or two months, the attack is considered to have ended, and restoration of full activity may then be permitted. In the presence of carditis, full activity cannot be permitted until several months after the absence of murmurs has been confirmed. Residual heart disease is treated in accordance with its severity and its type with digitalis, restricted activities, diuretics and a low sodium diet as indicated.

Recurrences

Recurrences were formerly considered to be nearly inevitable, with the possibility of additional heart damage with each attack. Understanding that attacks recur as responses to fresh streptococcal infections has resulted in a strict adherence to a prophylactic regimen of penicillin, with a resultant marked decrease in recurrent attacks.

The American Heart Association recommends the administration of penicillin or streptomycin for an indefinite number of years to all persons who have had one or more attacks of rheumatic fever. Specifically, recommendations include prophylactic medication for all patients who have a *well-documented history* of rheumatic fever or of chorea, or who show a *definite evidence* of rheumatic heart disease.

They state that the safest procedure is that of continuing the prophylaxis indefinitely, particularly in the presence of rheumatic heart disease. It is recognized, however, that some physicians may wish to terminate prophylaxis in certain adult patients who have been free of attacks for several years and who have no present involvement. Adolescents, who are generally negligent in regard to prophylactic medications, are urged to continue protection.

Prophylactic Program

Initially, a full therapeutic course of penicillin is given to eradicate the streptococci, regardless of whether their presence is detected by culture tests. Prophylactic therapy is maintained by the use of benzathine penicillin G, oral penicillin, or oral sulfadiazine. The public health nurse in the community should encourage adherence to the prophylactic program. She should be aware of the merits and of the disadvantages of each type of program in her support of the physician and his patient.

Intramuscular injections of benzathine penicillin G have given the most consistently reliable results. Benzathine penicillin G (marketed as Bicillin) is injected in a dosage of 1,200,000 units once a month. The physician is thus assured that his patient is receiving the proper medication. Oral penicillin is equally as effective, but is too often omitted or taken haphazardly by a patient in good health.

A careful history of allergic reactions to penicillin should be obtained before the program is started. Sulfadiazine may be subsituted if penicillin intolerance is present.

Oral penicillin is given in dosages of 200,000 to 500,000 units daily. Reactions from this administration probably occur less frequently than do those from intramuscular penicillin, but similar precautions are necessary. The temptation to be careless about continuing medication for a well child is great, especially if there is a financial problem once the home supply has been used up.

Oral sulfadiazine is cheaper than oral penicillin and is as effective. Reactions are infrequent, but then should be watched for. Chief reactions are skin eruptions, an associated sore throat or fever, and leukopenia. Weekly white blood cell counts are recommended for the first two months of prophylaxis with this drug, after which the occurrence of leukopenia with agranulocytosis is extremely rare.

NURSING CARE

Home Care

A child who has developed rheumatic fever may be hospitalized for diagnosis and beginning therapy, and may then be returned home for continuing care, depending on the particular circumstances.

The severity of the condition, the home circumstances, and the availability of care outside the home should all be considered. If the family is able to provide adequate physical care and emotional support, and if medical supervision is obtainable, home care would appear to be the best method of meeting the child's needs.

The nurse involved in helping the family to prepare for their child's care as well as the other family members, must have a clear understanding of the physician's definition of strict bed rest. Must the patient be positioned with pillows, turned and fed by others and not allowed to hold books or toys? Is he to be lifted onto the bedpan, and is the urinal to be held for him? Consideration of the various gradations of meaning in the terms strict bed rest, bed rest with bathroom privileges, and so on, is well outlined in an article in Nursing Research.*

A child may be willing to accept total dependency when he is in pain and is acutely ill, but any prohibition of all activity when he feels better may be extremely traumatic emotionally—with the trauma possibly out-weighing the adverse physical effects. Not only the nurse and the family need to understand the physical limitations imposed, but a child patient must have the need for any limitations clearly explained to him in terms suited to his understanding and his ability to accept.

Preparation for home care includes the selection of a room for the temporarily bed-ridden child. If at all possible, he should have his own room, within easy accessibility by his mother. If a hospital bed cannot be rented, blocks placed under the bed legs will raise it to permit easier care, and a back rest can be improvised. Although an ill child needs quiet, his surroundings should be cheerful, with colorful objects of interest spread about the room. Limits for watching television, reading, and for visits from other persons, as well as the resumption of his schoolwork are set by the physician in accordance with the child's condition.

The tendency to overindulge a chronically ill child and to relax dis-cipline is quite understandable. It is not in the child's best interest. He would shortly become a serious burden to his family, and to himself, if guidance is withheld from him and if discipline not enforced as neces-sary.†

If schoolwork is permitted, homebound teachers are available in most communities. Some communities have two-way closed television circuits that allow the child to participate in classroom instruction from his bed.

Convalescent Hospitals

Many children in need of this type of home care may not be able to receive it because of his mother's employment outside the home, or from an inability to provide the necessary environment caused by over-crowd-ing, insanitary conditions or financial difficulties, or from a lack of moti-vation on the part of the family to observe the necessary rules and pre-cautions. Convalescent homes for chronically ill children are available in many localities. Excellent care, consideration for the child's emotional health, and open-minded acceptance of the current philosophy of child care generally characterize these homes. However, at best, they are dreary substitutes for a warm, close family setting.

* Roose, J.: Interpretation of bed rest by doctors and nurses. Nurs. Res., *12*:111, 1963.

† An excellent portrayal of aspects of discipline and home care for a child with rheumatic fever is given in the film *The Valiant Heart*. Obtainable on loan from the American Heart Association, or from state heart associations.

Preventive Health Services for School-Age Children

Because rheumatic fever is a condition that has its peak of onset in school-age children, health services for this age group assume an added importance. The overall approach is one of the promotion of continuous health supervision for all children, including the school-age child. The establishment of well child conferences or clinics, with an encouragement among the general population for their use is one opportunity of which more advantage should be taken. Well infant and child conferences are quite well established throughout the United States with attendance fairly evenly divided between infants and preschool children. An expansion of these services to include school-age children is viewed by many health authorities as the most satisfactory method of providing a continuity of care.

School nurses, public school teachers and public health nurses now have the responsibility for health teaching, for observation, and for case finding and referral of children for diagnostic services. The streptococcal infection that precedes rheumatic activity is transferred much more easily in densely populated areas. Typically, studies have shown that children who migrated from Puerto Rico to New York City were particularly susceptible to rheumatic fever, although the disease was rare in the tropical climate of their homes. Recently, however, because of the growth of tourism in Puerto Rico, the incidence of rheumatic fever there has grown to at least the proportions found in New York. This has led to some speculation concerning the role played by climate versus the effect of greater exposure to the causative factor.

This finding does not, of course, explain the significant decline of this disease's incidence in northern areas. Socio-economic factors, hygienic practices and vigorous campaigns directed toward case finding and prophylaxis have played a significant role. One can scarcely claim, however, that overcrowding no longer exists, or that a majority of children live under optimal sanitary conditions.

Clinic services in the area of prevention and treatment are available from several sources. Crippled children's agencies function with the support of the Children's Bureau. Public health agencies and the Heart Association, through its state associations, are also sources of support.

Registration with a state heart association is a helpful way of keeping in touch with persons who have had one or more attacks of rheumatic fever. Through the association, prophylactic drugs may be purchased at wholesale prices, a service that also makes possible guidance and encouragement during the continuation of self-care.

WHAT IS THE MEANING OF THIS TYPE OF ILLNESS TO A CHILD?

Six-year-old Billy was home with a cold, with a fever and a cough, a moderately sore throat. His mother worried, but Billy was not too ill, and, in two or three days he appeared to be quite well again. It was not until several weeks later that his mother worried again—Billy was so irritable and touchy, and had developed a strange, repetitive head jerking. A visit to the pediatrician provided a considerable shock when a "probable chorea" was the verdict.

Billy was put to bed and was placed on elixir of phenobarbital twice daily. All of the well-developed theories concerning the needs of such children are excellent, but fall somewhat short of being adequate when the family is desperately poor, and when the mother must work full time outside the home. Well-intentioned neighbors helped, but Billy was alone a great deal, and received a minimum of support from a mother who desired only to come home to peace and quiet.

Eventually Billy progressed to full activity, but a few months later, a second attack of considerably greater severity made such haphazard care entirely inadequate, and Billy entered a children's convalescent home. Here the hours and the days stretched endlessly. Eventually some degree of ambulation was attained, but the development of a rapid pulse and a suggestive heart murmur put an end to all activity for months to come.

No residual heart condition developed, however, and Billy was beginning to find his place in the community when a third attack of lessened intensity sent him back to bed. This was the final recurrence, and eventually the time came when Billy was sent back to school with no restrictions placed on his activities.

No restrictions imposed—so they said. What restrictions are imposed on a child by the effect of two years of nearly total exclusion from the healthful activities of his peers? Especially for a boy, who is expected to compete in physical activities at school and on the playground. Billy could not swim, and his coordination was poor. He did not know how to throw a ball or how to perform any athletic feats. His schoolmates laughed at his clumsy attempts, and his physical education directors were impatient. Billy's efforts became almost totally concentrated on academic study and on means for avoiding all physical recreational pursuits. His self-consciousness and previously enforced isolation made him excessively shy, and greatly multiplied his adolescent problems.

Billy's situation was not unique. Rheumatic fever is declining in incidence and in severity, but our pediatric wards have large numbers of children who are repeatedly admitted for treatment of the exacerbations of chronic illnesses that keep them from participating in activities appropriate for their age group. Larry, the six-year-old whose recurrent laryngeal papillomas necessitate a permanent tracheotomy and frequent excisions of the recurring growths; Ruthie, whose nephrosis fails to respond to treatment; the children with hydronephrosis who are chronically ill; these are a few who, without outward deformities, are still unable to live the full life of childhood. Nursing these children must mean much more than giving them bedside care.

BIBLIOGRAPHY

American Heart Association: Prevention of Rheumatic Fever. New York, American Heart Association, 1964.

————: The Jones Criteria (revised) For Guidance in the Diagnosis of Rheumatic Fever. New York, American Heart Association, 1965.

————: The Valiant Heart, film, 29 minutes. M.P.O. Productions, 16 mm., sound, 1954. (Distributed by the American Heart Association.)

Roose, J.: Interpretation of bed rest by doctors and nurses. Nurs. Res., *12*:111, 1963.

Stollerman, G.: Treatment and prevention of rheumatic fever and rheumatic heart disease. Pediat. Clin. N. Amer., *11*:213, 1964.

Wallace, H.: Health Services for Mothers and Children, chap. 25. Philadelphia, W. B. Saunders, 1962.

SUGGESTED READINGS FOR FURTHER STUDY

Feinstein, A. R., and Spagnuolo, M.: The duration of activity in acute rheumatic fever. J.A.M.A., *175*:1117, 1961.

Saslow, M. S., and Vieta, A. G.: Prevention of rheumatic fever: limitations. J. Pediat., *64*:552, 1964.

23

Handicapped Children

HEARING PROBLEMS IN THE CHILD

It has been estimated that of the 40 million school children in the United States, 200,000 have a serious hearing loss. A hearing loss presents a definite handicap to a child, a handicap that has a profound effect on his development, on his emotional stability and on his vocational ability as he grows older.

An explanation of some of the terms used to describe hearing difficulties may permit a better understanding of the problem.

A hard of hearing child is one who has had a loss of hearing acuity, but his hearing has been sufficient to enable him to learn speech and language by imitation of sounds.

A deaf child is one who has no serviceable hearing.

The failure of an infant or a young child to react to sounds does not necessarily mean that simple deafness is the cause. A child may fail to respond to sound or may fail to develop speech for several different reasons. Some of these are mentioned here.

1. CONDUCTIVE HEARING LOSS. In a conductive hearing impairment, the middle ear structures fail to carry sound waves to the inner ear.

2. SENSORY-NEURAL (OR PERCEPTIVE HEARING LOSS). This may be caused by damage to the nerve endings in the cochlea, or to the nerve pathways leading to the brain.

3. CENTRAL AUDITORY DISORDERS. This child may have normal hearing, but because of damage or faulty development of the proper brain centers, he is unable to use the auditory information he receives.

4. MENTAL RETARDATION. This condition or a severe emotional disturbance may prevent the child from responding to auditory stimulation. His hearing may not be impaired, however.

The discussion in this section is limited to true hearing loss, whether it is partial or complete.

Causes of Deafness

Conductive hearing impairment is most commonly the result of otitis media of long standing. Serous otitis media is a condition in which fluid is present in the middle ear, possibly because of an allergy or as the result of a protracted ear infection that has not been completely treated. The child complains of "fullness in his ear," but has no real pain or fever. Drainage relieves the symptoms and improves his hearing, but repeated recurrences, if they are not treated, may cause a permanent hearing loss. Long standing middle ear infections that have destroyed part of the ear drum or the ossicles lead to conductive deafness. (Other causes may include congenital ear deformities.) Deafness is seldom complete, and improvement through treatment is frequently possible.

Perceptive, or sensory-neural losses are generally severe and unresponsive to medical treatment. Diseases such as meningitis or encephalitis, hereditary or congenital factors, or toxic reactions to certain drugs (such

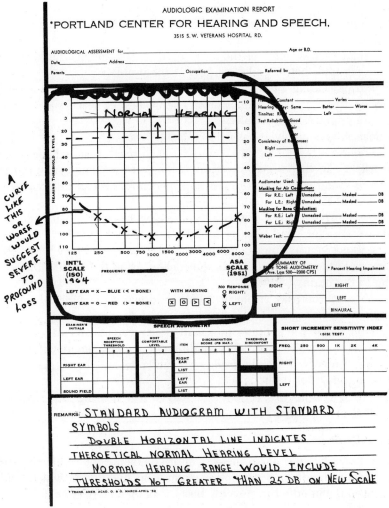

Fig. 112. Audiogram.

as streptomycin) may cause perceptive hearing losses. It is believed that maternal rubella may be the largest single cause of perceptive nerve deafness in children.

Discovering the Defect

A child should not have to wait until he is in difficulty at school before anyone discovers his poor hearing—yet this happens to many children. He may have had a gradual hearing loss, and yet have been so skillful at lip reading that neither he nor his family have become aware of his partial deafness. His teacher is frequently the first person to recognize the child's trouble. She may not be alert to this possibility, however, and may

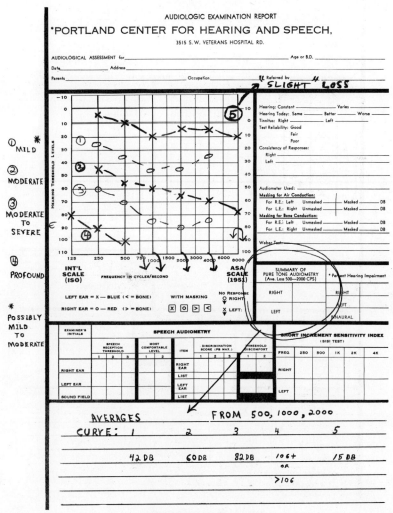

Fig. 113. Audiogram.

scold him for inattention. Children who are noisy or who create a disturbance in class may be expressing resentment over their inability to understand, but may not realize that they are not hearing correctly.

Certain reactions and mannerisms should alert the parent, a teacher or a school nurse to the possibility that the child is not hearing well. He may not be able to localize sound. He may turn his head to one side when listening; he may fail to comprehend when spoken to, or he may appear inattentive or give inappropriate answers. A child who has never heard may also go undetected until his parents realize that he is not responding to sounds or learning to talk.

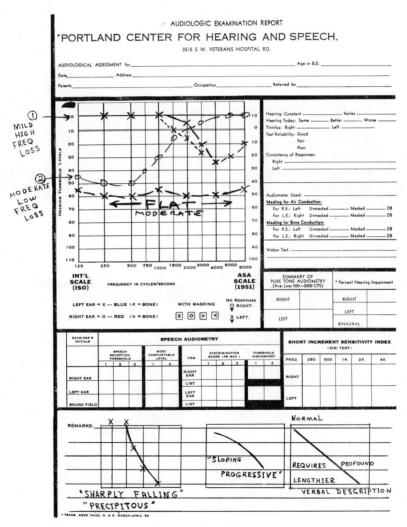

Fig. 114. Audiogram.

Diagnosis and Evaluation of Hearing Problems

The child who is suspected of having a hearing loss is entitled to an audiological assessment. This includes pure tone audiometry testing, speech reception loss and speech discrimination tests. Persons with perceptive nerve impairment have, as a rule, a greater loss of hearing acuity in the high pitched tones. The loss may vary from slight to complete. Persons with a conductive loss are more apt to have equal losses over a wide range of frequencies (pitch). (Figs. 112–114)

A child's hearing level should be tested at all frequencies in a soundproof room by a pure tone audiometer. Speech reception and speech discrimination tests measure the amount of hearing impairment for both speech and communication. Accurate measurements can usually be obtained from children of five years old or more.

Infants and very young children must be tested differently. An infant with normal hearing should be able to localize a sound at 28 weeks, be able to imitate sounds at 36 weeks, and associate sounds with people or objects at one year. A commonly used screening test employs noisemakers of varying intensity and pitch. The examiner stands to the side or to the back of the child who has been given a plaything of interest. As the examiner produces sounds with a rattle, a buzzer, a bell, or with some other noisemaker, a hearing child is usually distracted from his play, and turns to discover the source of the new sound, whereas the deaf child pays no heed. More discriminating tests help to distinguish the deaf child from an autistic, a brain damaged or from a retarded child.

The Child Who Has Never Heard

The deaf infant not only does not hear, but if he has never heard, he has no language concept. One has only to consider the amount of time it takes a hearing child to learn to communicate with language, to get some idea of a deaf child's handicap. Although persons feel and experience emotion, they *think* in words, and a congenitally deaf child has no words. A deaf child has to learn to communicate and to use the language if he is to develop a well-adjusted personality or if he is to share his thoughts and his feelings with others. It is a terrific problem, but deaf children can and do acquire language. This is not saying that a deaf child does not have ideas and concepts: he simply lacks the words to express them. The child who has heard and has learned to talk has an immense advantage—even if he should lose all hearing—because he has learned expression.

The children who learn sign language rather than lip reading and speech suffer a communication disadvantage because this is a talking world. His parents must be their child's first teachers until he is old enough to venture away from home. The parents need to be aware of all phases of a child's development—physical, emotional, social, intel-

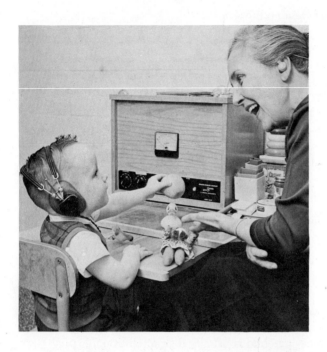

Fig. 115. Learning to talk with use of visual aids.

Fig. 115a. APple!

Fig. 115b. SHoe!

Fig. 115c. Learning color and form.

Fig. 115d. Helping a child to make use of his residual hearing.

A

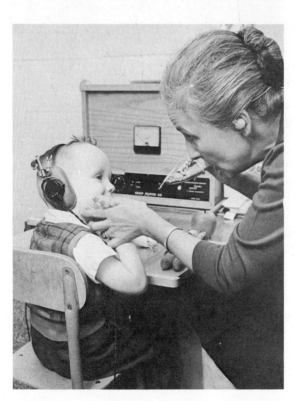

B

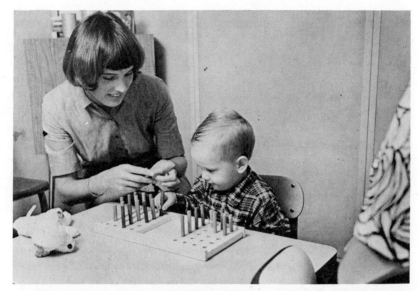

C

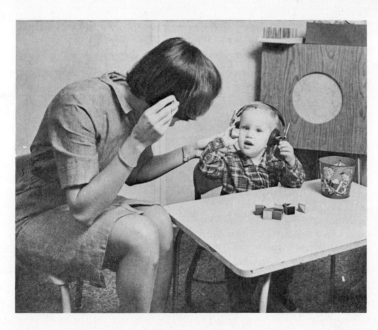

D

lectual and communicative, and then to seek ways to aid this development if a lack of hearing impedes his progress.

For a deaf child, sight and not hearing is the main "way in" by which words can reach his brain. Because the first five years of life are the years of learning and perfecting speech, these are the years when speech reading (lip reading) can most readily be learned.

Personnel who work with preschool deaf children advise parents to "talk-talk-talk" to a young child. Of course a deaf child can not understand all or perhaps any of what is said, but neither does a hearing baby understand his mother's words until he is able to make a connection between what is done and what is said. A deaf baby learns to lip read in the same way, only it takes him much longer. His mother's interaction with him, as she directs his attention to the movements of her mouth, to her facial expressions, and to the way she moves and acts, all are part of his training. (Fig. 115)

Sense perception training (in matching colors and shapes and later figures) is another basis of any readiness program. Training in the use of all his senses, sight, smell, taste, heat, and vibration, make him better able to make use of whatever hearing he may have, and it is believed that most children do have *some*.

Preschool classes for deaf children seek to create an environment in which a deaf child can have the same experiences and activities that normal preschoolers have. Children are generally enrolled at the age of two-and-a-half years and are expected to attend all sessions. Enrollment in the Preschool Deaf Classes at the Portland Center for Hearing and Speech carries the requirement that the child have a hearing loss significant enough to preclude normal speech and language development, and that he have the mental and physical capacity to benefit from the program.

Parents are encouraged to take the Tracy Clinic Correspondence Course for Parents of Little Deaf Children while their children are attending the Preschool Deaf Classes. The Tracy Correspondence Course is designed to be used with preschool deaf and hard of hearing children between the ages of twenty months and five years. It includes first lessons in lip reading, sense training, and in language and speech preparation. The clinic also suggests ways in which parents can help a younger child until he reaches the age of twenty months.*

Education for the School-Age Deaf Child

There are certain advantages for the deaf child who can attend day school. He is not segregated from people who can hear and talk, but can go home each afternoon to a normal home setting, where he can participate in the activities of his home and his neighborhood. Some public school systems have established such day classes. If these classes are held adjacent to the regular school, the children may participate in certain activities with the hearing children, particularly in the higher grades.

For many children, such opportunities are not available, however, and placement in a residential school is necessary. School education continues to provide speech therapy, lip reading and auditory training. Group hear-

* John Tracy Clinic, 806 West Adams Boulevard, Los Angeles, California.

ing aids with individual earphones are used in classes, and various types of visual aids are utilized as well. One class of five-year-olds in a public day school had been prepared for a visit from a group of student nurses by a picture of a nurse in uniform cut out and posted on a placard. Most of the children had been in a hospital at some time, so identification was not difficult, although the student nurses were not in uniform. One mischievous little boy—rather bored perhaps with the obvious—identified the picture readily enough, but when he was asked to name it, he replied, with a sparkle in his eye, "witch!" (Perhaps he was remembering those "shots.")

THE CHILD WITH A VISUAL DEFECT

"There are still many problems. She is going to have to learn to be helped a little, to have people give her a hand crossing streets and show her around in new places. She'll have to learn to fight the pity and vain hope that sighted people too often extend to the blind. She will have to convince teachers and employers that being blind does not necessarily mean being helpless, sad or stupid.

"In my mind I can see her walking confidently into that world with a smile on her face."*

No one, certainly, has to be convinced that blindness is a severe handicap, and that to have been blind from birth is to miss all of the light and the color, the beauty and the majesty of the world about us. Yet, to quote again from *Our Daughter is Blind:* "We began to think about her blindness in a clearer way: We've never heard a dog whistle. There must be a whole universe of sounds above and below what we can hear. And there are myriads we will never know. Yet we never grieve for these lost sounds and colors. She knows nothing of what we see, so why assume she will feel any loss?

"This was the first step in our emancipation. We began to forget that we were the parents of a *blind* baby. We were parents of a happy, bouncy little girl, who was incidentally, blind."

Definition of Blindness

The legal definition of blindness is a visual acuity of 20/200 or less in the better eye after correction. It has been found, however, that many children with a visual acuity of less than 20/200 can see well enough to make use of the equipment and special educational media provided for the partially sighted.†

PARTIALLY SIGHTED CHILDREN. These are children with a visual acuity between 20/70 and 20/200 in the better eye after all necessary medical or surgical treatment and correction.

SIGHTED CHILDREN WITH EYE PROBLEMS. Such children have a visual acuity of 20/20 or more after any necessary correction.

* Johnson, M.: Our Daughter is Blind. McCalls, Dec., 1953. (Copies of this article may be obtained from The American Foundation for the Blind, 15 W. 16th St., New York, New York.

† Hathaway, W.: Education and Health of Partially Seeing Children. P. 17. 4th ed. New York, Columbia University Press, 1959.

Causes of Eye Problems

Myopia (nearsightedness). Among sighted children with eye problems, errors of refraction are the most common. This appears in the early school years and progresses until the early twenties, after which it may remain stationary. The common belief that eye strain causes nearsightedness or increases its progression is a fallacy. When proper lenses are fitted, vision is corrected to normal. This is a type of defect that may label a school child as being inattentive or retarded, simply because he cannot decipher blackboard writing or distinguish objects at a distance.

Hyperopia (farsightedness). Farsightedness is a common condition of young children, and frequently persists into the first grade of school, or even longer. Whether corrective lenses are needed must be decided on an individual basis by the specialist examining the child. His teachers and his parents should be aware of the considerable eye fatigue that may result from efforts at accommodation for close work.

Astigmatism. Here there is a difference in the refractive power of the various meridians of the eye that results in a distorted image. Astigmatism is usually combined with myopia or hyperopia. Slight degrees often do not require any correction; moderate degrees usually require glasses for reading, television and movies; severe degrees require that glasses be worn constantly.

Partially sighted children also have a high incidence of refractive errors, particularly myopia. Eye injuries are also responsible for the loss of vision, as well as those conditions that can be improved by treatment but result in diminished sight, as is the case in many instances of cataract. Nemir[*] states that about one in 500 school-age children needs special attention because of defective vision—children whose vision cannot be improved with glasses.

The causes for *blindness* have been brought under control in those areas in which medical and surgical care have been adequate, and readily available for those who need it. We still have children in our schools for the blind who are blind by legal definition, however, and we will continue to have them for a long time to come.

Case Finding and Visual Testing

Behavior patterns such as squinting and frowning while trying to read a blackboard, holding work too close to the eyes while reading or writing, and rubbing the eyes to see better are all possible signs of visual difficulty. Simple screening tests are routine in many schools and can be performed by either a teacher or a school nurse. The *Snellen test* is commonly used for children who can read, and the *Snellen E test* is used for younger children who have not yet learned to read.

[*] Nemir, A.: The School Health Program. P. 73. 2nd ed. Philadelphia, W. B. Saunders, 1965.

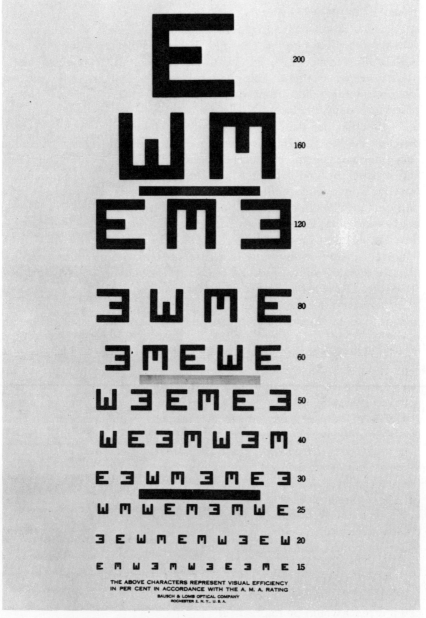

THE ABOVE CHARACTERS REPRESENT VISUAL EFFICIENCY
IN PER CENT IN ACCORDANCE WITH THE A. M. A. RATING
BAUSCH & LOMB OPTICAL COMPANY
ROCHESTER 2, N. Y., U. S. A.

Fig. 116. The Snellen E chart for sight testing in small children.

The Snellen chart. This is the familiar one on which the letters in each line are smaller than those in the preceding line. If the child can read the lines when standing 20 feet away from the chart, his visual acuity is stated as 20/20. If he can read only the line marked 100, his acuity is given as 20/100. The chart should be placed at eye level, with good lighting, and in a room free from distractions. One eye is tested at a time, with the other eye covered. A child should be allowed to take his time reading the letters.

The Snellen E chart. This chart has a series of E letters, with their "fingers" pointing in various directions. The child first learns what is expected of him by placing his fingers over the letter on the chart in the same direction. He then takes his stand at 20 feet, and indicates in which direction the E points by extending his own fingers in the same direction. Some children are apt to become confused, in which case a child may find it easier to hold a large E, and turn that letter in the appropriate direction. Some young children who have a poorly developed sense of direction, or who are confused about what is expected, profit from a little practice at home. One little boy could not make up his mind about which direction he wanted, so a motherly girl his own age promptly took him in charge, and a few days later he passed the test with no difficulty. Such practice does not alter results of the test. (Fig. 116)

Picture charts for identification may be used, but are not considered to be so accurate. It is quite easy for a bright child to memorize the pictures and to guess from the general shape without seeing distinctly.

Long-Term Planning

A child able to associate with normally sighted children is at an advantage, whether he has poor sight or has none at all. The trend is to provide the special education needed by a child with a visual handicap within the context of a regular school. This may be by means of a special class plan, in which a special classroom is his base, and from which he goes out to join the normally seeing children for activities not requiring intensive use of his eyes. A specially prepared teacher directs the work done in the special classroom.

A second plan enrolls a partially sighted child in a regular classroom. He leaves this classroom for concentrated eye work in a specially equipped classroom with a specially prepared teacher.

Another plan, called an *Itinerant Teacher Plan* provides a specially prepared teacher, who acts as consultant for the regular classroom teacher. Together, they work and plan to meet the child's needs. This later plan is especially useful in small communities where a special room and a teacher would be impractical.

Special equipment for the use of children with sight impairment includes printed material with larger type, pencils with large leads for darker lines, cream colored writing paper, tape recordings (which the entire class can enjoy), magnifying glasses and typewriters. The class is inclined to think of these as special privileges rather than in terms of any handicap.

For the children who have a serious impairment and whose participation in regular activities is sharply curtailed, talking books, raised maps and braille equipment is needed as well. Such programs prevent a child from being isolated from the community and do much to minimize his differences from the rest of the children.

Residential schools have played an important part in the education and adjustment of children with severe visual handicaps, and their value should not be minimized. Although it is desirable to keep children in their own homes and in their own community, this is not always possible —or in the child's best interest.

A *blind child,* particularly a child who has never seen, may profit greatly from close contact with sighted children. Children are normally attracted to everything they see about them, and are quite vocal in their enthusiasm. Their spontaneous observations can do much to enrich the life of a blind child, who sees through the eyes of the others. These children can learn to develop their other senses to a degree where they learn to take their place quite confidently among their friends.

In localities in which facilities are available, the same kind of program described for the partially sighted child may be used to advantage. Residential school personnel also realize the disadvantages of isolation from sighted persons, and promote opportunities for community experiences.

CEREBRAL PALSY

Cerebral palsy is a term used to denote a group of disorders arising from a malfunction of motor centers and nerve pathways in the brain. A difficulty in controlling voluntary muscle movements is one manifestation of this organic brain damage, and other manifestations occurring in conjunction with the motor defect may include seizures, mental retardation, various sensory defects and behavior disorders. The condition may be very mild, moderate, or perhaps severe enough to be totally disabling. Training and individual therapy help an affected child to take advantage of every bit of his residual ability, but there is no cure, and some children are too severely affected to respond to treatment. Cerebral palsy may have its origin in the prenatal, the natal, or in the postnatal period. Heredity is a factor in some cases, as are prenatal infections in others. Adverse factors at birth can be traced in many affected children. Anoxia caused by respiratory obstruction, atelectasis, placenta praevia and breech delivery with a delay of the aftercoming head are frequently cited causes. Maternal toxemia, dystocia, and premature separation of the placenta are mentioned as well.

Postnatal causes include trauma, infections of the central nervous system, kernicterus, and a variety of other nervous system affections.

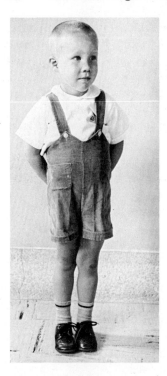

Fig. 117. A five-year-old girl with athetosis uses a walker. She cannot stand alone and does not talk. Two healthy brothers (above left and below right) accept her naturally. Although heredity may be a factor in this condition, note that the posture and general appearance of the siblings indicate normal muscular control.

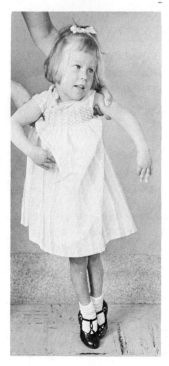

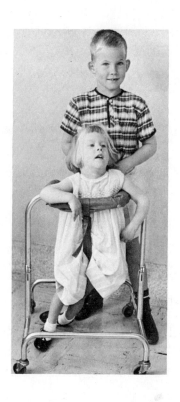

Types Most Commonly Seen

1. ATHETOID. Athetosis is marked by involuntary incoordinate motion with varying degrees of muscle tension. These are the cerebral palsied children who are constantly in motion, described as the whole body being in a state of slow, writhing, muscular contractions whenever voluntary movement is attempted.*

2. SPASTIC. This is the most frequent type. There is a hyperactive stretch reflex in associated muscle groups, an increased activity of the deep tendon reflexes, clonus, and contractures affecting the antigravity muscles and scissoring. When *scissoring* is present, the child crosses his legs and points his toes when he is set on his feet.

3. ATAXIA. This is essentially a lack of coordination caused by disturbances of the kinesthetic and the balance senses.

4. RIGIDITY. This type is characterized by rigid postural attitudes.

5. MIXED TYPES. These are seen, but one form usually predominates.

Treatment

Treatment is directed toward helping the child make the most complete use of his residual abilities, and toward helping him achieve satisfaction and enrichment to the full limit of his capacities.

Three Children With Cerebral Palsy

The first child, whom we shall call Mary L., is a petite, blue-eyed 5-year-old with a sweet smile and happy, friendly disposition. Mary has severe athetosis. She has two sturdy, active brothers of six and three years of age, and understanding, loving parents.

Case 1. Mary was born about two weeks after the expected date, with a birth weight of 6 pounds, 8 ounces. There was no history of any hereditary condition, maternal infection or birth injury. Mary's mother noted that at about the age of one to two months that her baby smiled, cooed, and followed objects with her eyes, but did not kick or use her arms freely as her brothers had.

At 13 months of age, she was examined in the crippled children's division at a medical center. At that time she was unable to sit, to hold her head erect, or to roll over. Her babbling and her vocal play was limited—she echoed some vowel sounds but had no true words. She appeared to be alert, reacting differently to various words, and responding visually with facial expressions. At this time a diagnosis of cerebral palsy, athetoid type, was made.

At the age of five, Mary is an appealing little girl, shows an interest in the world about her, and adapts well to functional situations. She has no speech, and no functional use of her arms or her legs. Her "yes" response is a smile, and her "no" is a crying response or puckered lips.

With the aid of short leg braces and a walker, Mary is able to attain an upright position. She loves to be with people, especially with other children, and appears content to watch their play. Because of her severe physical handicaps an accurate assessment of her intellectual ability is impossible. Swallowing presents some difficulties, but she is progressing from strained to solid foods.

* Woods, G.: Cerebral Palsy in Childhood. P. 70. Bristol, England, Wright, 1957.

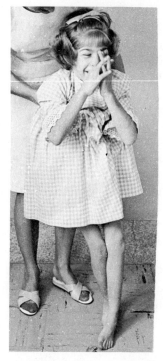 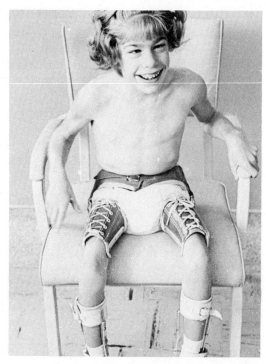

a.   b.

Fig. 118a. Cerebral palsied seven-year-old with severe spastic diplegia. Note scissoring without braces and forward thrust of head.

Fig. 118b. Same child showing hip and leg braces.

She is partially toilet trained, and functions adequately if placed on the toilet, but she is not always able to make her needs known.

Mrs. L. states that the diagnosis of her daughter's condition was difficult for her to accept. She feels that her husband's strongly supportive role has helped her greatly, and she has learned to accept Mary as she is, and has learned to appreciate her gentle, lovable personality. The relaxed, accepting attitude of the family is quite apparent, and undoubtedly plays a considerable role in the child's own adjustment. Mrs. L. is concerned about Mary's future, and is anxious for her to have speech therapy. Mary is thought to be too immature, however, to accept a planned program of instruction at this time.

Case 2. Louise C. is a 7-year-old with severe spastic diplegia. No maternal infection or other difficulties were apparent at birth, but she was cyanotic at birth, and stained amniotic fluid gave evidence of fetal distress. She received oxygen during the first 24 hours after her birth, and was kept in the hospital for two weeks. Thereafter she had an uneventful postnatal course.

Her mother became aware of her slow development, when, at the age of six months, she did not coo, did not grasp objects and was unable to sit with support. A diagnosis of cerebral palsy, spastic type, was made at the age of eight months. At the age of one year, Louise commenced having grand mal seizures that ultimately became frequent. At the present time, her seizures occur less frequently now that she takes Dilantin and Mebaral.

Louise commenced therapy at a crippled children's center at the age of two years. She had an increased tonus with stretch reflexes of the spastic condition, with an evaluation of a motor quotient of six or seven month level. Her mother was taught methods of speech therapy to carry out at home in conjunction with therapy at her regular sessions at the center.

At the age of six years, surgery was performed for a right hip flexor release, and long leg casts were applied. At present she wears hip and leg braces to help her maintain an upright position and to help her place her feet squarely on the floor. She does not stand unsupported, but must use a wheelchair instead.

Louise is the second child in the family, with both older and younger brothers. Her parents give her support and understanding care, and have been able to adjust to her disabilities. She attends a special day school three times weekly, and has a moderate mental deficiency. Her voice has a hypernasal quality. She rarely initiates speech, using a few words but not in connected sentences.

Case 3. Sharon H. is an 11-year-old girl in a family of six children, a beautiful collie, a cat, and a litter of kittens. She has brothers aged thirteen, nine, seven and four, and a busy sister of toddler age.

Sharon has cerebral palsy, athetoid type. She was born prematurely (caused by placenta abruptia) was lethargic and had postnatal breathing difficulties. She was given oxygen and intravenous fluids for a few days, but appeared to be in good condition at discharge.

Mrs. H. states that she was told she might expect Sharon to show some brain damage, but she did not know how this would be manifested and feared that the term meant severe mental deficiency. A diagnosis of athetosis was made at the age of nine months. Mrs. H. found it is not easy to accept a handicap in one's child, even when one has been alerted to the possibility. Both of Sharon's parents set about with faith and persistence, however, to help her develop to the limit of her potential.

Sharon had difficulty sucking and taking baby foods because of the reverse tongue thrust common in athetosis. She eventually achieved control, but her drooling is a problem, and she has to make a conscious effort to swallow.

As Sharon grew older, her parents wished to enroll her in a school for handicapped children, but psychological testing gave indecisive and conflicting results, and the question was raised as to her ability to profit from such schooling. This was very discouraging to Mrs. H., who believed that Sharon's ability was not accurately reflected in her test scores. A teacher was obtained to teach her at home for two years, after which she was accepted at school where she has shown remarkable progress. Testing now reveals her intelligence to be within normal range.

Sharon is a girl of great determination, with a strong desire to be independent. She has consistently accepted challenges, achieving beyond the predictions of her probable ability. She is able to stand alone momentarily with the use of braces, can take several steps with crutches, and she frequently succeeds in turning herself around. She achieved fair control of her random movements, dresses herself except for buttons and zippers, and takes care of her own toilet needs with the aid of specially built appliances. (Figs. 117–119)

Sharon was greatly pleased to be interviewed at home with her family, because, as she said, "I want to help other children." Speech is difficult for her because an effort may produce a spasm, but she is persistent and very patient. The family atmosphere is casual; Sharon realizes her difficulties and no one glosses over them or hides them. They are accepted the same way any disability might be. She is hard to understand, but this does not deter her from talking. Her mother may say, "I didn't get any of that," and Sharon will try again—and again; beaming with pride when things get across. Sometimes, when things are too difficult, she goes to her typewriter and types out the message.

The family loves camping, and Sharon joins in with zest, although her mobility is considerably more difficult than in the atmosphere at home or in school. She attends Easter Seal camp and wishes it lasted longer. Her greatest interest is school, however, and she "can hardly wait for school to start," for the fall term.

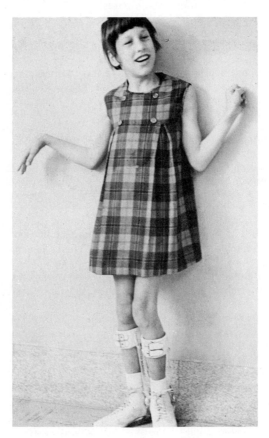

a.

Fig. 119a. Eleven-year-old with athetosis. She wears short leg braces, and special shoes to keep her feet fairly flat on the floor.
Fig. 119b. The same child, showing the random movements of athetosis.

She became somewhat excited during the evening, but when the interviewer remarked that an entire evening of being talked about was hard to take, she giggled and relaxed. When she was asked about how she felt about her difficulties she said wistfully, "I would like to be able to walk," but in other respects, she has accepted herself as she is and lets nothing interefere with her enjoyment of life.

Mrs. H. worries somewhat about the future as Sharon matures, and is rather apprehensive about the problems that face this severely handicapped girl. Sharon, with her stubborn determination, may still have some surprises for everyone.

General Discussion

These three girls have several points of similarity. They all have severely handicapped speech and motor abilities, and they all have parents who show tenderness and affection toward them. The outstanding factor, however, is the manner in which they are simply accepted as a part of the family unit, each with her own unique problems, but not

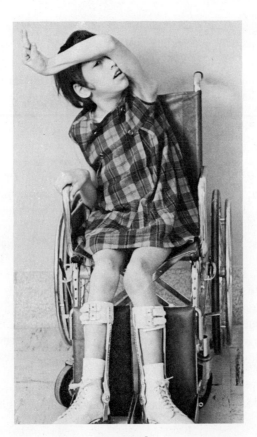

Fig. 119b

someone who is "different" or an outsider. They differ in their personalities as any persons do; Sharon, with her intense drive to succeed, and Mary, with her quiet acceptance of a passive role.

Each child exemplifies some reaction that frequently appears among children with cerebral palsy. One author mentions the "occasional abnormal fears," that are found in many children with cerebral palsy.* Sharon's parents were somewhat puzzled by the existence of totally unreasonable fears in an otherwise well-adjusted child, until they were informed that they are not uncommon. As a small child, Sharon was thrown off balance by the exuberant greeting of a large puppy. Her subsequent fear of dogs grew into fear of furry toy animals, and then into a fear of music boxes! Her parents reason that the inability of a handicapped child to run away from a fear-provoking object may help account for this persistent conditioning.

Mary appears to be the sort of child who accepts her limitations and finds her satisfaction from the affection of her family. Her active brothers, absorbed in the normal pursuits of their age, certainly show no indications of rejection.

The manner in which each set of parents has met the problem, has undoubtedly been the basis for the total family integration and adjustment. The parents who had been able to attend parent-group meetings and who had been able to talk over their mutual problems had felt they profited considerably.

Treatment and Special Aids

The control of the body, needed to carry out physical activities, is learned automatically by a normal child, but must be consciously learned by a physically handicapped child. Physical therapy attempts to teach such a child to carry out an activity that he has not previously been able to accomplish. The methods must be suited to the needs of the individual child, as well as to the general needs arising from his condition. Such methods are based on principles such as conditioning, relaxation, utilization of residual patterns, stimulation of contraction and relaxation of antagonistic muscles, and on other pertinent principles.

Braces are used as supportive and control measures to facilitate muscle training, to reinforce weak or paralyzed muscles, or to counteract the pull of antagonistic muscles. They are of various types, designed for specific purposes. Orthopedic surgery may improve function and correct deformities in many instances. (The release of contractures and the lengthening of tight heel cords are just two examples.)

Helpful appliances for home care and training. A child who has had difficulty maintaining balance while he sits may need a high backed chair,

* Illingworth, R., (ed.): Recent Advances In Cerebral Palsy. P. 120. Boston, Little, Brown & Co., 1958.

with side pieces and a foot platform. If a child has serious difficulty, straps may be needed to help hold him in place. The addition of casters or wheels behind the back legs make it possible to move the chair about. Specially constructed toilet seats also help the child achieve independence.

Feeding aids include spoons with enlarged handles for easy grasping, or with bent handles allowing the bowl of the spoon to be brought easily to the mouth. Plates with high rims and suction devices to prevent slipping (such as those used for infants) enable a child to feed himself. Covered cups, set in holders, with a hole in the lid to admit a plastic drinking tube, help a child who does not have hand control.

An improvement in manual skill can be aided by games such as peg boards, or by cards that must be manipulated. The ability to use a typewriter is an enormous morale booster for a child whose handicap is too severe to permit him to write legibly. A shield placed over the keyboard, with round holes over each key, allows the child to strike the desired letter key with a rubber-tipped stick. This has even been successful for those children with poor hand coordination and has proved valuable as a means of self-expression.

Prognosis

The basic defect is a fact that must be accepted. The child's future is dependent on so many variables that no flat statements can be made about his future. Some children, given the amount and type of help necessary, and the important emotional support they need, are able to achieve a satisfactory degree of independence. Vocational training with employment in a sheltered workshop may furnish an opportunity to many who otherwise might never achieve independence. Some of them will always need a significant amount of nursing care, with the possibility of residential care in an institution when their parents can no longer care for them.

When the significant advances that have been made and the present interest in these children are taken into consideration, the future for the children presents a more optimistic picture than formerly.

BIBLIOGRAPHY

Hathaway, W.: Education and Health of Partially Seeing Children. 4th ed. New York, Columbia University Press, 1959.
Illingworth, R., (ed.): Recent Advances in Cerebral Palsy. Chap. 12, P. 120. Boston, Little, Brown & Co., 1958.
Johnson, M.: Our Daughter is Blind. McCalls, (Dec.) 1953.
Katzin, H., and Wilson, G.: Rehabilitation of a Child's Eyes. 3rd ed. St. Louis, C. V. Mosby, 1961.
Moriarty, M.: How the Deaf Child Learns to Talk. Chicago, Hearing Aid Division, Zenith Radio Corp.
Nelson, W., (ed.): Textbook of Pediatrics. 8th ed. Pp. 820, 1244–1247. Philadelphia, W. B. Saunders, 1964.

Nemir, A.: The School Health Program. Chap. 6, 2nd ed. Philadelphia, W. B. Saunders, 1965.

Oregon School for the Deaf: The A B C's For Parents of Preschool Deaf Children. Salem, Oregon School for the Deaf.

Roper, K.: Referral to the opthalmologist: when and why? Clin. Pediat., 3:451, 1964.

Scheie, H.: Disorders of children's eyes: notes on early recognition of disturbances. Clin. Pediat., 2:91, 1963.

Silver, H. K., Kempe, C. H., and Bruyn, H. B.: Handbook of Pediatrics. 6th ed. Los Altos, California, Lange Medical Publications, 1965.

Utley, J.: How to Help the Deaf Child at Home. Distributed by Chicago, Hearing Aid Division, Zenith Radio Corp.

Wallace, H.: Health Services for Mothers and Children. Philadelphia, W. B. Saunders, 1962.

Woods, G.: Cerebral Palsy in Childhood. P. 70. Bristol, England, John Wright & Sons, 1957.

SUGGESTED READINGS FOR FURTHER STUDY

Battin, R., and Haug, C. O.: Speech and Language Delay. Springfield, Illinois, Charles C Thomas, 1964.

Crothers, B.: The Natural History of Cerebral Palsy. Cambridge, Harvard University Press, 1959.

Denhoff, E., and Robinault, I. P.: Cerebral Palsy and Related Disorders: A Developmental Approach to Dysfunction. New York, McGraw-Hill, 1960.

DiCarlo, L.: The Deaf. Englewood Cliffs, New Jersey, Prentice-Hall, 1964.

Dougherty, A. L., and Cohen, J. L.: Auditory screening for infants. Nurs. Outlook, 9:310, 1961.

Fraiberg, S., and Freedman, D. A.: Studies in the ego development of the congenitally blind child. Psychoanl. Stud. Child, 19:113, 1964.

Gay, M.: A preschool program for children with cerebral palsy. Children, 12:105, 1965.

Harris, G.: Language for the preschool deaf child. 2nd ed. New York, Grune & Stratton, 1963.

Minear, W. L.: A Classification of Cerebral Palsy. Pediatrics, 18:841, 1956.

Pendleton, T., and Simonson, J.: Training children with cerebral palsy. Amer. J. Nurs., 64:126, (May) 1964.

Spock, B., and Lerrigo, M.: Caring for your disabled child. New York, Macmillan, 1965.

Steele, S.: Physical education in a rehabilitation center. Nurs. Outlook, 14:41, (May) 1966.

UNIT 7

THE ADOLESCENT

24

Normal Growth and Development

A child moving from middle childhood into adolescence moves from a climate of security into a new sphere. This is a transition period in which physiological changes, as well as society's expectations, bring about uncertainty in his mind as to the role he should play. This uncertainty frequently extends to the adults in his environment as well. Quite literally, the rapid changes in his physical development make him a stranger to himself.

Some Descriptive Terms for this Age Group

Some clarification of terms is necessary. The *pubescent period* denotes the time from the onset of the adolescent changes and ends in puberty itself. It is marked by a spurt in physical growth, changes in body proportions and by the maturation of the secondary sex characteristics. This period, lasting approximately two years, may be called the prepubescent or the preadolescent period, although the latter term is not strictly accurate.

Puberty. This is the point at which the biological changes reach a climax, and mark the termination of the pubescent period. It is marked by the appearance of the *menarche* in girls, and the production of spermatozoa in boys.

Adolescence. This period begins with a growth spurt and ends when the individual has reached his full physical and his full social maturity.

Menarche is the term used for the first menses. *Secondary sex characteristics* include breast development, widening of the pelvic girdle, the appearance of axillary and pubic hair (in girls) and, in boys, an increase in the size of the external sex organs, the appearance of axillary and pubic hair, voice changes and eventually, the appearance of facial hair.

In our culture, the adolescent period is culturally as well as physically oriented. For a painfully long time the adolescent is neither child nor adult, and he has a great uncertainty as to his appropriate responses. His uncertainty is not helped by adults, whose laws, customs and individual treatment of him reflect their own ambivalence toward him. He is all too apt to hear, today, "Don't act so childish," while yesterday, he heard "You are not old enough."

In some cultures, puberty rites separate the boys, and often the girls as well, from their childhood, so that after a period of weeks or months of ceremony, he becomes an adult, with all adult privileges. Vestiges of these rites remain in our own culture with confirmation, Bar Mizvah, and coming-out ceremonies. The complexities of modern western culture, however, appear to make this transition period one of increased tension and turbulence.

In large part, of course, a child's own maturing body and personality changes are responsible for his bewilderment. His new body, his feelings and emotions, do not fit his self-image and he must go through a period of intense self-awareness—in other words—a period of self-absorption.

Physical Changes

The physical changes commence in a girl with the beginning of breast development, and with the beginning of the growth spurt. These changes commence approximately two years before the appearance of the menarche. This period of rapid growth in both height and in weight is the second such period during a child's life, the first occurring during the first year of life.

The average age for the first menstrual period of American girls is between 12 and 13 years, but there is a wide variation among individuals. It appears as early as the age of 9 in some girls; in others it has been delayed as late as the age of 15 or 16.

An average boy begins his growth spurt at the age of eleven, with an early growth of his external genitalia at twelve. Pubescence, signaled by the production of spermatozoa, cannot be pinpointed as easily as can the menarche in girls, but occurs in an average boy between the ages of fourteen and fifteen. Although it is correct to say that adolescence appears

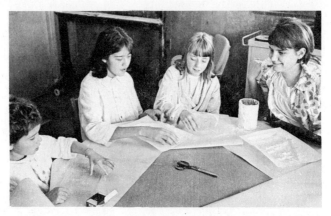

Fig. 120. Adolescents in the hospital, ages 12 to 13. (The small child is 11.) Note the different degrees of development.

approximately two years later in boys than in girls, there is actually much overlapping. Because of the wide variance between individuals in their rate of growth and maturation during this period, one may see children of the same age in all stages of development. Within a group of thirteen-year-old girls there are some who are small and thin, with flat breasts and narrow hips. Others may show quite womanly figures with developing breasts, widened hips and tall stature. (Fig. 120)

A young girl may become embarrassed about her budding breasts, but she is secretly often pleased about this evidence of her femininity. Sometimes, however, she may really resent that she is a girl, and may try to resist development. Similarly, a girl experiencing delayed puberty may feel left out of her more rapidly maturing age group. She is apt to feel that she is not normal, and that something has gone wrong.

A boy, however, suffers most keenly over his delayed development. His ideal is to become manly, and in our culture, short stature in the male (or any feminine characteristics) are traits ridiculed or disapproved of by the majority. A virile looking male is the ideal. Therefore, the despair of a boy is very real if he believes that he is not developing the appropriate characteristics.

These young people need someone to listen to their fears and someone to be sympathetic to them. They need to be reassured that many people are slow to develop, and that in but a few years, they will have achieved normal growth. As a matter of fact, the late developers have the best possibility for becoming tall because an early closure of the epiphyses also marks the end of bone growth. Perhaps the father could show that he too was slow in maturing. Some parents need to be reassured, however, and may need to have pointed out to them that their concern is only fixing the idea more firmly in their boy's mind that something is wrong.

A young person grows and develops with great rapidity after pubescence has started. He may grow unevenly, perhaps one arm may be temporarily shorter than the other, or his legs may be growing out of proportion to the rest of his body. A girl may develop breasts that are large in proportion to her size. Many boys develop "feminine" breasts because of an increase in hormones and suffer agonies because they feel they are abnormal. They need to be assured that this, too, is normal, and, in nearly every instance, is no cause for concern. Some boys ask for surgery if this period is prolonged—but unless the boy's emotional life is seriously disturbed, his breasts are better left alone.

Developmental Tasks of Adolescence

Because of the rapid changes in body development, a young person has difficulty in forming a clear image of himself. This accounts for much of his seeming awkwardness. Actually, adolescents can be very graceful and well co-ordinated, as are figure skaters and athletes.

An adolescent's glandular changes make him seem like a new person to himself as well. He must learn to be an effective person all over again, and the developmental demands of this period are unique. These include achieving an emotional independence from adults, establishing satisfying relations with both boys and girls, choosing and preparing for a vocation, building social, ethical and spiritual values, developing socially responsible behavior, and reaching forward to maturity.

As he leaves his childish self behind him and tries on his new adult role, he naturally wishes to be considered by others as adult. The transition cannot be as abrupt as this, however. These new forces appearing are so powerful and so little understood by him, that often he is secretly terrified by them, even while he strongly desires to act as an adult. He sometimes is desperately afraid that he cannot control them. Although he almost certainly grumbles and rebels, he is often relieved when his parents put the weight of their authority behind his own inadequate control, in much the same manner as when he was a toddler exploring his strange, bewildering universe.

Indeed, in spite of his maturation and his changing status, he is the same person he was at two or three. Unquestionably, the foundations laid down during early childhood are the factors that can help either to smooth or trouble his present development. This realization is extremely important in child rearing practices, but it brings cold comfort to both the parents and their offspring when, because of any number of circumstances, the child's early environment was somewhat less than ideal. Parents are human and make mistakes just as anyone else does. It seems to make little sense to say to a troubled parent "This is the result of your rejection, or your possessiveness, or your over-protection." If the parent is at all intelligent or sensitive, he already has some awareness of his own failure, and a confirmation does not ease his sense of guilt, or aid him in facing the present situation. Also, for a maturing child, the sense of failure on the part of the parent may become a rationalization of his own inadequacies, and, in a very real way, prevent him from facing and conquering his problems.

What are the problems and tasks of this period? The most important is finding oneself and discovering what sort of person one is. The youth is actually "trying on for size" different types of personalities in an effort to discover one that fits his present idea of himself. As his self-concept is constantly changing, his conscious personality is changing with it. He can discard last week's concept easily and expects you to do the same.

If he is to develop an individuality, he must have independence and the freedom to *be* independent. Hence his intense, fierce rebellion against parental restraint even while, secretly, he would like to be back in that simpler period when he could conform without question. Although he would be relieved if he could occasionally surrender his independence, his need to achieve status with his peer group forbids it.

The Hospitalized Adolescent

What does all this have to do with nursing an adolescent? We find here too that we cannot function in a situation that we do not understand, or that we only partially comprehend.

When an adolescent enters the hospital, he brings his own personality structure with him. It may be quite difficult for a young nurse, who is too near this age herself, to feel comfortable or to function effectively under these circumstances. She may become too involved, and find any objectivity very nearly impossible.

An adolescent may also find the situation difficult when the nurse is so near his age level. Because of his increased self-consciousness, his body becomes a source of embarrassment. Although the adolescent depends on his peers for approval and acceptance, he senses that a mature adult is the kind of person he needs when he is made dependent by an illness. He can now dare to indulge his need for "mothering" because of the imposed dependency.

The authority and status conferred by the nurse's uniform and by the title of Nurse may help a young nurse or a student nurse to achieve this role of authority figure, both for herself and for her patient.

If a nurse is functioning in the situation that still prevails in a majority of hospitals, she will not have much choice as to whether she cares for adolescent patients. Practices vary, but a large number of hospitals set the upper age for patients in their pediatric departments as anywhere between twelve and fourteen years. In such situations, adolescent patients are scattered throughout the hospital, on the adult wards. While this may seem unrealistic in terms of development, it is often necessary in terms of the hospital's physical facilities which may not be geared to handle an adolescent in the pediatric department.

A newer trend, which is becoming increasingly popular, is to establish adolescent wards. These may consist of a few rooms set aside at one end of the pediatric department or, more probably, an entire adolescent wing. Because of the fascinating possibilities for the improved care of teen-agers in such an arrangement, this idea is dealt with in some detail later in this chapter.

To return to the patient himself, and to the problems that illness and hospitalization bring, we find that because of his absorption in his body image and in its changes, illnesses also have an increased interest for him. He is apt to have a large fund of information, much of which is incorrect or distorted. He probably has many fears about the effect of his illness on his appearance or on his future adequacy.

This intensified interest, as well as the alert and curious nature of a teen-ager provides a wealth of opportunity for the nurse, if she can rec- ognize it. The way is open for some sound health teaching.

Miss Brown was busy behind the bed-side curtains while she was caring for a twelve-year-old boy, while four other boys in the ward were discussing life in general. Ignoring her presence, they were busily discussing menstruation. They were honestly puzzled, especially as to the effects of "all that bleeding." Finally Johnny suggested, "Why don't we ask Miss Brown?" which they promptly did. Startled, but rallying bravely, Miss Brown gave an elementary lesson in the physiology of menstruation, which satisfied the boys. One needs to be prepared for all eventualities when working with young people.

The adolescent, of course, is experiencing a renewed interest in sex, and is trying to chart a course for himself in an area in which he finds very little guidance. Often he is quiet about this and gives little indica- tion of any need for help. On the other hand, he frequently does throw out clues. One fourteen-year-old boy repeatedly attempted physical inti- macies while receiving his morning care (which included a bed bath) from the student nurse. The nurse was confused and troubled. She knew that Jerry was from a deprived, broken home, and she fancied that she would be showing him more "rejection" if she refused the kiss he de- manded. She began to dread her clinical experience. When she was asked why she had not sought advice, she admitted a reluctance to do so for fear that she would be considered "squeamish," or unable to work out her own problems. In this case, both the patient and his nurse were con- fused. A student should be willing to accept her own inexperience and lack of background. This young woman simply did not have the maturity to handle the situation alone, and should have sought help from someone competent to give it to her. Undoubtedly Jerry had been a rejected child, but the student could not undo the years of environmental deprivation in a matter of days, nor did she have the experience to try. A young nurse should have a very clear idea of her role. She is not a psychiatrist, a medi- cal doctor, a social service specialist, nor is she a priest. She is a nurse, and does all that she can to bring a child back to health, and undoubtedly draws on all these resources. She should also know her limitations very clearly.

It would seem that at this point Jerry needed firmness. He probably needed an older person for his nurse, because a young woman giving him intimate care confused him. It was a situation that should not have been allowed to continue.

Adolescent Clinics

An adolescent has worries and fears that may seem childish to an adult, and because an adolescent fears that he may seem childish, he often keeps his troubles to himself. Gallagher, commenting on a youth's reluctance to discuss his problems with his parents, says, "For this reason if the physician will present as a strong, warm, interested person—non-authoritarian, neither approving or disapproving—he will gain their confidence and he can be of great help."*

Adolescent clinics seem to provide the ideal setting for an exploration of the needs and the anxieties of adolescents. There are a number of these unique clinics in the United States, and they are proving to be very successful. An adolescent clinic is a place set apart for young persons only. Personnel and doctors are sympathetic to their problems. The young person has reached a phase of his life in which he has an intense interest in his own body. This is also an age at which his desire to identify with his peers is paramount. This is all preparation for his maturity and should thus be respected.

One great difficulty that an adolescent seems to experience is that no one appears to want to listen to him. He may talk, worry and question, but it seems to him that adults are not really listening. The attitude strikes him as one of, "These things do not mean anything. You will soon get over them. This is just a phase you are going through."

We go through phases all our lives, and it would be too bad for us if no one ever took them seriously. Perhaps we do think that adolescents take themselves too seriously. They need to do this to find themselves. We must respect them and listen to them, if we want them to grow into confident, responsible people.

An adolescent clinic is a place in which they can be heard, in which their worries are respected, and in which they and their doctors together can try to work out problems. Adolescent patients make their own appointments and go unaccompanied to the clinic, where they find all the other patients are of their own age group.

One girl has acne, which worries her greatly, but she hesitates to talk to her mother about it because she boasts about the beautiful complexion she had when she was young. A boy is concerned about his slow development, while another worries over a functional heart murmur that has convinced his mother that he should not play football. Still another is puzzled about his severe headaches which are worse during the sports season (in which he is active) but at which time his grades "are not so good."†

All of these persons need and must receive consideration, not only of their ailments, but also of their confusing personal problems. At the clinic they have careful physical examinations, and are shown their X-rays and the results of laboratory tests. The entire setting is geared to a consideration of a young person's problems.

---

* Gallagher, J. R.: Medical Care of the Adolescent. New York, Appleton-Century-Crofts, 1960.

† From the film *Medical Care for the Adolescent,* 16 mm., sound (color) 30 min. Philadelphia, Merck, Sharp and Dohme.

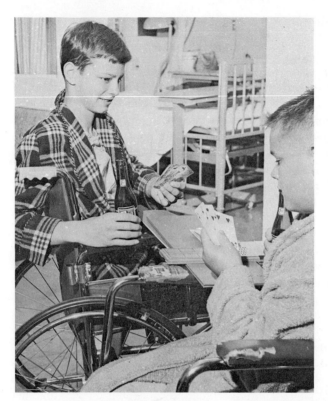

Fig. 121 (Top). The adolescent ward provides atmosphere suited to this age.

Fig. 121 (Bottom). Two adolescent girls playing a game.

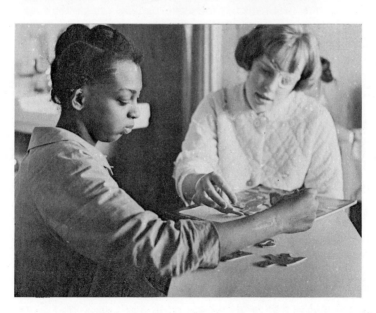

Adolescent In-Patient Care

For a young person who must be hospitalized, a separate adolescent unit seems so right that one wonders why it has taken so long to get them started. Virtually any hospital should be able to set aside at least a small unit for this purpose. (Fig. 121 and 122)

Some hospitals that have done so have found the experiment very successful. The director of one hospital had his attention drawn to the unhappy situation of teen-age patients scattered throughout the hospital, by the experience of his own son. Here, as in many hospitals, teen-agers were assigned to adult wards according to the nature of their ailments. A young boy in a ward with older men found them quite free with unwholesome stories. A young girl had for roommates senile, withdrawn patients; another was in a room with women suffering from gynecological troubles, who freely discussed their ailments. To the administrator, this did not seem to be the best setting for learning "the facts of life." In fact, he was shocked by the situation and resolved to do something about it.

The "doing something about it" took the form of a unit of care just

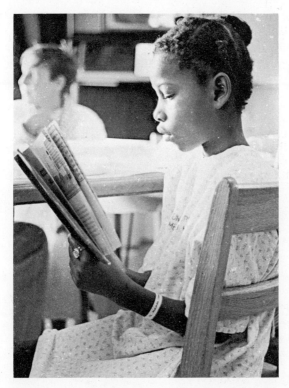

Fig. 122. A thirteen-year-old in the adolescent ward.

for teen-agers. A wing adjacent to the children's ward was utilized, and it has been an outstanding success.

In such a setting, enthusiastic young visitors do not annoy older, sick persons. The patients are sympathetic and understanding toward each other. Their interests are similar, their school work is shared, and the staff is chosen from among those who have a sympathetic understanding of this age group. Rules are enforced, of course—but they are written with this age group in mind. Meals are nutritious, and the food is plentiful, geared to adolescent appetites. The unit has now passed the experimental stage and is an integral part of the hospital.

Young nurses may gain both insight and competence if they are assigned to care for patients in an adolescent ward, but some caution is indicated. Most young males feel embarrassed about having personal services performed by someone near their own age, and they may occasionally show this by aggressive behavior. They may also attach too much personal meaning to the attention given them. Girls in this period of development are also very shy about their bodies and may prefer an older, motherly person to care for them, or perhaps an older, impersonal woman.

A student or a young nurse should be quite secure in her own role. She can do much to put a patient at ease, in any situation, with her professional manner and her impersonal ministrations, and thus the experience can have great value for both the nurse and her patient.

BIBLIOGRAPHY

Blos, P.: On Adolescence. Chicago, Free Press of Glencoe, 1961.

Breckenridge, M., and Vincent, E.: Child Development. 5th ed. Philadelphia, W. B. Saunders, 1964.

Gallagher, J. R.: Medical Care of the Adolescent. New York, Appleton-Century-Crofts, 1960.

Merck, Sharp and Dohme: Medical Care for the Adolescent: (film) 16 mm., sound, (color) 30 min. Philadelphia, Merck, Sharp and Dohme, Film Library % Ralph Lopatin Productions.

Pediatric Clinics of North America: Symposium on Adolescence. Pediat. Clin. N. Amer., 7, (Feb.) 1960.

Watson, E. H., and Lowrey, G. H.: Growth and Development of Children. 4th ed. Chicago, Year Book Publishers, 1962.

SUGGESTED READINGS FOR FURTHER STUDY

Chapman, A. H.: On managing adolescents. J.A.M.A., *174*:1954, 1960.

Eisenberg, L.: A developmental approach to adolescence. Children, *12*:131, 1965.

Erikson, E.: Challenge of Youth. New York, Basic Books, 1964.

Hurlock, E. B.: Adolescent Development. 2nd ed. New York, McGraw-Hill, 1965.

Peckos, P. S., and Heald, F. P.: Nutrition in adolescence. Children, *11*:27, 1964.

Rule, J. T.: The parental dilemma. Pediatrics, *35*:486, 1965.

25

Emotional Development
of the Adolescent —
Conditions of Adolescence

When considering the various aspects of adolescent care, it is important to keep in mind that an adolescent "was not always and will not always be an adolescent," as Gallagher states.* His problems are those of someone who has *been* a child and who *will be* an adult. Certain aspects of life have particular importance for him now, but they occur in the context of his development as a child, and influence his future.

It is true that adolescents have reached a stage of development that presents special problems that cut across both physical and emotional areas. They may be called "adolescent problems" because they are nearly universal for that age group. The manner in which they are met is determined largely by the personality of the individual confronting them. Various conditions, medical or emotional, do have a special meaning for an adolescent, however, because of the particular stage of development that he has reached. One particularly annoying condition is acne.

ACNE VULGARIS

Acne is a condition that is so common among young people that it may be considered as one of the hallmarks of adolescence. This does not make it popular, nor does it diminish the seriousness with which teen-agers regard it. Young people wish to be popular and need to be attractive. An unsightly skin condition can decrease their self-confidence, and can cause shyness and social withdrawal. A young person with acne may consider the blemish to be much more severe than do others, which causes a disproportionate amount of anxiety. This trait of concentrating on one defect—to the extent of ignoring one's own assets is not, however, limited to adolescents.

Acne vulgaris is characterized by the appearance of blackheads, white-

* Gallagher, J.: Medical Care of the Adolescent. P. 3. New York, Appleton-Century-Crofts, 1960.

heads, papules or pustules on the face, and to a lesser extent on the back and the chest. The sites of these changes are the follicles into which the sebaceous glands empty sebum, the lubricating fluid secreted by the sebaceous glands. The inflammatory lesions appear to be a result of the irritant action of sebum, and impaction of these follicles cause the comedones (or blackheads) of acne.

Predisposing Causes

Adolescent acne is primarily an expression of the endocrine imbalance that occurs at this time of life—but a variety of factors contribute to its production. Hereditary factors seem to be involved, as well as emotional conflicts, infection, poor hygiene and diet. The acne may be mild, characterized by an oily skin and by blackheads; it may be more severe with papules, pustules, and some scarring, or it may be a severe type with rope-like cystic lesions, with scarring a common feature. Because the condition may become severe, it is well to give it early attention.

Local Treatment

Washing and cleansing of the skin two or three times a day (or oftener) makes the face feel drier and more comfortable. Vigorous scrubbing causing irritation should be avoided. Antisepsis may be achieved by the application of 70 per cent isopropyl alcohol following washing.

Comedones should not be squeezed, but should be removed by a comedo extractor—generally by a physician. Lotions containing sulfur and resorcin are useful for drying the skin.

Severe acne that does not respond to these measures may be treated by the dermatologist with systemic antibiotic therapy. Ultraviolet light therapy has also brought improvement. Roentgen therapy and dermabrasion are generally not recommended during adolescence.

General Management

Sufficient sleep and exercise, recreation and social activities are all beneficial. The role of diet is inconsistent, but certain foods such as chocolate, nuts, fried foods and sea foods may aggravate the condition. A young person may have fantasies about the cause of his condition, and encouragement to discuss it with a physician *or the school nurse may help him understand* the nature of this skin infection. Of even more importance, the understanding, interested manner of a nurse or a physician may give him the courage to discuss some of his anxieties. Young people frequently find it difficult to discuss personal, emotionally charged matters with their parents because they need to be emancipated from their role of childhood dependency. An adult who listens objectively, with the emphasis on *listen,* may be able to give the most help, whether this is a nurse, a teacher, a counselor or a physician.

OBESITY

Obesity is another condition that can have an adverse effect on an adolescent's self-image. Obesity means, quite simply, an excessive accumulation of fatty subcutaneous tissue. It is a common problem in adolescence—a particularly unwelcome problem to girls in American culture—where to be fat is to be unattractive.

Obesity undoubtedly is caused mainly by overeating, but the problem cannot be solved by commanding a young person to use will power and to eat less food. Many factors enter into the problem and should be considered.

Activity is of major importance in controlling adolescent obesity. An active adolescent may eat large amounts and still not gain weight, while his sedentary counterpart may have a relatively low caloric intake but remain fat. Many obese young people do not eat excessively, but instead lack enough activity to burn up the food they eat.

Excessive food intake does necessarily need correction, but correction usually means something more than following a low calorie diet. Why does this person eat too much? Does he turn to food for emotional relief, because of unpopularity, low self-esteem, or because he is unsuccessful? Unless he can be helped in these areas, a dietary restriction may take away his only source of satisfaction and may only make his emotional difficulties worse.

Some shy, anxious adolescents retreat into obesity as a way of avoiding the world's competitive challenges. Other factors may, of course, enter into the causes of obesity. Heredity may be one, and a nurse or a physician should be careful not to make a young person feel that his obesity makes him unacceptable. Heredity does not mean that the condition is untreatable, but an obese person is not inclined to cooperate if he feels that he is being rejected because of a condition for which he had little responsibility.

Regulation of Diet

An adolescent may be getting the greater amount of his caloric intake from carbohydrates and fats, with a low intake of proteins and minerals. A record of his total food intake for a few days may be important in determining whether he should change his eating habits. He may be well versed in the "basic four," but not until he can relate it to his own problems will it mean much to him.

THE HANDICAPPED ADOLESCENT

A mentally retarded child, or a physically handicapped one, or an emotionally deprived one can be expected to develop into a deprived, a retarded or a handicapped adolescent.

As a handicapped child reaches adolescence, his problems take on an added seriousness. The obstacles to his physical and emotional independence may be overwhelming. A young person with severe cerebral palsy may present physical problems that are beyond the capacity of his parents to solve. The same holds true for a severely retarded, or a crippled child. For many of these, residential care in an institution may be the only solution. This is a traumatic decision for parents to have to make.

A handicapped adolescent with enough residual ability to become productive deserves an early referral to vocational training agencies. His preparation should begin long before this, however, preferably at home and at school. Counseling and a serious evaluation of his potential is of great importance. Many young persons may learn to achieve satisfaction in supervised employment or in sheltered workshops who might otherwise spend their lives in frustration and discontent.

EMOTIONAL PROBLEMS

No one would actually believe that the emotional problems of adolescents could be adequately discussed in a few pages of a textbook. Certain facets of today's adolescent world are interesting, and it might prove useful to discover a fraction of what those people who work with young people are especially concerned about.

Rabinovitch* says that many of our aggressive teenagers have not "achieved a sense of competence through the elementary school years" and thus have a real need to prove themselves further. He states that today's teenagers need to clarify their role in their family, their role in school, and their future. He states that adults must communicate values, standards and morals to teenagers, and intimates that teenagers are looking for much more leadership than they are getting.

This appears to be true. Probably everyone has had the experience of admiring a teacher or other adult for some particular trait. Such a person does not inspire the admirer to rebellion, to show defiance, but rather to an attempt to learn, even to conform to his values.

An interesting experience is provided in a certain study group that cuts across age limits, and includes young and older teenagers as well as older persons. In a relaxed atmosphere, the young people ask penetrating questions and make shrewd observations. They are willing and very eager to talk about their problems and to discuss their feelings. Unfortunately, the adults are too often inclined to become pedantic, to "set them straight" without ever hearing what it is they are saying, and the young person goes away with the strengthened conviction that the older person is not interested in him or in his opinions.

Perhaps emphasis today is placed too heavily on the need of all adolescents to rebel. Certainly the adolescent has a need to free himself

---

* Rabinovitch, R.: Psychology of adolescence. Pediat. Clin. N. Amer., 7:65, 1960.

from childhood controls in order to establish himself, but the question arises as to whether we need to make a cult of "adolescent rebellion." Beards and long hair do not make boys into delinquents. Instead they would seem to be innocuous enough as symbols of "rebellion." Some researchers have questioned the rebellion image as the characteristic pattern of adolescence. There are many indications that there is a strong tendency for young people to accept parental values, even when adolescents are becoming absorbed in their peer groups. A difference exists between the fads, the special language and the tastes of a group, and the values of its individual members. Granted that one may be an expression of the other, but they are not automatically interchangeable.

A young person from a deprived home, who has never had his needs satisfied; a child who has been confused by the values of his home as against those of society, or who has seen lip-service only given to professed values, is much more likely to turn to antisocial behavior, but he will not be so free to verbalize his "rebellion."

Antisocial Behavior in Adolescence

The 1960 White House Conference (in which young people themselves participated) gave considerable attention to the problems of juvenile delinquency. In all, 22 recommendations for study, prevention, and for reforms in the handling and treatment of juvenile delinquency were made. One interesting recommendation was: "That in designing preventive programs, organizations listen to suggestions and recommendations made by delinquents themselves."* It is unlikely that many forum participants anticipated the extent to which the helped would become helpers in the programs that have followed.

Many of the recommendations for the prevention of delinquency through youth conservation camps, improved school facilities, and improved employment services have been implemented by the Economic Opportunity Act of 1964.

Emphasis on economic opportunity alone does not cope with the problem of delinquency. Many background experiences make up the character of the delinquent and there are a good many unknown factors. Neglect, emotional deprivation, conflict of cultures in the home, and excessive permissiveness or inconsistency of discipline—these are but a few of the background characteristics. Still, all children with such backgrounds do not grow up to be delinquents.

In his message to Congress on the nation's youth in 1963, President Kennedy said:

A common subject of discussion in midcentury America is assigning the blame for our mounting juvenile delinquency—to parents, schools, courts, com-

---

* *Recommendations*—Composite Report of Forum Findings. 1960 White House Conference. P. 65. Washington, U. S. Government Printing Office, 1960.

munities, and others, including the children themselves. There is no single answer—and no single cause or cure. But surely the place to begin is the malady which underlies so much of youthful frustration, rebellion, and idleness; and that malady is a lack of opportunity.

The serious problem of adolescent antisocial behavior, in the area of juvenile delinquency, is receiving much study and consideration. Another problem that has a great impact on the young as well as the old is that of the adolescent unwed mother.

PROBLEMS OF THE UNMARRIED TEENAGE MOTHER

The conflict in today's culture about the acceptance of sex as a basic drive, and the disapproval of pregnancy out of wedlock, is most confusing to teenagers, as it is to the older members of our society who attempt to meet their responsibilities to these younger people. As one writer put it: "There seems to be widespread tolerance of extramarital sexual intercourse—as long as there is no baby."*

Consider the extent of the problem. In 1960, there were 91,700 illegitimate births to teenage girls, of whom 48,300 were girls of school age.† Contrary to popular belief however, the highest rate of pregnancy out of marriage is not among teenagers, but among women in the 20 to 30 age group.

Why illegitimacy? There have been many attempts to pinpoint the reason, but the truth is that there is no one answer. Social and emotional immaturity, faulty child-parent relationships, and weak, confused moral standards no doubt contribute. A feeling of rejection, and of never having been accepted may lead a girl to seek affection and acceptance in relationships outside of her home. She becomes involved in highly emotional romantic relationships that have little contact with reality. It may not seem to her to be immoral as long as affection is involved. To have sexual relationships may seem the thing to do: the others tell about their experiences—she just happened to be "unlucky." There is little understanding or social maturity.

Other generalizations, such as membership in a socioeconomic class or ethnic group, a broken home, and dependency needs are offered as reasons for behavior unacceptable to the prevailing culture, but no one theory gives the entire answer. We must study this problem a great deal more. Those who make studies must first free themselves from stereotyped ideas and from bias, and give consideration to individuals rather than to general groups, or social classes.

* Garland, P.: The community's part in preventing illegitimacy. Children, *10*:71, 1963.

† Adams, H., and Gallagher, U.: Some facts and observations about illegitimacy. Children, *10*:43, 1963.

Prenatal Care for the Teenager

An adolescent girl does not have the motivation to seek antepartal medical care that is normal for an older, married woman. Pregnancy means being excluded from school, rejection from her family, and a strange, frightening immediate future. She thinks of herself as a young girl, not as an expectant mother. She may even deny her pregnancy. Small wonder then that she lacks enthusiasm for traveling across the city to an impersonal prenatal clinic, to join a group of patients with whom she feels no bond whatever.

The lack of prenatal care that many (but not all) unmarried teenagers receive accounts for much of the high rate of prematurity and infant mortality found in this group. A greater effort must be made to reach these young people and provide them with the necessary medical care as well as with counseling and guidance. A school nurse may be a person with a real opportunity to initiate a sound course of action. If she has established a good relationship with the students, a troubled girl is very likely to take this problem to her as she has done with other problems. The nurse, the teacher, the social worker, and the girl herself, may work as a team to arrange for physical care, for an emotional adjustment, as well as for continuing education.

States differ in their application of compulsory education laws to pregnant girls. Some states require that they be dropped from school as soon as their pregnancy is known, but not all school systems provide any alternate educational opportunities. Some school systems provide special classes for girls in maternity homes, and a few have special programs of instruction for girls living at home. In these situations, the girls are encouraged to reenter school after the delivery, and no mention of the pregnancy appears on their school record. Other pilot projects have been set up for continuing their education during the first months of their pregnancy.

An unmarried adolescent father needs counseling and guidance as well. Those who have worked with teenage fathers have found that they feel more responsibility and concern than had been thought. Someone is greatly needed to help them work out their confused, troubled feelings.

A Nurse's Role in Counseling

A young nurse may have difficulty relating to a young unmarried patient in the postpartum department, unless she has been able to resolve her own feelings. Her understanding of her professional role will help her; her need to be of service and her desire to assist her patient in achieving physical and emotional health should provide the necessary stability.

An adolescent mother must choose whether she keeps her baby or gives him up for adoption. The position that adoption is the best answer has been widely held. A normal home life for an infant and a healthy future are more likely than with the uncertainties of life with a mother who is herself immature. A girl may put an end to this unfortunate phase, complete her schooling and later make a successful life for herself.

The question is now being asked as to whether this is inevitably the right solution. Again, we have been dealing in generalities. Many mothers have kept their children and have been able to provide them with satisfactory lives. These mothers need services and support from the community in greater measure than they have received in the past.

NORMAL, ADJUSTED TEENAGERS

If adolescence is a time of rebellion, it is also a time of idealism. It is the time of life, perhaps more than any other, when enthusiasm, an eagerness to be of service to others, and a dedication to a cause are strongly present. Maladjusted young people, who rebel against accepted standards simply because they are standards, are still a minority group in spite of the attention they receive.

Young people need to be active, and need to keep busy. Most of them are eager for purposeful, meaningful employment. Some of them are high school girls who help in the hospitals as "candy-stripers," or who are "play ladies" in the children's division. Projects such as helping in neighborhood centers, visiting nursing homes, helping to care for migrant worker's children and other social service activities have been well accepted.

Young people not only need to be busy, but for many, the ability to earn some money determines whether they can stay in school. Summer or part-time employment is in very short supply for high school students, and is, in large measure, obtained through personal contacts. One of the major contributions of the 1960 White House Conference was the focusing of national attention on the problem of finding jobs for adolescents and young adults to enable them to finish their education, or enable them to take their places as contributing members of society.

Several training projects (government sponsored or set up by private employers) have been inaugurated. The Neighborhood Youth Corps, created in 1964, has grown with great rapidity. This is a project to provide work experience in a young person's community, enabling him to stay in high school through a work-study program, or to find full-time training and work opportunity for those out of school. It affects youths between the ages of 16 and 24. Hospitals have benefited from this program because positions have included nurses' aides, orderlies, cafeteria workers and others. The expected enrollment during the year of 1966 is 290,000.

Other Federal projects such as the Job Corps, and the opportunities for older young people in Vista, the Peace Corps and similar experiences have not suffered from lack of applicants.

BIBLIOGRAPHY

Adams, H. M., and Gallagher, U. M.: Some facts and observations about illegitimacy. Children, *10:*43, 1963.

Chapman, A. H.: Management of Emotional Problems of Children and Adolescents. P. 204. Philadelphia, J. B. Lippincott, 1965.

Gallagher, J.: Medical Care of the Adolescent. P. 3. New York, Appleton-
Century-Crofts, 1960.

Garland, P.: The community's part in preventing illegitimacy. Children, *10:*71,
1963.

Nelson, W., (ed.): Textbook of Pediatrics. 8th ed., pp. 405, 1444. Philadelphia, W. B. Saunders, 1964.

Oliver, R.: Acne vulgaris. Current Therapy, *6:*504, 1964.

Pannor, R.: Casework for unmarried fathers. Children, *10:*65, 1963.

Pochi, P., and Strauss, J.: Treatment of acne. Mod. Treatment, *2:*847, 1965.

Rabinovitch, R.: Psychology of Adolescence. Pediat. Clin. N. Amer., *7:*65,
1960. Recommendations—Composite Report of Forum Findings. 1960
White House Conference. P. 65. Washington, U. S. Government Printing
Office, 1960.

Ross Laboratories: The Adolescent Unwed Mother. Columbus, Ohio, Ross
Laboratories, 1965.

Symposium on Adolescence. Pediat. Clin. N. Amer., *7:*, (Feb.) 1960.

SUGGESTED READINGS FOR FURTHER STUDY

Auerbach, A. B., and Rabinow, M.: Parent education groups for unmarried
mothers. Nurs. Outlook, *14:*38, (Mar.) 1966.

Bare, C., Boettke, E., and Waggoner, N.: Self-help clothing for handicapped
children. Chicago, National Society for Crippled Children and Adults, 1962.

Burton, M., and Holter, I.: Health education classes for unwed mothers. Nurs.
Outlook, *14:*35, (Mar.) 1966.

Claman, A. D., and Bell, H. M.: Pregnancy in the very young teen-ager. Amer.
J. Obstet. Gynec., *90:*350, 1964.

Gallagher, J. R.: Medical Care of the Adolescent. Pp. 138, 177. New York,
Appleton-Century-Crofts, 1960.

Godenne, G.: A psychiatrist's techniques in treating adolescents. Children,
*12:*136, 1965.

Hammer, S. L.: Adolescent Obesity—Nutrition News. Chicago, National Dairy
Council, *27:* Oct., 1964.

Herzog, E.: Unmarried mothers: some questions to be answered and some
answers to be questioned. Child Welfare, *41:*339, 1962.

Hunter, L.: Foster homes for teenagers. Children, *11:*234, 1964.

Kahn, A.: Planning Community Service for Children in Trouble. New York,
Columbia University Press, 1963.

Knight, E.: Conferences for pregnant, unwed teenagers. Amer. J. Nurs., *66:*
1758, (Aug.), 1966.

Konopka, G.: Adolescent delinquent girls. Children, *11:*21, 1964.

Massimo, J., and Shore, M.: Job-focused treatment for antisocial youth. Children, *11:*143, 1964.

Noshpitz, J.: The antisocial or asocial adolescent. Pediat. Clin. N. Amer., *7:*97,
1960.

Parsons, E., *et al:* Teenage pregnancy. J. Amer. Med. Wom. Ass., *20:*225, 1965.

Schima, M.: A better start for girls. Amer. J. Nurs., *66:*1758, 1966.

Symposium on Adolescence. Pediat. Clin. N. Amer., *7:*, (Feb.) 1960.

Tuttle, E.: Serving the unmarried mother who keeps her child. Social Casework, *43:*415, 1962.

UNIT 8

CHILDREN OF THE NATION
AND OF THE WORLD

26

Children of the Nation

A glance back over the road we have travelled in our concern for children shows that we have come a tremendous distance. There is still much reason for concern however, both in the United States as well as elsewhere in the world. Where do we stand at present, and in which areas do we need to become more aware of new or of continuing needs?

It seems logical to examine first the development of concern for the needs of children within the United States, and then to follow this with a consideration of world-wide services. People everywhere are coming to realize that children's problems are universal and that the welfare of the world's children knows no national boundaries. We must not ignore our needs at home, however, in the face of problems elsewhere.

A brief outline of national progress in the awareness of children's needs should give us perspective and understanding.

THE CHILDREN'S BUREAU—YESTERDAY AND TODAY

As recently as 1903, in the United States, the question was asked "Why is it so many children die like flies in the summertime?"[*]

The question was pertinent indeed. Inspection of dairies was not required, milk was not pasteurized, and tuberculosis was present in the dairy herds. Ignorance of home sanitation was also a large factor. An accurate gastroenteritis called summer diarrhea (or cholera infantum) appeared every summer in the cities, especially among infants with poor resistance to infection, and the mortality rates were high. Predisposing factors, believed by many to be "causes," were stated as a lack of refrigeration, flies, hot weather, and the improper care of both food and utensils.

Two women, dedicated to the promotion of the health and welfare of children, were so disturbed about these conditions that they believed that action on a nation-wide scale was necessary. Miss Lillian Wald, founder of the Henry Street Settlement in New York City, knew the conditions very well. Her friend, Florence Kelly of the National Consumer's League was also well informed. The National Government, they said,

[*] United States Department of Health, Education and Welfare. It's Your Children's Bureau. P. 2. Washington, U. S. Government Printing Office, 1964.

479

had established a bureau to safeguard the nation's crops. Why shouldn't there be a bureau to safeguard the rights of children? They were concerned with not only the incredibly high infant mortality rate, but with child labor, illegitimacy, orphanages, birth registration, and a number of other related questions.

Eventually, President Theodore Roosevelt heard about their work and invited them to Washington to discuss their concern with him and with other concerned leaders. He gave them whole-hearted support, and much time was spent in planning the functions and the scope of such a national child-oriented bureau. Both President Roosevelt, and his successor, William Howard Taft, urged adoption of this proposal, but it was not until 1912 that public pressure prevailed upon Congress, and the Children's Bureau was formed.

Chiefs of the Children's Bureau are appointed by the President of the United States. Miss Julia Lathrop was its first director, with Miss Wald, Mrs. Kelly and with Jane Addams among the board of advisers. The first subject to be considered by the newly formed bureau was the high incidence of infant mortality. Nation-wide studies of causes, rates and of similar data were instituted. The Bureau proceeded with the discovery and validation of facts, followed fact-finding with the wide dissemination of expert advice on child care and child welfare; and finally became the chief agency for dispensing financial (as well as technical) aid for the betterment of child welfare.

The Children's Bureau has been one of the greatest powers ever developed for children's well-being—serving the well child and the sick; the rich child and the poor. There is no aspect of child health or welfare that is not within its range of responsibility. It has always been in the forefront of the nation in its fight for children's rights, the inauguration of research projects, in its search for new and better means of solving perplexing problems.

It might be profitable to cite an example of the extremely high mortality rates that were so disturbing in the early 1900's. No accurate statistics were collected in 1913, but it was estimated that out of 2,500,000 babies born each year in the United States, 300,000 died before their first birthday, a ratio of about 124 deaths per 1,000 live births.* Studies conducted by the Children's Bureau to discover the causes of that high national figure were instrumental in bringing about improved sanitation, the general pasteurization of milk, and a greatly improved knowledge among the general population concerning the principles of child care. Infant mortality rates, still too high, had declined to 24.8 deaths per 1,000 live births in 1964.

---

* *Five Decades of Action for Children.* Children's Bureau publication #352, p. 6, 1962.

Children's Bureau Publications

The popular pamphlet *Infant Care*, first published in 1914, was considered to be an innovation, and quickly became a best seller. When the eleventh edition was published in 1964, nearly 48,000,000 copies had been distributed since the appearance of the first edition.

Authoritative, up-to-date, practical pamphlets discussing nearly every aspect of child welfare have been published since 1914.* It would be difficult to estimate the value of these publications. The bi-monthly magazine *Children* is published for professional persons serving children.†

Present Day Focus

The Children's Bureau is the focus of all concern for children in the United States, but is not limited in its vision. It works actively with international organizations such as UNICEF, WHO, FAO, and others as the need is indicated. It is the U.S. Government appointed organization for the administration of grant-in-aid programs in the fields of maternal and child health, crippled children, and child welfare. Pilot projects for the study of mental retardation have been set up throughout the country, with the aid of federal grants administered by the Children's Bureau. The problem of child neglect and abuse is another area in which the bureau is actively working for better legislation, as well as for preventive and treatment measures.

White House Conference

In 1909, President Theodore Roosevelt called a conference for the purpose of considering the manner in which the welfare of the nation's children could best be served. The first White House Conference took for its theme, *The Care of Dependent Children*. The major recommendation to come out of this conference was that of the formation of a Children's Bureau, which, however, did not take place until 1912.

In 1918, a children's year was proclaimed by the Children's Bureau, culminating in a second White House Conference in 1919. This conference, on *Standards of Child Welfare*, set up regional conferences on matters of child welfare, child labor, and on maternal and child health. The influence of the regional conferences appeared to be very effective.

White House Conferences have been called every ten years by the President, and have been useful opportunities to discuss current child-related problems. The 1950 Midcentury White House Conference on Children and Youth was especially noteworthy. Its focus was on considera-

---

* A list of Children's Bureau publications may be obtained from the U. S. Department of Health, Education and Welfare, Children's Bureau, Washington, D. C. 20201.

† Subscriptions to *Children* can be made through the Superintendent of Documents, U. S. Government Printing Office, Washington, D. C. 20204. The subscription price is $1.25 per year.

tion of the emotional development of the child, and considered the question of what is needed to give every child a good chance to develop a healthy personality. Over sixty resolutions for implementing action were formulated, and were carried back to the states by their representatives for discussion and use. This was the conference at which the Pledge to Children was written.*

The Golden Anniversary Conference on Children and Youth in 1960 was attended by over 14,000 persons, among whom were 1400 high school and college age youths and 500 foreign visitors. Little White House Conferences were held in the various states in preparation for the Washington conference, and follow-up state-wide conferences studied the recommendations and set up programs.

The theme of the 1960 White House Conference expresses the concern of everyone interested in children: "To promote opportunities for children and youth to realize their full potential for a creative life in freedom and dignity."

Child Labor

Mention was made in an earlier chapter of the manner in which children were exploited by long, heavy work in unhealthy surroundings. It seems incredible that it took until 1941 for the United States to establish a national standard for child labor, as well as to provide a means for its enforcement.

The Children's Bureau began to explore conditions of child labor in 1913. Boys were found working in mines, small children were working in home workshops until late at night, and children were working in factories. Many states had some laws—with varying degrees of enforcement—but there was no federal law.

As a result of these and other findings, a National Child Labor Law was passed in 1917. Many states formulated enforcement measures, but after only nine months, the law was declared unconstitutional.

A second study in the 1920's and 1930's found larger numbers of children working. Boys of 13 years were in coal mines, children under 11 years in industrial homework, and most of the beet sugar fieldwork was done by children of 6 years of age and over. Children under 16 worked long hours in fish canneries, and many did not even attend school. In such places the illiteracy rate rose to 25 per cent.

A constitutional amendment passed by Congress in 1924 failed to be ratified by the necessary three-fourths of the states. Finally, in 1938, the Fair Labor Standards Act was passed by Congress. This set the minimum age as 16 years for employment in interstate or in foreign commerce, or in employment for any producer engaged in interstate or foreign commerce.

* This Pledge to Children is at the end of this chapter.

In 1941 the Supreme Court found this law constitutional, and rendered the former verdicts against similar laws unconstitutional and invalid.

The Children's Bureau administered the Child Labor Law until 1941, when the responsibility for its administration was taken over by the Department of Labor.

At present, federal standards for child labor prevail in all interstate commerce, while each state sets up its own standards and practices for child labor within the state. Age laws within states for the employment of minors during school hours have minimum ages ranging from 14 to 16 years. In a majority of states, these laws do not cover agricultural and domestic service. All states make some provision for special protection in hazardous occupations.*

CHILD CARE OUTSIDE THE HOME

Institutional Care

We have come a long way from the foundling homes and orphanages of the past. One has only to read some of the writings of the early 1900's to become acquainted with bare dormitories housing 30 or more children in one room; files of children dressed alike, walking two by two to school, and returning to scrub, wash, and do all the menial labor around the big, bare institution. Such orphanages no longer exist in the United States. Institutions for the care of dependent or neglected children still numbered over 1,000 in 1965; these included temporary shelters for children. The trend is away from institutional care, however, because it seems clear that children do not thrive in large institutions. Foster homes, day care centers, as well as homemaker services in the child's home would seem to be preferable. Unfortunately, the demand far exceeds the supply.

Present day institutions for the care of healthy children stress the need for small groups. Many are set up in cottage style, with each unit under the care of cottage "parents." Even some institutions that have been obliged to use large, older buildings, have used both imagination and ingenuity in dividing their population into small units. The children are dressed attractively, and cannot be distinguished from their schoolmates by their appearance.

A number of institutions have become residential or treatment centers for mentally retarded, emotionally disturbed, delinquent or otherwise handicapped children. Experimentation with day care facilities for these children as well is being carried out with promising results. Institutional care for infants is avoided whenever it is possible, a few states having

* The handbook *State Child-Labor Standards* (Bulletin 158) (1960) is prepared by the U. S. Department of Labor and may be purchased from the Superintendent of Documents, U. S. Government Printing Office, Washington, D. C. This gives "A State-by-State summary of laws affecting the employment of minors under 18 years of age."

passed laws against such placement except on a temporary basis, until homes can be found. Placement in foster homes or in adoptive homes for healthy, attractive babies does not present the problem that confronts a young, handicapped child.

The prospect is not so cheerful as we would like to believe, however. In 1966, nearly 700 children live in a crowded public institution in Washington, D.C., while in New York City, nearly 2,000 await placement, some of whom have stayed in "temporary" shelters for as long as three years.*

Foster Homes

As we have become more sensitive to children's needs, we have begun to look for foster homes for those who must leave their own homes. We have come to recognize the importance of a family setting and have come to believe that an institution, no matter how well organized and administered, cannot take the place of a warm, well-integrated home. We must admit, however, that not all foster homes supply the atmosphere that a child needs. Good foster homes are not easy to find. It takes a person with a true love of children and a sensitivity to their needs, to provide a good foster home. It also takes broad vision and often a real sacrifice on the part of the foster parents, to let these children go when they are ready to go home again, or ready to be placed for adoption.

Many children in foster care go through the traumatic experience of being moved from one home to another, often many times. A most moving look into a little girl's heart has been portrayed in the story of one such child. She had gathered into herself all of the hurt and the criticism that she had received in her moves from one home to another, until she was afraid to respond naturally to anyone. Always she was the outsider. "In this home, do they want me to make my bed as soon as I get up, or will I be scolded for not letting it air? Should I offer to help with breakfast, or will I be in the way? It took long, patient understanding and acceptance in a home where she was really wanted before her barriers could finally come down."† For some children, it is too late.

All states require the licensing and the inspection of foster homes. Usually the number of children in a single home is limited, and the standards for hygienic practices and health measures are predetermined. Foster families must have a sufficient income to meet their living needs without the board payments on behalf of the child.

Efforts to find foster homes in which handicapped or disfigured children can also receive loving physical care and emotional support are meeting with considerable success as concerned people become aware of the need.

* Garrett, B.: Meeting the crisis in foster family care. Children, *13*:2, 1966.
† Winter, A.: Only People Cry. Woman's Day. P. 48. Sept., 1963.

Child Care Centers, Day Nurseries, and Nursery Schools

The terms child care centers and day nurseries are defined as facilities whose primary purpose is the care and the protection of children. A nursery school is a pre-kindergarten school whose main purpose is education of young children. In practical terms, however, today's distinction is far less clear.

Child care centers, in order to accommodate the families of working mothers, are generally open throughout the day, and provide meals and rest periods for the children. Some centers that function in depressed areas have discovered that many of the children under their care have come without having had breakfast. The centers thus serve that meal too.

Opportunities for education and for cultural enrichment are not neglected, particularly because society has come to realize that children from poor homes are the very ones who can profit most from such services. In today's culture, however, the number of mothers working outside the home is steadily increasing, again making the distinction between the different child care programs of less importance.

A large number of nursery schools accept children for periods of two to three hours daily, placing an emphasis on a young child's limited capacity for structured learning experiences; many others, however, are providing additional hours of day care for those who need it.

One research-oriented day care center has been set up for the care of children as young as six months of age, from low income families. The purpose is to test whether a planned environment can offset any of the detrimental effects of maternal separation, and perhaps add some enrichment to an environment that might otherwise not be available to a family with limited resources.* The results of such a program should prove to be of great interest.

Nursery schools and day care centers naturally differ in their ability to meet a child's needs. Parents would do well to spend some time and effort when they choose a place where their child is going to spend considerable time. Child care facilities are inspected and are licensed according to state laws, and thus they must meet certain standards. Hygienic measures, such as the ratio of wash basins and toilets to the number of children, individual towels, and provisions for isolation of a sick child until he can be taken home, are specified. In addition, safety measures, adequacy of play space and of play materials, and provision made for rest periods must meet approval.

The parents should see for themselves that requirements are met and maintained. There are other considerations. Are there provisions for individual initiative and for free play, or is the program strictly regi-

* Caldwell, B., and Richmond, J.: Programmed day care for the very young child—a preliminary report. Child Welfare, 44:134, 1965. (A special issue on day care.)

mented? Are teachers able to maintain discipline with guidance and understanding, or do matters get out of hand? Is there an adequate number of teachers and assistants with the necessary background experience and training for this work? Satisfactory answers to these and to other questions are important for the well-being of the child and the parent's peace of mind.

Homemaker Services

Homemaker service has, in many instances, become an attractive alternative to foster home placement. A child who has recently suffered the loss of his mother from death, illness, hospitalization, or from some other cause, may be a poor candidate for a foster home. His loneliness may be further intensified by the unfamiliar surroundings of a strange home, a school or a strange neighborhood, and undoubtedly he will find it more difficult to adjust than he would if left in the security of his own home.

In a home in which the mother must be the breadwinner of the family, a homemaker may make it possible to keep the family intact. Sometimes added burdens on the mother, such as a new baby, an ill child, or her own temporary illness, make such a service welcome. A severely retarded child, or one suffering from a severe chronic illness may absorb all of the mother's time, to the exclusion of sufficient time to care for the rest of the household, or of any rest and recreation for herself. Here a homemaker can take over some of the tedious housework and perhaps help take care of the child.

Potential homemakers are accepted for qualities such as reliability, adaptability, kindness, maturity, and home management skills, rather than their educational background. Training courses are offered by the employing agencies in the health or welfare fields, and continuing supervision is important for support and counsel.

Adoption

Popular ideas about adoption practices are still based, too often, on misunderstandings or confused ideas, or possibly on past attitudes that have been outgrown by the agencies responsible for placing children in the adopting homes.

The concept that children available for adoption are in short supply is not entirely correct. It is true that most prospective parents want infants, preferably young infants, who are appealing, healthy, and "normal." Too few of the children with handicaps—emotional or physical—are offered the opportunity to become family members. Children of mixed races or of minority groups find placement extremely difficult.

Adoption agencies are awakening to their responsibilities to these unfortunate children, and very real efforts are being made to find homes for them. The number of people willing to accept the responsibility of adopting a handicapped child may be greater than expected as people discover that placement for these children is now seriously considered by adoption agencies.

Interracial adoptions may also be accomplished with marked success, if they are seriously undertaken. Older concepts of the foredoomed failure of any such adoption have not been verified.

As official adoption agencies have re-examined their placement policies and have developed more realistic practices, there appears to be less justification for independent adoption. Authorized agencies are best qualified to deal with the emotional factors involved in adoption, and are better equipped for handling success-ensuring details.

Age limitations for adoptive parents are still a factor, although standards are in general not so rigid as they have been in the past. Young parents are considered to be better able to rear children from infancy successfully. Matching for coloring and body characteristics is no longer considered to be a major factor; rather, the tendency is to weigh those characteristics that would seem to promise successful parenthood, and to assess the potential for adjustment for each separate case. Certain state laws, individual preferences and agency policies may set particular standards, however, such as not allowing the placement of a child in a home of a different religious faith than that of the child's natural parents.

The prevailing belief today is that a child should be told about his adopted status in a simple, matter-of-fact manner—much the same as one would tell a child about his birth. Problems may arise in either case, but a child who has known from the beginning of his ability to understand, that he is adopted, probably adjusts to this much easier than one who finds out from the neighborhood, and who then wonders why there has been secrecy.

Nurses caring for hospitalized infants, or for adoptable newborn infants, must learn to use discretion. It is never professional behavior to discuss the private affairs of patients, but too often we forget this, and do discuss them. It is usually in the best interest of a mother and her child (when a child is offered for adoption) if a complete break with the past is accomplished.

Specialized Services for Children

Specialized services for children and for their parents are numerous. A nurse should know what services are available in her area, whether they give practical care, financial assistance, information, or are mainly engaged in research. Parents' groups exist throughout the country, to enable the parents of handicapped or of ill children to talk over their problems together, and to learn more about the care of their children. A few of these specialized services are listed below.

> Child guidance clinics.
> Schools and centers for emotionally disturbed children.
> Day care centers and classes for the mentally retarded.
> Sheltered workshops and rehabilitation centers.
> Well child clinics and diagnostic clinics.
> State heart associations.
> National Foundation—March of Dimes.
> Schools for crippled children.
> Cystic fibrosis parents' groups.
> Mentally retarded parents' groups.
> Child welfare agencies—protective services.
> Cystic fibrosis research centers.
> Schools for blind and for deaf children.

CHILDREN OF MIGRANT WORKERS

We may at times feel satisfied in the United States that we do not have the problems found elsewhere in the world, of which it still is said that over half goes to bed hungry. Even in our favored country, however, there are many children who have a minimum of the benefits that we take for granted.

The children of migrant workers present one example. Over 500,000 migrant families, including 350,000 children under the age of 18, are "trapped in a vicious circle of unending poverty and rootlessness," according to a report prepared by the Children's Bureau in 1961.* At that time, there were only 24 state-licensed day-care centers primarily serving migrant children. More states are awakening to their responsibilities to these children, but only a small fraction of them receive day-care or health services.

Migrant families, following the crops from place to place, represent the lowest economic level of any major group in our country. Cultural differences (and language barriers for many) mobility and non-resident status, and distances from child clinics all hinder adequate participation in health programs. The only way in which a majority of mothers can care for their small children is to take them into the fields with them. Older children can ill be spared to act as baby sitters.

Children of migrant workers find school attendance discouraging. The frequent moves necessitate a continual changing of schools. When a child *does* attend, he is often a stranger to the culture and possibly an unwelcome one. Also a child ten years old or over is needed to help in the fields in order to augment his family's income, and law enforcement is lax in many areas. States reporting that migrant children are accepted into their schools may add such comments as "children are socially

* Children of migrants. Children, 8:115, 1961.

accepted only with difficulty; there are still crop vacations"; and "they are not encouraged to attend."

The country is finally awakening to the seriousness of the conditions affecting the people who do a real service in harvesting our crops, but who have been shamefully exploited. The average earning wage for migrant workers has improved, housing provided by employers comes closer to meeting sanitary requirements, but a great deal is still to be done.

Women's organizations, particularly church women, and migrant ministry leagues, have led the way in publicizing the plight of these people, and in attempting to meet their needs. They have given outstanding service to many, and have established friendly relationships and have worked together with the parents for improved child welfare. As various states accept their responsibility, they often find it advantageous to make use of the experience and knowledge these workers have acquired from their volunteer services. Colleges located near areas in which migrant labor is employed have, in several instances, set up centers for child care and for study, furnishing interesting summer employment for college students.

CHILDREN OF THE AMERICAN INDIANS

According to the Bureau of Indian Affairs, there were 552,228 Indians and Alaska Natives in the United States in 1960. (As a matter of historical interest, the number of Indians in this country when Columbus discovered America is estimated to have been about 846,000. The number decreased to approximately 243,000 late in the 19th century but since then has steadily increased.)

American Indians are full United States citizens with privileges and responsibilities indistinguishable from those of other citizens. Those living on reservations, under the jurisdiction of the Bureau of Indian Affairs (of the Department of the Interior) make up about two-thirds of the Indian population. The remainder are members of the general population and receive public services as do the other members of their communities.

The responsibility for providing medical care and health services belongs to the Division of Indian Health of the Public Health Service, Department of Health, Education and Welfare. The Division of Indian Health works in cooperation with tribal leaders and tribal representatives in working out health plans, and trains and employs Indian men and women in health services as qualified Indian men and women are available for training.

Infant mortality rates continue to be high among Indians; the rate in 1961 was 43 per 1000 live births, as contrasted with 25 per 1000 live births in the general population. The tuberculosis rate among Indians is four times that of the general population; even this amount is a great reduction over previous rates. The Public Health Service has intensified its program in maternal and child care, sanitation and in health education.

Indian children attend public schools (or federal schools if public schools are not available), and mission schools. Indian children living outside of reservations are subject to the school attendance laws of their state. Tribal governing bodies on reservations must approve enforcement, and many have done so, but school facilities are still inadequate on some reservations. The Bureau of Indian Affairs encourages higher education through loans and grants to those high school graduates who need financial help to enter college.

PLEDGE TO CHILDREN

To you, our children, who hold within you our most cherished hopes, we, the members of the Midcentury White House Conference on Children and Youth, relying on your full response, make this pledge:

From your earliest infancy we give you our love, so that you may grow with trust in yourself and in others.

We will recognize your worth as a person and we will help you to strengthen your sense of belonging.

We will respect your right to be yourself and at the same time help you to understand the rights of others, so that you may experience cooperative living.

We will help you develop initiative and imagination, so that you may have the opportunity freely to create.

We will encourage your curiosity and your pride in workmanship, so that you may have the satisfaction that comes from achievement.

We will provide the conditions for wholesome play that will add to your learning, to your social experience, and to your happiness.

We will illustrate by precept and example the value of integrity and the importance of moral courage.

We will encourage you always to seek the truth.

We will provide you with all opportunities possible to develop your own faith in God.

We will open the way for you to enjoy the arts and to use them for deepening your understanding of life.

We will work to rid ourselves of prejudice and discrimination, so that together we may achieve a truly democratic society.

We will work to lift the standard of living and to improve our economic practices, so that you may have the material basis for a full life.

We will provide you with rewarding educational opportunities, so that you may develop your talents and contribute to a better world.

We will protect you against exploitation and undue hazards and help you grow in health and strength.

We will work to conserve and improve family life and, as needed, to provide foster care according to your inherent rights.

We will intensify our search for new knowledge in order to guide you more effectively as you develop your potentialities.

As you grow from child to youth to adult, establishing a family life of your own and accepting larger social responsibilities, we will work with you to improve conditions for all children and youth.

Aware that these promises to you cannot be fully met in a world at war, we ask you to join us in a firm dedication to the building of a world society based on freedom, justice, and mutual respect.

So may you grow in joy, in faith in God and in man, and in those qualities of vision and of the spirit that will sustain us all and give us new hope for the future.

BIBLIOGRAPHY

Caldwell, B., and Richmond, J.: Programmed day care for the very young child —a preliminary report, Child Welfare, *44*:134, 1965.

Children: Bi-monthly publication of the Children's Bureau. Superintendent of Documents, U. S. Government Printing Office, Washington, D. C. 20204.

Children of migrants. Children, 8:115, 1961.

Children's Bureau: Five Decades of Action for Children. Washington, U. S. Government Printing Office, 1962.

————: It's Your Children's Bureau. Washington, U. S. Government Printing Office, 1964.

Garrett, B.: Meeting the crisis in foster family care. Children, *13*:2, 1966.

U. S. Department of Labor: State Child-Labor Standards Bulletin No. 158. Washington, U. S. Government Printing Office, 1960.

U. S. Department of Health, Education and Welfare: The Indian Health Program. Washington, U. S. Government Printing Office, 1963.

U. S. Public Health Service: Nursing Careers Among the Indians. Washington, U. S. Government Printing Office, 1964.

White House Conference: Recommendations: Composite Report of Forum Findings 1960, Recommendation Washington, U. S. Government Printing Office, 1960.

Winter, A.: Only People Cry. P. 48. Woman's Day, 1963.

SUGGESTED READINGS FOR FURTHER STUDY

Aponte, H. J.: Children of society's ills. Amer. J. Nurs., *66*:1749, (Aug.) 1966.

Bernard, V. W.: Adoption. New York, New York Child Welfare League of America, 1965.

Brittain, C.: Preschool programs for culturally deprived children. Children, *13*:130, 1966.

Bureau of Indian Affairs: Answers to Your Questions on the American Indians. Washington, U. S. Government Printing Office, 1965.

Child Welfare: Special issue on day care. Child Welfare, *44*, (Mar.) 1965.

————: Child Welfare League of America, Standards for Day Care Service. New York, Child Welfare League of America, 1965.

Child Welfare League of America: Day Care: An Expanding Resource for Children. New York, Child Welfare League of America, 1965.

————: Day Care: A Preventive Service. New York, Child Welfare League of America, 1964.

Gordon, R.: A nursery school in a rehabilitation center. Children, *13*:145, 1966.

Hosley, E.: Culturally deprived children in a day-care program. Children, *10*: 175, 1963.

Johnston, H. L.: A smoother road for migrants. Amer. J. Nurs., *66*:1752, (Aug.) 1966.

Littner, N.: Some Traumatic Effects of Separation and Placement. New York, Child Welfare League of America, 1965.

Moss, S. Z.: How children feel about being placed away from home. Children, *13*:153, 1966.

Uhde, M.: Agricultural migrant families in New Jersey. Nurs. Outlook, *12*:46, (Mar.) 1964.

U. S. Department of Health, Education and Welfare: Facts About Children's Bureau Programs. Washington, U. S. Government Printing Office, 1965.

————: Northwest Indian Health Program. Washington, U. S. Government Printing Office, 1963.

————: Nurses in the United States Public Health Service. Washington, U. S. Government Printing Office, 1961.

————: Services for Children Fact Sheet: How Title V of the Social Security Act Benefits Children. Washington, U. S. Government Printing Office, 1964.

Waller, M. V.: Serving a nation on wheels. Nurs. Outlook, *12*:43, (Mar.) 1964.

Yankee, M.: Migrant Day Care Center. Amer. J. Nurs., *66*:1756, (Aug.) 1966.

27

Children of the World

The health of children throughout the world is everyone's concern. Many countries have well-developed maternal and child welfare programs that have lowered infant mortality rates and have raised child health standards to high levels. Among many of the developing countries, and among some of older cultures as well, conditions still prevail that are based on traditions difficult to overcome, and serious diseases with high mortality rates are common.

"Mankind must accept the challenge that this is one world, that however great the dangers of atomic destruction, there is the even greater danger of an unequally divided world that keeps on merely rolling along, some of its areas riddled with ignorance, poverty and disease."[*] These are the words of a physician who understands from personal observation and from practical experience what he is talking about.

CONDITIONS OF MALNUTRITION

The World Health Organization explains: "More than half the world's population—are victims of hunger or inadequate nutrition in one form or another. Over large areas of the world, people's everyday meals are insufficient; the children go without milk after they are weaned and child mortality between the ages of one and five is often fifteen times higher than it is in places where people are able to get proper food. All this is nothing new. It is probable that the world has never in its history fed all its people adequately. The difference is that today, thanks to the discoveries of science—we already have the knowledge and power to produce sufficient food, measured on a health standard for more than twice the population of the world."[†]

"Protein-Calorie Malnutrition" (Kwashiorkor)

The condition that assumes great importance for everyone concerned with child health is that called protein-calorie malnutrition. Protein deficiency accounts for most malnutrition among the world's children. It is known by various names in various countries, but the condition as it

[*] World Health Magazine. P. 6. May, 1963.
[†] Ibid. Pp. 5–6. March, 1963.

appears in Africa, called *Kwashiorkor,* serves as an example of any child-hood protein deficiency.

Kwashiorkor is a nutritional syndrome caused by a diet deficient in protein, with its highest incidence among children in the age period of six months to five years. An affected child develops a swollen abdomen, retarded growth with muscle wasting, edema, gastrointestinal changes, apathy and irritability. In untreated cases, mortality rates are 30 per cent or higher. Even when children are brought for treatment, the condition has often advanced sufficiently to keep mortality rates as high as 15 to 20 per cent at some treatment centers.

Children with mild or moderate protein-calorie malnutrition may not show overt signs but they fail to grow normally. This condition is common in many African countries, and although strenuous efforts are being made to prevent it, its causes are complex. Traditionally, these babies have been breast-fed up to the age of two or three years. The child is weaned abruptly and is then given the regular family diet, which contains mostly starch foods with very little meat or vegetable protein. Cow's milk is not generally available, and in places where goats are kept, their milk is not considered fit for human consumption.

A similar condition exists in Latin America where malnutrition is one of the most important medical problems. Wherever people cannot afford meat, fish, eggs or milk, or do not have access to these foods, a protein deficiency is found. If any such food does appear in the diet, it goes first to the father of the family. It is not solely an economic problem, however, but is one also of custom and belief—a situation that is extremely hard to change. In some areas meat is believed to cause worms, and milk to cause diarrhea. A reluctance to eat unaccustomed foods is not easily overcome, even among hungry people. Rice eaters in Asia have had difficulty accepting wheat when rice could not be obtained. It is said that during the potato famine in Ireland in 1845 and 1846, the Irish people, whose main dietary staple was the potato, went hungry and even starved before they would eat the maize (corn) sent from America. In some countries, snails are prized as dietary items, but it is difficult to get the average American to accept them.

It is unrealistic, however, to educate people about proper infant diets if the essential foods are not available to them. Milk is unattainable in many areas, or, if it is available, the general lack of refrigeration lends some substance to the belief that milk causes diarrhea. Some other, economical means of supplying protein must be found. The statement is made that "when it has been brought home to mothers that their children should be properly fed with protein-rich foods, it should be made possible for them to obtain foods of this kind that are cheap, similar to familiar foods in taste and texture where this is feasible and easily prepared. In this

TABLE 27–1. "ARTIFICIAL" PROTEIN-RICH FOODS OF PRIMARILY VEGETABLE ORIGIN*

LATIN AMERICA (INCAPARINA)		INDIA[a]		UGANDA	
Ingredient	Percentage	Ingredient	Percentage	Ingredient	Percentage
Corn	29	Chickpea		Wheat flour	12.5
Soya bean	29	(roasted)	24	Corn	25.0
Cottonseed		Groundnut Flour		Groundnut	
(de-fatted)	38	(low fat)	75	(toasted)	37.5
Torula yeast	3	Calcium carbonate	1	Cottonseed oil	6.5
Calcium carbonate	1			Sugar	18.5
Vitamin A	4500 units				
Protein	27.5%	Protein	42%	Protein	14%

[a] (This food is fortified with vitamins A and D, thiamine and riboflavine.)

connexion, it should be remembered (that) many African mothers are not used to buying food for their children."[†]

Dried skim milk has been furnished by UNICEF for the treatment of Kwashiorkor in Africa, and has been a means of reducing clinical symptoms. Some sort of acceptable protein-rich diet is necessary for the prevention and for continued use as a supplement to the usual diet. A vegetable protein mixture, made into a liquid that resembles milk in texture, and has an acceptable taste, was developed in Latin America and has proved its value. Called Incaparina, it is sold commercially, costs but a fraction of the price of milk. Its use is promoted by an educational campaign. India and Uganda have developed similar mixtures. All of these use soya bean or groundnuts mixed with cereals to provide a protein-rich food.

The nutritive value of mixed vegetable protein can be enhanced by adding skim milk powder of a fish protein concentrate.

These supplements are good if people will use them, but education to make use of *available* food supplements is of greater importance. Dr. Sai, a research physician in Ghana, says that children in fishing villages do not eat fish because their mothers believe fish is not good for children. Mothers should learn to use protein-rich beans by soaking them to remove their husks. Most of all he states, Ghana now needs a factory to produce its own baby foods.[‡]

Vitamin A deficiency with xerophthamia is prevalent in those countries where protein-calorie malnutrition exists. In fact, the two often occur together. The incidence of blindness or of reduced vision is high.

* WHO Chronicle, *19*:435, 1965.

† Malnutrition in early childhood: WHO Chronicle, *20*:86, 1966.

‡ Michaelis, A. R.: Science for him. World Health Magazine, p. 6, May, 1963.

COMMUNICABLE DISEASES AND SANITATION

A communicable disease that has been a common childhood infection in tropical countries throughout the world is *yaws*. This is a non-venereal spirochetal disease with acute and chronic relapsing phases. Lesions on the face, on the palms and the soles of the feet, and bony lesions, cause extensive suffering in children, adolescents and in adults, with permanent and disabling sequelae in as many as 1 per cent of those infected.

Treatment had been unsatisfactory until the discovery was made that a single dose of benzathine penicillin G would cure yaws in its initial stage, and would bring considerable improvement if it was given in the more advanced stages of the disease.

Mass campaigns have been worked out with technical advice from WHO, and with supplies of penicillin and equipment provided by UNICEF. Between 1948 and 1963, campaigns in 45 countries (with 135 million people examined and 45 million treated) reduced the incidence to a low level, less than one percent in many areas where sixty percent or more of the inhabitants had been infected. The reduction in these areas has made control possible by using surveillance methods from local rural health centers, and this in turn has paved the way for a more rapid establishment of rural health services in developing areas, thereby providing improved health care. There are, however, many areas where intensive efforts have still to be made.

Other problems concerning the health and the well-being of the world's children are in the areas of sanitation and clean water. These problems are intensified by the rapid growth of urban areas in every country, the cities in developing countries growing at a faster rate than those elsewhere.

Large numbers of urban dwellers in Latin America, Africa and Asia get their water from public outlets. Many do not have readily available public outlets. Diarrheal diseases are prevalent where clean water is difficult to obtain, and significant reductions in the mortality rate caused by enteric diseases have followed the establishment of clean water supplies. It is difficult to get people interested enough to demand clean water, however, if they have to pay for it. Water is man's birthright—like the air he breathes. It should always be free, they reason. If purification, filtration and distribution is costly, there is always water to be had from the local wells and ponds.

WHO has set a goal for piped water to be supplied to all people living in urban communities by 1977, by house connections, or by public outlets within a reasonable distance from each home. This is the first phase of a more ambitious program to make piped water available in every home, to provide it in adequate volume and to protect its sources from contamination.

Public health work in these fields is rapidly expanding as more people are educated to assume leadership. The difficulties involved in reaching people in widely scattered areas are tremendous and challenging. Modern communications media have proved useful, not only for teaching sanitation and hygiene, but also to awaken people to the possibilities of better living. In spite of this rather optimistic outlook, however, the number of trained health workers is still far short of the need.

THE WORLD'S CHILDREN

We can no longer afford to think in terms of a few of the world's children. Today we have come to realize that the theme of the 1960 White House Conference "to promote opportunities for children and youth to realize their full potential in freedom and dignity" applies to all children.

The World Health Organization (WHO)

The World Health Organization (WHO) is one of the special agencies of the United Nations. Through this organization, which came into being in 1948, the public health and medical professions of more than 100 countries exchange their knowledge and experience, and collaborate in an effort to achieve the highest possible level of health throughout the world. WHO deals with problems that can only be solved by the cooperation of all, or of certain groups of countries—the eradication of diseases such as malaria, the control of diseases that affect or are a potential danger to many, such as most of the infectious and parasitic diseases, some cardiovascular disease, and cancer. In many parts of the world there is need for improvement in maternal and child health, nutrition, nursing, mental health, dental health, social and occupational health, environmental health, public health administration, professional education and training, and in health education of the public. Thus a large share of the Organization's resources is devoted to giving assistance and advice in these fields and to making available—often through publications—the latest information on these subjects.

The achievements of WHO have been impressive. A world-wide program to eradicate malaria has been outstandingly successful. In 1966, WHO reported that of the population of over 1,500 million in the originally malarious areas of the world, 885 million now live in areas that have been freed from malaria, and that pre-eradication or full eradication programs are in progress in areas containing about 377 million more persons.* A full, detailed report of the progress in malaria eradication in 1964 is given in WHO Chronicle.†

WHO has worked intensively and extensively with UNICEF (United

* World Fight Against Communicable Diseases: a Progress Report. World Health Magazine. May, 1966.
† Malaria eradication in 1964. WHO Chronicle, *18:*339, 1964.

Nations Children's Fund) and with FAO (Food and Agricultural Organization) in devising methods for the prevention and the treatment of protein-calorie malnutrition, a condition causing high mortality rate among children in much of the world. Other deficiency diseases, such as beriberi and pellagra, infections such as diarrhea (and other diseases that are particularly disastrous to children) are vigorously treated.

There are several WHO publications. *WHO Chronicle* (published monthly for the medical and for the public health professions) provides a monthly record of the principal health activities undertaken in various countries with WHO assistance. The *Bulletin of the World Health Organization* contains technical articles in English or in French and is published monthly.

World Health is an illustrated monthly magazine for the general public, and gives an idea of WHO activities throughout the world. It is published in English, French, Portuguese, Russian and Spanish editions.

Other publications include a Monograph Series, a Technical Report Series, and Epidemiological and Vital Statistics Report, and others.*

WHO Headquarters is located in Geneva, Switzerland.

The United Nations Children's Fund (UNICEF)

In 1946 the United Nations General Assembly established the United Nations International Children's Emergency Fund (UNICEF) on a temporary basis to assist needy children, primarily in war-devastated countries. Its charter came to an end in 1953, but the General Assembly voted unanimously to continue the agency indefinitely as the United Nations Children's Fund, but retained the symbol UNICEF.

UNICEF is simply and completeiy concerned with the health and welfare of children and mothers. It works with any nation that requests service, without regard to race, creed or politics. Assistance is provided only upon request of a country, and is a cooperative venture. Assisted governments spend approximately two-and-a-half dollars for every dollar contributed by UNICEF, for materials, local personnel and facilities.

UNICEF works in cooperation with WHO, FAO, and UNESCO, the United Nations Educational, Scientific and Cultural Organization. In a new emphasis on child nutrition in 1958, an FAO—UNICEF Joint Policy Committee was established, with the United States as one of the countries representing FAO. UNICEF also undertook a study, at the suggestion of the chief of the Children's Bureau, of children in institutions and in daycare centers, with several countries now participating in programs set up as a result of the study. UNICEF is particularly concerned with helping governments help themselves, by offering incentive and material help to

* WHO publications, or information concerning them, may be obtained in the United States through the Columbia University Press, International Documents Service, 2960 Broadway, New York, New York 10027.

get them started. It is one organization that works to put itself out of a job, by training and by educating persons within their own countries to take over the projects. It has a proud record. It has participated in bringing such diseases as yaws and malaria under control, and is actively attacking trachoma, tuberculosis and leprosy. Millions of children have been rescued from deficiency diseases by supplies of dried skim milk, soybean and fish flour, and by new protein-rich foods now under development.

UNICEF's work is financed entirely by voluntary contributions from governments, private groups and from individuals. In the United States, the Trick or Treat for UNICEF Halloween Program is well known, and it receives hearty support from the nation's children. The sale of UNICEF Greeting Cards has furnished milk and medicine to needy children all over the world.

UNICEF believes that the future of mankind depends on the well-being of our chlidren. Its slogan is—The Child of Today for the World of Tomorrow.*

INTERCOUNTRY ADOPTIONS

An interesting service for the world's children is that concerned with finding homes for homeless children through intercountry adoptions. Placement of children needing homes is made in countries throughout the world. This short discussion is concentrated on placement within the United States.

An international family and children's agency, the International Social Service (ISS), with headquarters in Geneva, Switzerland, has assisted in the adoption of over a thousand children from abroad into American families, through its American branch, WAIF. The ISS has branches and offices in twenty countries, with cooperating agencies in eighty others, which makes it most helpful in guiding adopting families through the intricacies of international adoption. Other adoption agencies mainly interested in placement of Korean children, also exist in the United States.

Children of mixed parentage, particularly Korean-Caucasian or Korean-Negro, face severe prejudice in their native country; their mothers finding conditions nearly impossible for child rearing. These children, homeless, or gathered in large orphanages, constitute the largest group needing homes. Hong Kong children of Chinese origin (mostly girls) abandoned and living in orphanages, also need homes, particularly the older children up to the age of 14. Most of the Japanese children are placed in their own country, but there are some racially mixed and older children that no one seems to want.

* Additional information concerning UNICEF, its purpose, its scope and its functions, may be obtained from the United States Committee for UNICEF, United Nations, New York, or from one of the state United Nations Associations.

The need of European children for adoption out of their own countries has diminished considerably, although there are still some who have little prospect of finding a home.

An American family interested in giving a home to one of these children, initiates procedures by calling the child welfare department or adoption agency in their vicinity. The agency caseworker makes a "home study" of the inquiring family, assessing its ability to make a home for a foreign, homeless child. Intercountry adoptions have, on the whole, been remarkably successful. This is due in part, perhaps, to the families who have been involved—families with remarkable capacities for love, patience and for understanding.

Such adoptions are not to be undertaken lightly. These children, who have been homeless, rejected and deprived, come into a home where the language, customs, and the entire culture are strange and frightening. Further rejection in this new home is an unthinkable cruelty. The experience can be a happy one, deeply satisfying and rewarding for both child and for his new parents.

When a prospective child for adoption has been picked by an agency, details are provided for the adoptive parent's consideration. If all is satisfactory, application is made to the U. S. Immigration and Naturalization Service for the child's entry. The adoption agency assists in procuring documents from the country from which the child comes, such as a passport and departure approval. If the U. S. immigration quota from that country has been oversubscribed, a special petition for a non-quota visa (for the purpose of later adoption) is filed with immigration authorities. Rules must be followed governing the adoption policies of the foreign country, as well as those effective in the state in which the adopting parents live.

The adoption agency takes the responsibility for travel plans, proper escort enroute to the United States, and for assistance through immigration procedures, and delivers the child to his new parents at the port of entry nearest their home. The agency also assumes a large portion of the cost.

Completion of the adoption procedures is carried out through the assistance of the local child welfare or adoption agency, following the requirements of the state in which the family lives. The local agency also assumes the responsibility for assisting the new parents and the child as desired and needed.

Families wishing to adopt a child of friends or relatives abroad, or a child whom they have located independently, may also use the services of intercountry adoption agencies.*

---

* WAIF Adoption Division, International Social Service. American Branch, Inc. 345 East 46th St., New York, New York 10017.

BIBLIOGRAPHY

Brock, J., and Autret, M.: Kwashiorkor in Africa. Geneva, WHO monograph series no. 8, 1952.

Jelliffe, D.: Infant nutrition in the subtropics and tropics. Geneva, WHO monograph series no. 29, 1955.

World Health magazine: Against hidden hunger. P. 12, (Mar.) 1963.

————: Diseases of hunger as seen by the doctor. P. 8, (Mar.) 1963.

————: Half the world goes hungry. P. 5, (Mar.) 1963.

————: Industry: baby food: health. P. 6, (May) 1963.

————: World fight against communicable disease: a progress report. P. 3, (May) 1966.

WHO Chronicle: Malnutrition in early childhood. WHO Chronicle, 20:86, 1966.

Zottola, G.: Tortillas and beans. World Health magazine, 15:24, (Sept.-Oct.) 1962.

SUGGESTED READINGS FOR FURTHER STUDY

Brock, J. F., (ed.): Recent Advances in Infant Nutrition. Chap. 23. Boston, Little, Brown & Sons, 1961.

Curry, M.: A Chilean clinic. Nurs. Outlook, 12:52, (Jan.) 1964.

Egbert, J. P.: Experiences in Mexico. Nurs. Outlook, 12:38, (Jan.) 1964.

Houwer, D. Q. R. Mulock: Children—a universal concern. Children, 9:91, 1962.

James, H.: African nurse. Nurs. Times, 58:1295, 1962.

Jelliffe, D. B., and Bennett, F. J.: Cultural problems in technical assistance. Children, 9:171, 1962.

Longo, L. D.: Medicine and medical education in Nigeria. New Eng. J. Med., 268:1044, 1963.

Loughlin, B. W.: Pregnancy in the Navajo culture. Nurs. Outlook, 13:55, (Mar.) 1955.

Monteith, M. C.: International aspects of nursing. Nurs. Outlook, 12:56, (Jan.) 1964.

Saba, V.: A nurse goes to Saudi-Arabia. Nurs. Outlook, 14:58, (May) 1966.

Sinclair, A.: The world's deprived children. Children, 9:84, 1962.

UNICEF Board Meeting. Children, 11:120, 1964.

United States Department of State: Food for Peace. Washington, U. S. Government Printing Office, 1963.

Voorhies, E. F.: Public health nursing in India. Nurs. Outlook, 12:43, (Jan.) 1964.

28

The Role of the
Nurse in the Community

The role of the nurse today cannot be defined in narrow terms. She is beginning to see herself as a practitioner in her own field of nursing, and she is now trying to define for herself what nursing really is. For this, she needs a clear head and broad vision.

It is not enough for a nurse to be proficient in bedside nursing skills. Important as this is, it is but one dimension of nursing. A nurse may keep a young patient clean and physically comfortable. She may protect him from infection and dress his incision, but if he still remains only a *patient* to her, she is not giving him the nursing he needs. How does she become a competent nurse? By becoming involved, by seeing her patient as someone with a background, and as someone with a future.

The boy who came into the hospital as a result of a bicycle accident, and who insisted that he had no father and no one to visit him, could have been considered to be a liar by the nurse who had seen a deeply concerned father with him the evening before. Instead, she saw him as a boy who was struggling to handle his guilt—he had been strictly forbidden to ride his bicycle on a busy highway, and the only way he could come to terms with himself for the moment was to deny reality.

The nurses in the pediatric ward who cared for scared and homesick Indian boys from the reservation (and who sent them home with a toy, new socks and with jeans) did not do this solely to see their faces light up. They knew these children came from a desperately poor tribe, that they were frightened and bewildered, and never completely understood why they were in the hospital. Perhaps, if they took back with them a remembrance of kindness, it might help.

In preparing to be a good nurse, the student must have a broad knowledge to draw from. Theoretical knowledge of growth and development is of course essential, and it is one of her greatest assets. Her knowledge, however, is not enough. She must also acquire empathy, as well as an understanding of child behavior. Does Jimmy cover his eyes, sulk, and refuse to recognize even his best friends when the nurses make early morning report rounds? Isn't it about time he got over such nonsense? After all, he is nearly six years old, and he should be well adjusted to the hospital on this his twentieth admission. Or could it be that he is so completely disillusioned by waking every morning to find himself still in the hospital, still unable to run and play like other children, that it takes him a while to remember that these are his friends?

A nurse's role in the community is many things. She is a case finder, a health educator, a research worker, a teacher, a counselor and a skilled nurse. It is an absorbing profession and one that provides excitement and deep satisfaction. Let us look at some of the ways in which she may serve.

The School Nurse

A school nurse has a unique opportunity to employ many and varied talents. She may be employed full-time by a board of education, and may be required to meet certification requirements formulated by state school boards. In other situations, particularly in smaller cities and towns, a school nurse is a public health nurse with a district in her care—one that may include one or more schools.

Her services also vary in different settings. She may spend much of her time in conducting screening tests, assisting with health examinations, and so on. She may be a member of a team that includes a child psychologist, a social worker and a guidance counselor. These roles tend to overlap, and the nurse's guidance and counsel will be respected. Unless a child's emotional and social adjustment, as well as his physical well-being and intellectual potential are the concern of every member of the team, the child's best interest is not served.

A school nurse needs a well-integrated background of knowledge. She must know what to do if Johnny needs glasses or if Susie is in great need of dental work—if family resources cannot meet the strain. She is the person to inform the teachers about what to watch for if she has a diabetic child or a child with seizures or with other problems in her class. One cannot expect a teacher to have expert, up-to-date medical knowledge. A school nurse should have it.

A school nurse may initiate or carry out a sex education program, and she may find herself the target for much criticism, because it is difficult to avoid stepping on a few toes. The fifth grade pupils may be too young, or the sixth grade pupils may be too old. Some parents object to any sex education in the schools, and some would wish it all be given there. Probably a nurse could have her greatest success if she follows some simple rules. She should herself be well adjusted, and she should understand the children's need for sex knowledge at different age levels and with various family backgrounds. Then, if she and the school system are in accord, she may find that obtaining the cooperation and the active assistance of the PTA works out to everyone's best advantage.

Camp Nursing

Camp nursing presents excellent opportunities for worthwhile summer employment. Regular children's camps have seldom had difficulty recruiting nurses for the season. An interesting trend is to provide camp experience for children with various handicaps that limit or prevent their participation in normal camp activities.

Camps for diabetic children are quite well established. Such a child can finally believe that he is not alone with his problem when everyone in camp lines up for urine tests, insulin and for blood tests. Many camps find this an excellent opportunity to help a child correct any misunderstandings, or errors in technique, concerning his tests, his diet, and his insulin.

A unique camp, held for the first time, proved very successful and will be repeated on a larger scale. This was a camp for children with cystic fibrosis. Sixteen children between the ages of 6 and 14 attended camp for one week and enjoyed it immensely. Two resident doctors, one nurse, a pediatric social worker, a therapist and a dietician were in attendance. The children received their daily inhalation and postural drainage therapy, had chest examinations, and received diet and medications as they did at home. No restrictions on their activity were imposed other than any child might impose upon himself. The children thrived, and went home at the end of the week in excellent spirits.

Children with cerebral palsy, muscular dystrophy, and with orthopedic handicaps have special camps in which there are plentiful activities geared to the child's ability. Young nurses have found work in these camps stimulating and greatly helpful in increasing their knowledge of the handicapped child.

Nursing Careers Among the American Indians

A challenging, satisfying career is available for nurses who would like to contribute to the health of this portion of the American population.

The Division of Indian Health of the Public Health Service has the responsibility for health services to the American Indians and to Alaska Natives. The Division operates more than 50 hospitals, over 200 health stations and clinics, and several school health centers. These are located in 25 states, mainly on the reservations.

Clinical nurses work in Indian hospitals and field clinics, while public health nurses provide services on a family-centered basis. A nurse may join through Federal Civil Service, or through the Commissioned Corps of the Public Health Service. Nurses work in close relationship with local health departments, and through them find provision for additional services for special conditions.

Project Head Start

Project Head Start has given public health nurses interesting experiences. This project, sponsored by the Office of Economic Opportunity, seeks to help deprived children develop better concepts of themselves through preschool enrichment programs. Health education has been incorporated into the program, and public health nurses have had the responsibility for health supervision and for education. Health education for the children has included handwashing, dental hygiene and elementary nutrition. An involvement of parents has, in some areas, taken the form of Mother's Clubs, as well as voluntary assistance for the project staff from some of the mothers.

The Nurse in the Child Health Conference

Health supervision of infants and preschool children has the objective of assisting and counseling parents, preventing disease, the early detection of health problems, and the basic objective of keeping the well child well.

A Child Health Conference is that part of a public health program offering health supervision for healthy young children.* It is the name given to the clinics that serve well infants and preschool children. Although the title indicates children of all ages, it rarely includes those of school age. The services include health appraisal and discussions with mothers on aspects of their children's health, immunization, special services as needed (dental, nutritional, etc.), and referral to community agencies when necessary.

Functions of the nurse. The nurse in a Well Child Conference usually is the first to see a mother and her child, the first to obtain data such as height, weight, the baby's condition at birth, his health history, his growth and development landmarks, and his immunization history. If the nurse is a warm, friendly, interested person, and inquires whether the mother has any special problems, it is quite likely that she will bring out many things that a mother hesitates to mention to a busy doctor, because she thinks they are too unimportant. A nurse may be able to discuss her problems to their mutual satisfaction, or she may suggest that it would be a good thing to talk over with the doctor.

The doctor follows this with a physical examination of the child and with a conference with the mother, at which the nurse may also be present. In this way, she can follow up with explanations and with guidance. She also is responsible for arranging consultations with a nutrition expert, a social worker or with a child guidance worker as this

* Health Supervision of Young Children. P. 96. Committee on Child Health of the American Public Health Association, 1960.

is needed. A nurse who shows a personal interest in guiding the parents and their child to the proper help, and who shows a sensitivity to their needs, is a nurse who will build confidence and respect for medical consultation.

These are a few of the opportunities for nurses interested in child welfare. There are hosts of others. Research into many aspects of child care is needed, and nurses should be interested in preparing for a role in future care programs. Many nurses are interested in specializing in one aspect of child care—the mentally retarded, the crippled child, or the child requiring thoracic surgery. The field of maternal and child nursing is drawing the attention of nursing specialists. To many, helping to guide and to educate young persons in other parts of the world is an attractive prospect: and for many, the satisfaction found in helping a hospitalized child achieve health is the greatest of any.

BIBLIOGRAPHY

Brittain, C.: Preschool programs for culturally deprived children. Children, *13:* 130, 1966.
Clark, J. H.: A head start for preschoolers. Nurs. Outlook, *13:*55, (Nov.) 1965.
Cromwell, G. E.: The child in the school. Nurs. Outlook, *13:*27, (Feb.) 1965.
The American Public Health Association: Health Supervision of Young Children. P. 96. New York, The American Public Health Association, 1960.
Radke, M. L.: What does the teacher expect of a school nurse? Nurs. Outlook, *13:*33, (Feb.) 1965.

SUGGESTED READINGS FOR FURTHER STUDY

Furman, S.: Suggestions for refocusing child guidance clinics. Children, *12:*140, 1965.
Lindberg, H. G.: A community health potentiator. Nurs. Outlook, *14:*43, (Sept.) 1966.
Steele, S.: Physical Education in a Rehabilitation Center. Nurs. Outlook, *14:*41, (May) 1966.

APPENDIX

Table of Contents

PART 1

TABLES; PREPARATION FOR LABORATORY TESTS

Abbreviations Commonly Used 511
Average Normal Blood Values 512
Average Urine Excretion in Healthy Children 512
Average Pulse Rate (Resting) 512
Average Respiratory Rate (Approxmiate) 513
Equivalent Centigrade and Fahrenheit Temperature Readings 513
Conversion of Avoirdupois Body Weight
    to Metric Equivalents 513
Conversion of Linear Height to Metric Equivalents 514
Metric Doses with Approximate Apothecary Equivalents . . 514
Equivalent Weights in Metric and in Apothecary Scales . . 514
Preparation for Laboratory Tests 515

PART 2

PROCEDURES

Blood Pressure Readings 519
Emergency Treatment for Cardiac Arrest ("Code 99") . . . 520
Isolation Procedure for Communicable Diseases 523
Protective Technique for Highly Susceptible Patients . . . 529
Nasopharyngeal Suction (for Children and for Older Infants) 530
Tracheotomy Care 531
Water Seal Suction for Chest Drainage 533
Tube Feeding (Gavage) 535
Peritoneal Dialysis 537
Mist Tent Therapy 539
Methods for Computing Fractional Doses of Medications . . 541
Burn Bath (Tub Bath when Ordered) 543
Collection of Clean Urine Specimen 545
Enema (Cleansing) 545
Medication Administration for Small Children and for Infants 546
Instillation of Ear Drops 551
Instillation of Nose Drops 551
Rectal Medications (Suppositories) 552
Procedure for the Use of the Z Tract Method in the
    Administration of Iron Dextran (Imferon) 552
Positioning an Infant or a Child for Treatment 554
Tepid Sponge Bath (to Reduce Fever) 555

Part 1

Tables and Preparation for Laboratory Tests

TABLE APPENDIX–1. ABBREVIATIONS COMMONLY USED

ABBREVIATION	MEANING	DERIVATION
aa	of each	ana (Greek)
a.c.	before meals	ante cibum (Latin)
ad lib	as desired	ad libitum (Latin)
A.P.	apical pulse	
b.i.d.	two times daily	bis in die (Latin)
B.P.	blood pressure	
C.	centigrade	
c̄	with	
cc	cubic centimeter	
cm.	centimeter	
D.C.	discontinue	
F.	Fahrenheit	
fl.	fluid	
Gm.	gram	
gtt.	drop, drops	guttae (Latin)
(H)	hypodermically	
h.s.	at hour of sleep	hora somni (Latin)
I.M.	intramuscularly	
I.V.	intravenously	
kg.	kilogram	
L.	liter (1000 cc., or 1 qt. approx.)	
mg.	milligram	
mm.	millimeter	
O.D.	right eye	oculus dexter (Latin)
O.S.	left eye	oculus sinister (Latin)
O.U.	both eyes	oculus unitas (Latin)
oz., or ℥	ounce	
p̄	after	
P.O.	by mouth	per os. (Latin)

511

TABLE APPENDIX–1. ABBREVIATIONS COMMONLY USED *Cont.*

ABBREVIATION	MEANING	DERIVATION
p.r.n.	as necessary	pro re nata (Latin)
q.s.	as much as necessary	quantum satis (Latin)
R.B.C.	red blood count	
s̄	without	
s̄s̄	one-half	
W.B.C.	white cell count	
X	times	
℥	dram	

TABLE APPENDIX–2. AVERAGE NORMAL BLOOD VALUES*

	NEW-BORN	14 DAYS	1 YEAR	4 YEARS	8–12 YEARS
Red cells/cu.mm. (in millions)	5.5		4.6	4.8	5.1
White cells/cu.mm. (in thousands)	15	12	9	8–10	8
Hemoglobin Gms./100 ml.	17.6	17	12.2	13.1	14–15
Platelets/cu.mm. (in thousands)	350	300	250	250	250

* from various sources.

TABLE APPENDIX–3. AVERAGE URINE EXCRETION IN HEALTHY CHILDREN

AGE	HOURLY	FLUID INTAKE PER 24 HOURS
0–12 months	8–20 cc.	200–500 cc.
1–4 years	20–24 cc.	500–575 cc.
4–7 years	24–28 cc.	575–650 cc.
7–10 years	28–30 cc.	725–800 cc.
Adult	50 cc.	1500–2000 cc.

TABLE APPENDIX–4. AVERAGE PULSE RATE (RESTING)*

AGE	RATE (TAKE FOR FULL MINUTE)
Birth–3 months	140–130
4–12 months	130–120
1–2 years	120–115
2–8 years	100–90
8–12 years	90–80
12–16 years	80–76

* Adapted from Behrendt, H.: Diagnostic Tests in Infants and Children. 2nd ed. Philadelphia, Lea & Febiger, 1962.

TABLE APPENDIX–5. AVERAGE RESPIRATORY RATE (APPROXIMATE)

Age	Rate Per Minute
Birth	30 – 50
Infancy	30
Toddler, preschool age	20 – 30
School age	18 – 20

TABLE APPENDIX–6. EQUIVALENT CENTIGRADE AND FAHRENHEIT TEMPERATURE READINGS

Centigrade	Fahrenheit
35	95.0
36	96.8
37	98.6
38	100.4
39	102.2
40	104.0
41	105.8

To convert centigrade readings to Fahrenheit, multiply by 1.8 and add 32.
To convert Fahrenheit readings to Centigrade, subtract 32 and divide by 1.8.

TABLE APPENDIX–7. CONVERSION OF AVOIRDUPOIS BODY WEIGHT TO METRIC EQUIVALENTS

LB.	KG.	KG.	LB.
10	4.5	10	22
20	9.1	20	44
30	13.6	30	66
40	18.2	40	88
50	22.7	50	110
60	27.3		
70	31.8		
80	36.4		
90	40.9		
100	45.4		

One pound = 0.454 Kilograms
One Kilogram = 2.2 pounds

TABLE APPENDIX–8. CONVERSION OF HEIGHT TO METRIC EQUIVALENTS

INCHES	CM.
18	46
24	61
30	76
36	91
42	107
48	122
54	137
60	152
66	168

One inch = 2.54 cm.

One cm. = 0.3937 inch

TABLE APPENDIX–9. METRIC DOSES WITH APPROXIMATE APOTHECARY EQUIVALENTS*

LIQUID MEASURE

Metric		*Apothecary*
4000	ml.	1 gallon
1000	ml.	1 quart
500	ml.	1 pint
30	ml.	1 fluid ounce
4	ml.	1 fluid dram
0.06	ml.	1 minum

Note: a milliliter (ml.) is the approximate equivalent of a cubic centimeter (cc.).

* When prepared dosage forms such as tablets, capsules, and pills are prescribed in the metric system, the pharmacist may dispense the corresponding approximate equivalent in the apothecary system, and vice versa.

TABLE APPENDIX–9a. EQUIVALENT WEIGHTS IN METRIC AND IN APOTHECARY SCALES

METRIC		APOTHECARY
30	Gm.	1 ounce
15	Gm.	4 drams
1	Gm.	15 grains
60	mg.	1 grain
30	mg.	½ grain
15	mg.	¼ grain
1	mg.	1/60 grain
0.4	mg.	1/150 grain
0.25	mg.	1/250 grain
0.2	mg.	1/300 grain
0.12	mg.	1/500 grain

PREPARATION FOR LABORATORY TESTS

Test of Renal Function

Addis Sediment Count*

Purpose: To estimate the concentration power of the kidney.

Preparation: (For children)

4 P.M.	Give the child his usual evening meal, include fluids up to a quantity of 200 cc.
4 P.M. to 8 A.M.	No fluids allowed.
8 P.M.	Child voids, urine discarded.
8 P.M. to 8 A.M.	Save all urine as a single specimen; 0.5 cc. of 40% formaldehyde may be added to the collecting bottle as a preservative. Send the entire specimen to laboratory.

The normal values of formed elements in concentrated urine after a period of fluid restriction:

R.B.C. upper normal 1,000,000
W.B.C. upper normal 1,000,000
Casts   upper normal   10,000
Protein upper normal   35 mg.

In inflammatory renal disease, there is a sharp rise in formed elements and in the quantity of albumin.

Test of Carbohydrate Metabolism

Glucose Tolerance Test

Preparation:

1. Give regular diet for 4 to 5 days before test.
2. Fasting period directly preceding test: children for 12 hours, young infants for a maximum of 9 hours, and newborn and premature infants for 7 hours.
3. On the morning of the test, a capillary blood specimen is taken (fasting).
4. A urine specimen is obtained (fasting).
5. A glucose solution is given orally. It may be flavored with a few drops of lemon juice. The amount of solution is determined by body weight.
6. Capillary blood is taken half, 1, 1½, 2 and 3 hours after the ingestion of glucose.
7. Urine is collected 1 to 2 hours after the ingestion of glucose.

Average normal response is a rise in blood sugar of 30 to 40 mg. per 100 cc., reaching a peak 30 to 45 minutes after the ingestion of glucose. The blood sugar level returns to normal within 2 to 2½ hours.

* Adapted from Behrendt, H.: Diagnostic Tests in Infants and Children. 2nd ed. Philadelphia, Lea & Febiger, 1962, (and from other sources).

An abnormal response may consist of an elevation of blood sugar above 150 mg., a failure to return to normal levels in 3 hours, and glycosuria.

Test for Tryptic Activity in Duodenal Fluid (Assay for Pancreatic Enzyme-Diagnostic Test for Mucoviscidosis)

Duodenal Aspiration

Preparation:

1. Explain the procedure to the child if he can understand.
2. Apply restraints as needed. A mummy restraint may be necessary while the tube is passed.
3. A number 10 or 12 French catheter, containing three to four openings at the distal end, is passed through the child's nose, is guided through the stomach and into the duodenum. The catheter is lubricated with water only.
4. The fluid is aspirated and tested for reaction. If the tube is in the stomach, the reaction will be acid: duodenal fluid is alkaline.
5. The tube may be guided into the pyloric antrum under fluoroscopic control, and cautious efforts to push it through may be made by the physician.
6. After the tube has entered the duodenum (as indicated by aspirated fluid having a pH of 6 or 7 or higher), the tubing is anchored to the child's face with adhesive tape.
7. Pancreatic fluid is obtained by gravity, or by occasional gentle suction with a Luer syringe.
8. Fluid is allowed to drain into a test tube, which is preferably kept standing in ice during collection. If fluid drips freely, fractional samples may be obtained.. The tubes must be changed at frequent intervals and placed immediately on ice.
9. Frequent testing of pH reaction is essential. Samples with a pH of less than 6 are not used for analysis.
10. Collection of 5 to 8 cc. of pancreatic fluid is necessary for analysis. If pancreatic failure is present, the flow may be unusually slow, and the amount collected within 60 minutes may have to suffice.
11. The aspiration procedure is extremely uncomfortable. The nurse may give support by her presence, by reading to child or by talking in soothing tone and giving assurance by her gentle touch. She may also release the restraints when she stays with child during this procedure, thus alleviating some of his discomfort.
12. After a specimen is collected, and the tube is removed, the child is comforted and given fluids, or food if he desires it.
13. Specimens are sent to the laboratory immediately and are examined within the hour. If mucoviscidosis is present, the pancreatic fluid has a high viscosity, and in some cases, it may not flow at all. The

fluid is tested for the presence of trypsin by observing (in the laboratory) the effects on a gelatin substrate, using varying dilutions of pancreatic fluid.

Urinary Tests to be Done by Nurses or by the Parents of Child Patients

Urine Albumin

1. Place 2 cc. urine in a test tube.
2. Add 4 drops reagent (20% sulfosalicylic acid).
3. Rotate the tube.
4. Estimation of the amount of albumin present:

   0   — clear urine
   Trace — slight turbidity
   1 +   — cloudy
   2 +   — quite cloudy
   3 +   — precipitate formed
   4 +   — urine becomes white, milk-like

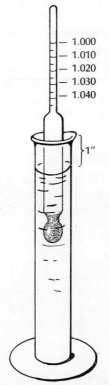

Fig. 1. A urinometer used for determining the specific gravity of urine.

Specific Gravity Determination

1. Fill the cylinder with urine to within one inch from the top (25 cc.). Grasp the float at the tip and insert slowly until it is immersed in the urine to near the top of the graduation marks. Give the float a slight twirl, and note the reading as it comes to rest. While reading, keep the float away from the sides of the container. Avoid wetting the stem above the water line because this gives an inaccurate reading. A normal specific gravity is 1.015–1.025. (Fig. 1) (urinometer)

pH of Urine

1. Dip nitrozine paper in urine, and compare the color of the paper with the chart.
2. The normal pH of urine is 6. Subtract 0.2 pH units from the indicated pH value.

Ferric Chloride Tests (for Phenylketonuria)

1. Put 5 cc. of urine in a test tube, and add two or three drops of 10% ferric chloride. The urine turns a blue-green color if phenylpyruvic acid is present.
2. The same results are obtained if a few drops of 10% ferric chloride are placed on a freshly wet diaper, or if *Phenostix* is dipped in urine or is pressed against a wet diaper. These tests are useful only if they are used with freshly voided urine. False positive results may occur.
3. A strip of ordinary filter paper may be saturated with urine, then dried, and then mailed to a laboratory, where it is tested the same way as in the diaper test.

Urine Sugar Test (Clinitest)

1. Put five drops of urine in a test tube, and add ten drops of water.
2. Add a Clinitest reagent tablet.
3. The solution will then "boil." After the boiling stops, wait 15 seconds, shake the tube and compare it with color chart.
   Negative — no change
   Trace   — blue green
   1 +   — light green
   2 +   — yellow green
   3 +   — yellow or orange green
   4 +   — orange

Part 2

Procedures

BLOOD PRESSURE READINGS

Accurate blood pressure readings are difficult to obtain from infants and from young children. Readings are taken usually only on specific order of the physician.

Principles

1. A child should be at rest for accurate reading. Excitement or exercise may significantly raise the systolic rate.
2. Fright, discomfort, or distrust of the examiner, causes resistance and excitement.
3. The proper size cuff is essential for an accurate reading. Too wide or too narrow a cuff gives an erroneously high or low reading. The cuff should cover two-thirds of the upper arm.
4. If strict accuracy is important, use of the same cuff for each reading will be necessary.

Technique

1. Ascertain the latest reading for comparison.
2. Choose the proper size cuff. If possible, use the same cuff each time.
3. Approach the child with a gentle manner and with slow, deliberate movements. Establish good rapport. Avoid tightening the cuff beyond a necessary point.
   For an older child, prepare him with an explanation, and with an opportunity to explore the equipment. Give the reasons for the procedure.
4. Apply the cuff to arm. Raise the manometer gradually to a point above the obliteration of the radial pulse.
5. Deflate the cuff slowly. The *systolic* pressure reading is made when the first sound is heard with each heart beat. The *diastolic* pressure reading is made when the sound suddenly diminishes in volume. A sudden muffling of the sound denotes a pressure equal to the diastole.

519

6. Compare this reading with previous readings. If there is a significant discrepancy, have the pressure checked by second person.
7. Remove the cuff. Reassure and console the child as it seems necessary.
8. Report any significant variation from the previous reading.
9. Record the time and the reading on the patient's chart.

Table Appendix–10. AVERAGE BLOOD PRESSURES*

AGE	SYSTOLIC	DIASTOLIC
4 years	85	60
6 years	90	60
8 years	98	64
10 years	100	65
12 years	108	67
14 years	112	70
16 years	118	75

Blood pressure readings in infancy and in early childhood are essentially the same as those of a four-year-old.

EMERGENCY TREATMENT FOR CARDIAC ARREST ("CODE 99")

The World Health Organization recommends that every hospital should have a master plan for dealing with the emergency of cardiac arrest whenever it occurs. The suggested plan has been put into practice in various countries.

In the United States, the plan has been instituted under various titles, one of which is "Code 99."

General Principles for Emergency Treatment in Cardiac Arrest

1. A wide cross-section of the hospital staff should receive training in resuscitation methods.
2. The person finding a patient in cardiac arrest should begin resuscitative measures immediately and should also call for help.
3. A cardiac resuscitation team, consisting of medical residents, an anesthesiologist and a designated nurse should be available on call or, as an alternative, all available medical staff in the vicinity should respond to the telephone operator's call.
4. An emergency cart, containing all necessary equipment, should be readily available and kept fully equipped at all times.

* Adapted from Nelson, W., (ed.): Textbook of Pediatrics. 8th ed. Philadelphia, W. B. Saunders, 1964.

Specific Program

Programs vary in details, but a sample program may be given here.

1. The emergency cart kept on each hospital division, should contain:
   a. A small oxygen tank and a mask.
   b. A small suction machine, tubing, and catheters.
   c. An Ambubag, a mask and tracheal tube attachments.
   d. An emergency tracheotomy set.
   e. A Laryngoscope and endotracheal tubes.
   f. An emergency drug box with syringes, needles, an intravenous set, 5% dextrose in water solution, and airways of various sizes.
   g. A large board on which to place the patient for closed chest massage.
2. An EKG machine should be kept readily available.
3. On finding a patient in cardiac arrest, the nurse calls for help and immediately begins mouth-to-mouth breathing and closed-chest massage.
4. The person responding to a call for help, goes to the telephone, and tells operator "page Code 99 for (ward _____)."
5. Operator pages "Code 99, ward _____," every 20 seconds until she is notified that further paging is unnecessary.
6. All medical staff available respond to the call.
7. An assistant (or the first person responding) brings the emergency cart to the patient's unit and remains available to do errands and to get additional supplies.
8. One person takes the responsibility to prepare medications as ordered, sets up intravenous equipment and takes other needed measures.
9. One person takes the responsibility for keeping an accurate record of all procedures.

Method of Mouth-to-Mouth Breathing

1. Clear the patient's airway with a finger.
2. Tilt the patient's head back, and pull his jaw forward. Make certain that his tongue does not fall back and obstruct his breathing.
3. (For an infant.) Place your wide open mouth over the infant's nose and his mouth. Blow puffs of air from your *mouth only*.
   (For an older child.) Close the patient's nostrils with your fingers and place your wide open mouth over the child's mouth. Blow air into child's mouth gently, not forcefully.
4. Move your head back, and allow the patient to exhale.
5. Repeat step 3. Breathe rhythmically, approximately 16 to 20 times per minute.
6. Continue until the physician arrives and gives further instruction.

The Closed-chest Method of Cardiopulmonary Resuscitation

The statement issued by the American Heart Association and distributed by the American Nurses' Association regarding closed chest cardiopulmonary resuscitation reads as follows:*

External cardiac resuscitation is a proved and accepted life-saving technique and should be applied as an emergency procedure by properly trained individuals of the medical, dental, nursing and allied health professions and of rescue squads; and the undersigned urge that training procedures for respiratory and closed-chest cardiac resuscitation be widely disseminated to these groups.

(signed)   American Heart Association, Inc.
American National Red Cross
Industrial Medical Association
United States Public Health Service

Proper Training for Paramedical Personnel

1. Training and practice in mouth-to-mouth resuscitation.
2. Demonstration of closed-chest cardiac compression.
3. Practice in closed-chest cardiac compression, using models such as Resusci-Anne.
4. Understanding of "appropriate cases"—on whom resuscitation should be attempted.
5. Understanding that reported injuries due to closed-chest cardiac compression have included damage to the heart and the liver, rib fractures and other internal injuries. That many lives have been saved by this type of resuscitation, however, and that the risk of injuries is at an acceptable minimum if the resuscitator is well-trained and uses appropriate measures.

Points to remember when faced with an emergency involving sudden cardiac arrest:

1. Irreversible changes to the central nervous system occur in 4 to 6 minutes after cardiac arrest. Therefore, resuscitation efforts must be instituted promptly on recognition of cardiac arrest.
2. The airway must be cleared and kept open.
3. Mouth-to-mouth resuscitation must be started at once if there are no spontaneous respirations.
4. Absence of pulse should be verified before starting closed-chest resuscitation (palpation for femoral or carotid pulse).
5. A properly trained nurse should place a child on a firm surface, which may be a board laid over the mattress, a table, or on the floor if necessary.
6. The lower third of the sternum must be correctly located. Pressure is applied by using the heel of one hand only for children and 2 fingers only for small infants.

* Closed-chest method of cardiopulmonary resuscitation. Amer. J. Nurs., 65:105, (May) 1965.

7. This procedure is considered an emergency measure, to be continued only until a physician arrives to give further instructions.

RELATED READING ON EMERGENCY TREATMENT FOR CARDIAC ARREST

Cahill, D.: The nurse's role in closed chest cardiac resuscitation. Amer. J. Nurs., 65:84, (Mar.) 1965.

Deutsch, R., and Deutsch, P.: Public has role in cardiac resuscitation. The Modern Hospital, 106:129, (May) 1966.

Hoefler, O.: The management of cardiac arrest. J. Nat. Med. Assn., 38:159, (May) 1966.

Johnson, J.: A plan in cardiac arrest. J.A.M.A., 186:468, 1963.

Organized services for cardiac emergencies. WHO Chronicle, 30:79, (Mar.) 1966.

Closed-chest method of cardiopulmonary resuscitation. Amer. J. Nurs., 65:105, (May) 1965.

ISOLATION PROCEDURE FOR COMMUNICABLE DISEASES

Definition

A separation from contact with others of a patient having a *communicable* disease.

The nurses caring for the patient use aseptic medical technique; that is, they use proper measures to prevent transmission of the infection to other patients, to visitors or to personnel involved in the child's care.

Principles

Medical aseptic technique is effective in preventing cross-contamination only to the extent to which everyone caring for the child adheres to the rules.

Medical aseptic technique may be employed to protect susceptible persons from the infectious diseases of the patient, or to protect a highly susceptible patient from the hospital environment. (See *Protective Technique for Highly Susceptible Patients.*)

Protective Measures

A. Type of unit
   1. The unit for the care of a child with communicable disease should be a private room, a cubicle, or a multiple-bed room admitting children with the same type of infection.
   2. The unit should be equipped with running water, a wall container of liquid or powdered soap (hexachlorophene soap preferred), and wall container of paper towels.
   3. Furnishings should be attractive, with eye appeal, but simple and easy to clean.
   4. All utensils not necessary for the child's care should be removed from the unit before admission, i.e., the bedpan (if the patient is an infant) and similar articles.

B. Equipment in contaminated area
   1. A sign saying "isolation" or some other indication that special technique must be used, and readily observable from outside the room.
   2. An individual fever thermometer with its container, a solution for disinfection of thermometer (alcohol 70%, zephiran chloride, or an alcohol-iodine preparation) attached to wall out of reach of child.
   3. A linen hamper with bag for used linen (covered).
   4. A covered container for soiled diapers (as necessary). (A step-on can if possible, with a bag inside.)
   5. Waxed paper or a plastic bag lining the wastebasket.
   6. A blood pressure cuff and a stethoscope.
   7. The usual equipment for the care of a child.

C. Equipment in clean area should include a stand containing
   1. Laundry bags, especially marked for isolation (red tag, striped, or marked "isolation").
   2. Clean waxed paper or plastic bags, and brown paper bags.
   3. Clean wrapping for materials to be autoclaved. May include long boat for syringes, needles, and for instruments to be autoclaved.
   4. Masks (if used).
   5. Isolation gowns.

D. Additional equipment
   1. A jar containing gauze flats or rags soaked in disinfecting solution for wiping off a bed-side table, a bed, and window ledges. (Microphene, alcohol.)
   2. A door mat in the doorway. Two large trays lined with absorbent pads—one saturated with a phenolic solution, one dry. An alternative—clean cloth covers to be slipped over shoes when entering the room.

E. Procedure for entering unit
   1. Wash hands.
   2. Collect linen and equipment needed for care of the patient.
   3. Remove your watch. If your watch will be needed in the care of the child, wrap in plastic and take it into the unit with the rest of the equipment.
   4. Don mask (if used). Make sure the mask is securely tied, covering your nose and your mouth. Adjusting or replacing the mask while caring for a child invites the spread of infection.
   5. Put on a clean gown, using care to cover the back of the uniform completely. If the gown is long-sleeved, push the sleeves back to expose the forearms.
   6. Enter the unit with the understanding that all objects are considered contaminated.

7. Wash your hands and your arms for 2 to 3 minutes using friction. Use care to wash between the fingers. Clean under your nails with an orangewood stick.

Procedures Related to Patient Care

A. Care of food tray and dishes. (Children)
  1. The tray may be brought to the door of the unit by a clean nurse, the dishes handed to nurse in unit, and the tray returned to the serving room.
      (Alternative—a disposable tray may be used, taken into the room, and discarded after use.)
  2. Disposable dishes may be discarded after use. Attractive disposable dishes are now available, and no longer make food appear unappetizing.
  3. Silverware may be used in the room, washed, wrapped, and may be sent to be autoclaved with other equipment.
      (Alternative—plastic spoons may be used and discarded.)
  4. Variation. In hospitals where facilities are available and housekeeping personnel are properly instructed, regular trays and dishes may be used, removed from a unit and put in a dishwashing machine with other dishes.
B. Care of nursing bottles. (Infants, toddlers)
  1. Disposable bottles and nipples may be taken into the room and then discarded after use.
  2. Glass bottles and nipples should be washed in the room, wrapped and sent to be autoclaved with other equipment.
  3. Plastic bottles should be gas autoclaved (if possible) or boiled.
  4. Variation. In hospitals where facilities are available and personnel are properly instructed, bottles and nipples may be washed in a unit, returned to the bottle-washing room and sterilized with other bottles.
C. Weighing child
    (Infant.) The clean nurse should place the scale outside the doorway of the unit, cover the funnel with a clean sheet, and balance the scale. The nurse in the unit places the infant on the scale, and the clean nurse manipulates the weights. After weighing, the unit nurse takes the sheet and discards it in the linen hamper in the unit.
    (Child.) The clean nurse brings the scale to the doorway, places paper on the platform, and manipulates the weights. The paper is disposed in a wastebasket in the unit. If the child has touched the scale, wipe it with a disinfectant solution.
D. Transporting child. (To X-ray, etc.)
    Place two clean sheets on the wheelchair or on the stretcher. The nurse in the unit places the child on an inner sheet, and the clean

nurse wraps the sheet around him. Personnel must be informed of the infectious nature of the child's condition. On return, both sheets are taken into the unit and are placed in the linen hamper in the unit.

E. Obtaining specimens

The clean nurse stands outside the unit, and holds the receptacle. The nurse in the unit transfers the specimen. If only one person is available and the container must be taken into a unit, the outside of the container should be thoroughly washed with an antiseptic solution.

F. Disposal of wastes

Uneaten food may be scraped into a waxed bag in the wastebasket, and liquids may be poured into the sink.

Potties and bedpans may be emptied into the disposal system. If these must be taken to a common utility room to be emptied, the following procedure is acceptable:

The nurse should remove her mask and her gown, scrub and take the bedpan or the potty in one hand, keeping the other hand clean. She should use her clean hand for opening doors, handling the flusher and similar things. Return the bedpan or the potty to the unit, scrub and change into a new gown.

Note: If the patient is a small child who urinates frequently, it may be helpful to keep a urine specimen bottle or some other container in the room, thus avoiding too frequent trips to the utility room.

G. Nursing care of child

The child in isolation has a particular need of companionship, diversion and personalized care. He needs to be held, rocked, loved, and played with. Practically any toy may be taken into the unit, including books, papers, and plastic toys, if gas autoclaving is available. If it is not available, toys should be those that can be easily cleaned by soaking in a disinfecting solution or disposable.

Visitors. The presence of the child's parents is important for his emotional well-being, and they should be encouraged to visit. They will need to be instructed about wearing the isolation gown, handwashing, and the undesirability of stepping out of the room for any purpose without taking the necessary precautions. Printed instructions are useful, but they must not take the place of demonstration and personal instruction.

H. "Scrubbing Out."

Any equipment or material used in the unit must be made free from contamination before it is deemed safe for use with other patients.

Care of Used Linen

1. Place the diaper bag (closed) in the larger laundry bag in the unit. (Some hospitals may keep diapers separate.)

2. The clean nurse stands outside the doorway holding a clean isolation laundry bag open. The opening should be turned down into a cuff covering the nurse's hands.
3. The nurse in the unit closes the contaminated bag and drops it into the clean bag, using care to avoid contaminating the outside of the clean bag. The laundry bag in the room needs to be emptied before becoming so full that it presents difficulty when double-bagged.
4. The clean nurse turns the cuff up, closes the outer bag and makes sure that the laundry is identified as "isolation."
5. The bag is placed in the laundry chute, or in the area for the collection of soiled linen.

   Alternative. If only one nurse is available, a clean isolation bag may be hung in a laundry hamper in the doorway and the contaminated bag dropped into it. This presents the problem of leaving used linen uncovered in a clean area for the period of time it takes for the nurse to leave the unit.

Care of Wastebasket

1. The clean nurse folds the edges of a clean paper bag in a cuff, covering her hands.
2. The nurse in the unit closes the waxed bag holding wastes and drops it into the clean bag.
3. The clean nurse closes the outer bag and deposits it in a covered waste can in the utility room.

Removal of Watch from Unit

The nurse in the unit unwraps the plastic cover, and drops the watch into the clean nurse's hand.

Treatment Trays and Equipment from Central Supply

1. The nurse in the room washes equipment, drys it and places it in a wrapper or a small bag designated for this purpose.
2. The clean nurse holds a second bag and receives the contaminated bag in same manner as for linen or for waste.
3. The outer bag is properly labeled "isolation" and designated as being for steam or for gas autoclave.
4. If the boat for instruments and syringes is used, the outside is kept clean. Tape the cover to the boat, label it, and send it to central supply to be autoclaved.

Equipment to be Returned to Pediatric Ward

1. Wash, wrap and bag as indicated above. Label it to include the ward to which the articles are to be returned.
2. Articles for steam autoclave may include bath basins, emesis basins,

any monel, aluminum or stainless steel receptacles, glass bottles, rubber goods and steel or iron toys.

3. Articles for gas autoclave may include plastic utensils, paper, books, dolls, and plastic toys.
4. Materials that cannot be gas or steam autoclaved (or if gas autoclave is not available).

    a. Soak in a disinfecting solution (Dicrobe or Zephiran) if possible.

    b. Articles such as stethoscopes, blood pressure cuffs, and manometers should be aired before being used on other patients.

Leaving Unit

1. Before leaving the unit, place a fresh laundry bag on the holder and a fresh waxed bag in the wastebasket.
2. Untie the strings of the gown at the back of the waist.
3. Wash hands and arms thoroughly.
4. Untie the strings at the back of the neck.
5. Slip the right hand under the cuff of the left sleeve, and pull it over the left hand.
6. Use the left hand inside the sleeve to pull the right sleeve down.
7. Remove the gown, folding the outer side inward and avoiding touching the outer (contaminated) side.
8. Place the folded gown in the laundry bag in the unit.
9. Wash hands and arms thoroughly, using a paper towel to handle the faucets.

    Note: Reuse technique for gowns is not recommended because of the difficulty in keeping the gown free from contamination.
10. Remove mask, handling it by the strings only. Drop it into the bag for contaminated masks, or discard it if it is disposable.
11. Wash hands in clean area after leaving the unit.

Care of Room

1. The bedside table, the bedframe, the window ledges, and the shelves should be wiped off daily with microphene, alcohol, Zephiran or some other agent.
2. Floors should be wet mopped. Housekeeping personnel, if properly instructed, may clean the room.

Termination of Isolation

If isolation has been maintained only as a precaution until the communicability of disease has been determined, and until the cultures have proved negative, precautions may be discontinued and routine care may be resumed.

Removal of Patient from Isolation

When the child's condition is determined to be no longer infectious, the following procedure may be employed.

1. Collect a clean bath basin, soap, a sheet, a wash cloth and towels and a bath blanket.
2. Put on a gown, enter the unit with utensils, and wash your hands.
3. Undress the child, place him on a clean sheet, and give him a sponge bath and a shampoo.
4. Wrap the child in a clean blanket and hand him to the nurse outside the room.
5. The child should be dressed and moved to a clean unit.

Terminal Cleaning of Room

1. Bag out utensils in the routine manner for isolation.
2. Notify Housekeeping department that the room is ready for cleaning.

PROTECTIVE TECHNIQUE FOR HIGHLY SUSCEPTIBLE PATIENTS

A susceptible person is a person presumably without resistance against a particular pathogenic agent and who is therefore liable to contract the disease if exposed to it.

Certain child patients need protection against the hospital environment either because of their increased susceptibility to infection, or because of the nature of their own disease. Such patients may include the following:

Children whose leucocyte count becomes abnormally low, because of the drugs used in the treatment of their condition, or because of the nature of the disease itself.

Premature infants.

Burned children (these children will usually need both strict isolation and protective technique during the period of increased susceptibility).

Infants or children whose condition is such that any superimposed infection may have serious consequences.

Technique for Protective Measures

This technique differs from the isolation procedure in these particulars.

1. All articles going *into* the unit must be aseptically clean.
2. Articles coming out of the unit do not need to be sterilized, unless the patient has an infection.
3. Persons with infections should automatically avoid caring for sick children. If the patient is a highly susceptible child, this rule assumes paramount importance.

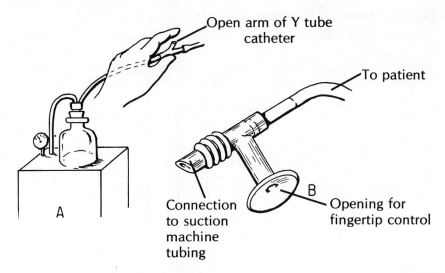

Fig. 2. Suction catheters used for tracheal and nasopharyngeal aspiration.

    a. Y—glass connector. Fingertip placed over open arm creates vacuum.

    b. Regu—vac suction catheter. Permits use of regulated suction technique by fingertip control.

NASOPHARYNGEAL SUCTION
(FOR CHILDREN AND FOR OLDER INFANTS)
Equipment

Sterile

    Nasal catheter.

    A labelled container containing one of the following solutions. Aqueous Zephiran 1:1000; iodine 1:500,000 (8 gtts. of 0.19% iodine in 200 cc. water); saline, water.

    Y connecting-tube.

    Fig. 2 (suction catheters and machine)

Non-sterile

    Suction machine.

Procedure

1. Turn on the suction machine.
2. Insert the catheter in the nose or in the mouth until the cough reflex is reached, with Y connecter open.
3. Rotate the catheter, control the suction by placing your finger over the open arm of the Y tube. Do not make poking or jabbing motions. Remove the catheter slowly.

4. Aspirate solution through the catheter to clear mucus.
5. Repeat the suction as necessary.
6. Leave the catheter in solution or wrap it in a sterile towel, or use a clean catheter for each suctioning.
7. Set up clean equipment every 8 hours when it is in use.

Suctioning for the Newborn

A DeLee mucus trap may be used, or a soft rubber bulb. If DeLee suction apparatus is used, the nurse places the catheter in the infant's mouth, takes the mouthpiece in her own mouth and applies gentle suction. The mucus trap holds mucus secretions from the infant, and prevents secretions from reaching the mouthpiece. Fig. 3 (DeLee mucus trap)

TRACHEOTOMY CARE

Equipment for Suctioning

Sterile

1 container (labelled) containing solution. Solution used: Zephiran Chloride 1:1000; or iodine 1:500,000 (8 gtts. 0.19% iodine in 200 cc. water); or normal saline; or sterile water.

1 container (labelled) containing hydrogen peroxide.

Whistle-tip catheter, size according to the size of the tracheotomy tube used.

Y connecting tube.

Sterile glove (if used). Note: procedures vary. Washing hands before suctioning may be considered sufficient.

Extra tracheotomy tube (to be kept at bedside).

2 Kelly forceps or a Trousseau dilator (to be kept at bedside).

Pipe cleaners.

Obturator from the tracheotomy set in use.

Non-sterile

A suction machine.

Procedure for Suctioning Tracheotomy Tube

1. Wash your hands and put on a sterile glove, if one is to be used.
2. Remove the inner cannula and drop it into hydrogen peroxide.

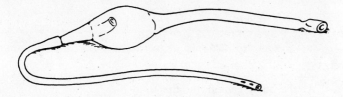

Fig. 3. A DeLee mucus trap.

3. With the suction turned on and with the Y tube open, use your gloved hand to insert the catheter to a point ⅛ inch beyond the cannula.

4. Control the suction by covering the open arm of the Y tube with your finger. Remove the catheter slowly, using a rotary movement. Limit aspiration to 15 seconds.

5. Aspirate solution through the catheter to clear mucus.

6. Pause between aspirations to allow the patient to rest and to allow air to enter the tracheotomy tube.

7. Repeat suctioning as necessary.

8. Clean the inner cannula, insert it and lock it in place.

9. Aspirate the solution through the catheter, and leave the catheter in solution or in a sterile towel, or remove and use a fresh catheter for each suctioning.

10. Remove your glove, and turn off the suction.

11. Comfort the child.

Suctioning the Bronchial Tree.

1. If "deep" suctioning is required, specific orders should be written indicating how deep the catheter should be passed.

2. To aspirate the left bronchus, turn the head to the right. To aspirate the right bronchus, turn the head to the left.

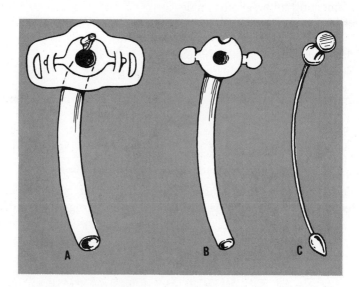

Fig. 4. A tracheotomy tube, showing the three parts.
A. the outer cannula of the tube.
B. the inner cannula of the tube.
C. the obturator, used for inserting the outer cannula.

Care of the Tracheotomy Tube

1. Unlock the inner cannula, remove it and clean it with hydrogen peroxide, using pipe cleaners to remove the mucus from inside the cannula. Rinse well under running water, and replace it in the outer cannula and lock it in place.
2. Check the ties on the tracheotomy tube to make sure that they are secure.

Fig. 4 (a tracheotomy tube)

Precautions

If the tracheotomy tube is displaced or removed, hold the wound open with a Kelly forcep or with a Trousseau dilator until the physician arrives to reinsert the tube. When suctioning, if the catheter meets with an obstruction at the end of the cannula or if the child appears to receive no benefit after suctioning (although tube appears free of mucus) the tracheotomy tube may actually be out of the trachea.

No child is to be left alone at any time with a tracheotomy tube in place, except on the written order of the attending physician.

Care of Equipment.

1. Set up clean sterile equipment every 8 hours and p.r.n.
2. Thoroughly wash equipment and return it to central supply. Most tracheotomy tubes do not have interchangeable parts; make sure that the correct outer cannula, inner cannula and the correct obturator are returned together.

Assisting Physician when Outer Tube is to be Changed

The nurse does not change the outer tube, but assists the physician when the tube is to be changed.

The equipment needed includes a sterile tracheotomy tube (inner and outer cannula, and obturator) of correct size.

Sterile gloves for physician.

Usual equipment for suctioning.

Procedure

1. Position child with neck hyperextended.
2. Restrain child as necessary; mummy restraint usually needed.
3. Standing at child's head, hold head securely between hands while tube is being changed.
4. Suction child following procedure.

WATER SEAL SUCTION FOR CHEST DRAINAGE
Purpose

To provide drainage of the pleural cavity following chest surgery, and to aid in the re-expansion of the lungs.

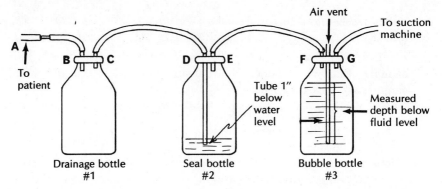

Fig. 5. Closed drainage of the pleural cavity, showing the use of the three bottle system.

Equipment

Sterile drainage bottles, tubing and stoppers.
Water-seal bottle holders.
Kelly forceps (2) kept at bedside.
Suction machine.
Measured amount of sterile water.

Procedure for Setting Up Closed Chest Drainage

1. Set up bottles 1, 2, 3 as in diagram.
2. Add a measured amount of sterile water to seal bottle number 2. Note the amount of water on a piece of adhesive tape on the side of the bottle.
3. Add water to the bubble bottle to cover the glass air vent to a depth ordered by the doctor.
4. Tape all bottle stoppers securely to prevent an air leak.
5. Secure the bottles to the floor, or place them in a holder on the floor.
6. Connect tubing A (patient's chest tube) to tubing B of the drainage bottle.
7. Connect tubing G of the bubble bottle to the suction machine.
8. Turn on suction.
9. Remove the clamp from chest tube (A).

Fig. 5 (water seal drainage diagram—closed drainage of pleural cavity with three bottles)

Nursing Care and Observation of Drainage

If it is draining properly, the fluid level in the long glass tube in the seal bottle fluctuates, and water in the bubble bottle will bubble during the respiratory cycle.

Check the tubing for kinks and compression. The tubing should not sag, but should be free from tension and should allow the child to move about.

Observe the drainage for its color, its amount, and its consistency. Note hourly the amount of drainage either by using a calibrated drainage bottle or by marking the level with a strip of adhesive on the side of bottle.

To Change Drainage Bottle

1. Double-clamp the tubing at A with forceps.
2. Clamp the tubing between E and F.
3. Turn off the suction.
4. Replace the drainage bottle, making sure to maintain sterility. Secure the stopper of the drainage bottle.
5. Turn on the suction.
6. Remove the forceps between E and F.
7. Remove the forceps at A.

To Transport Patient

1. Double-clamp the tubing at A before lifting bottles from the floor.
2. Disconnect the tubing at E.
3. Take all tubing and all bottles through the seal bottle number 2 with the patient.
4. Do not remove the clamps from tubing A unless the bottles are located below the chest level.
5. Do not disconnect the suction for any period of time without a written order.

Record

The amount of drainage and its character.

Fluctuation of the long tube in the seal bottle, and bubbling in the bubble bottle.

The patient's vital signs, any change in color, chest pain, restlessness and apprehension. Any change in well-being should be reported immediately.

TUBE FEEDING (GAVAGE)

Equipment for Gavage

Gastric tube.
Luer syringe.
Container of water.
Formula.

Procedure

1. Wash your hands and assemble the equipment.
2. Using the feeding tube, measure the distance from the bridge of the child's nose to the lower tip of his sternum. Mark the distance on the tube with adhesive tape.

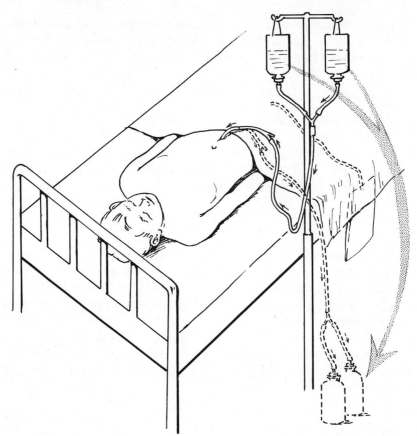

Fig. 6. The apparatus used for peritoneal dialysis. Following the flow of dialysing fluid into the peritoneal cavity, the bottles are placed on the floor to receive the return drainage. A Foley catheter and urine drainage bag are shown toward the foot of the bed.

3. Restrain the child. Usually, a mummy restraint is required for a small child.
4. Elevate the child's head with a small pillow or with a rolled blanket.
5. Dip the end of the tube in water for lubrication, and insert it through the nostril until the measured distance is reached. (If it is a young infant, insert the tube through his mouth.)
6. The child may struggle and choke because of apprehension. Allow time for him to quiet down.
7. Invert the free end of tube in water. Bubbles rising with respiration indicate that the catheter is in the respiratory tract rather than in the stomach. The tube must then be withdrawn.
8. If no bubbles appear, attach a 10 cc. syringe to the tube and aspirate

gently. The appearance of stomach contents in the syringe assures that the tube is in the stomach.

9. If so ordered, aspirate the stomach contents and measure the amount.
10. Remove the plunger from the syringe, and pour a small amount of formula into the barrel. Elevate the tube and let the formula run in slowly.
11. After the feeding has run into the tube, pinch the tubing and withdraw it quickly.
12. Position the infant or the child on his side with his head elevated to prevent aspiration if vomiting occurs.
13. Record the time, the amount suctioned, the amount given, and any other specific data.

PERITONEAL DIALYSIS

Peritoneal dialysis is a form of hemodialysis used in acute renal failure for the purpose of removing metabolic wastes from the blood stream. The peritoneal lining can be used as a dialyzing membrane for filtering out waste products from the blood plasma (by the process of osmosis) into a dialyzing solution on the other side of the membrane. Fig. 6 (peritoneal dialysis)

The procedure of peritoneal dialysis requires a strict aseptic technique and careful monitoring by both medical and nursing personnel. An accurate record of fluid input and fluid outflow must be kept, and the patient must be carefully observed for any adverse effect.

The physician should remain with the patient for one or more complete exchanges of the dialysis fluid. The nurse may then continue the exchanges. They may be continued for a period of 12 to 36 hours.

Equipment

Sterile

Dialysing solution (2 bottles).
A dialysis catheter.
A Y connecting set.
An abdominal paracentesis tray (including trocar).
A bladder catheterization tray (a Foley catheter may be inserted if not already in place).
Gloves.
Aqueous heparin and a broad spectrum antibiotic.
Potassium chloride as ordered.

Other Equipment

Masks (if worn).
A skin preparation set and novocaine.
A basin of water for warming solution bottles.

Procedure

1. Insert the Foley catheter if it is not already in place.
2. Warm the solution to body temperature.
3. Assist the physician as he introduces the trocar into the lower abdominal wall, inserts the catheter and applies a dressing around the catheter.
4. Attach the administration set to two bottles of solution using a Y connecting set. (Follow the instructions that accompany the solution and the equipment.)
5. Insert the ordered drugs into one or both bottles. Label the bottles with the name of the drugs and the dosage.
6. Flush the air out of the administration tubing with the dialysis solution, and clamp the tubing.
7. The physician will attach the administration tubing to the dialysis catheter.
8. Open the clamp on the administration tubing and allow the dialysis solution to flow into the peritoneal cavity as rapidly as possible (approximately 10 to 20 minutes).
9. Clamp the tubing before it is completely empty to prevent air from entering the peritoneal cavity.
10. Allow the fluid to remain in the abdomen for the prescribed length of time.
11. Prepare the next solution for use during this time. New tubing should be used for each dialysis.
12. When the time has elapsed, unhook the bottles and place them on the floor at the bedside. The bottles should be placed in a basin to catch any overflow if extra fluid is obtained.
13. Unclamp the tubing and allow the solution to drain back into the original bottles.
14. Connect a fresh administration set and fresh solution to the catheter and repeat the procedure.
15. Measure the fluid obtained from the previous flow while the second solution is running. Discard used bottles of the solution.
16. Repeat the exchanges for the period of time specified by the physician.
17. The physician remains with his patient for at least one complete exchange of dialysis fluid. The nurse may then continue the exchanges, reporting any change in child's condition.

Recording

Prepare a sheet giving the time that each exchange started, the amount of fluid inserted and withdrawn, the number of bottles used, and the medications added. Remarks should include vital signs, a description of the drainage, the rate of outflow, and the patient's state of well-being.

The urinary output should be measured in accordance with the doctor's order.

Sample Record:

		DIALYSIS FLUID			CUMU-			
Hour	*No.*	*In*	*Out*	BALANCE	LATIVE BALANCE	URINE	MEDICATIONS	NURSES' NOTES
9:20	1	start					5 mg. heparin	Started by Dr. Smith
9:30		1000 cc.					125 mg. tetra-cycline	B.P. 160/90, P. 100, R. 24
10:00			start					
10:10			900 cc.	in 100 cc.	in 100 cc.			Drainage clear
10:20	2	start					5 mg. heparin	
10:30		1000 cc.					125 mg. tetra-cycline	
11:00			start 1200 cc.	out 200 cc.	in 100 cc.			
11:10						10 cc.		

MIST TENT THERAPY

An atmosphere of high humidity is important to alleviate the distress of an infant or a child with respiratory difficulty. In the hospital, the use of cool mist has replaced that of hot steam and is gradually becoming popular for use at home. The cool mist tent has eliminated the danger of steam burns, and has made unnecessary the enclosed "croup tent," that isolated the small child from his environment.

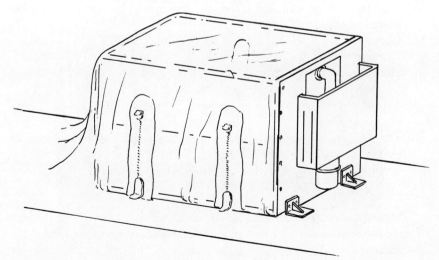

Fig. 7. A Croupette set up ready for use.

The mist tent may be used to provide high humidity and oxygen for the child, or it may be used to provide a humidified atmosphere when oxygen is not needed, by the use of an air compressor.

The Use of an Ice-Cooled Mist Tent (Croupette)

Fig. 7 (Croupette)

1. Make up the crib in the usual manner. Place a cotton blanket over the sheet to absorb the increased moisture caused by humidity in the croupette (optional).
2. Unfold the frame, and set it in the crib. Open the plastic canopy and fit it over the frame, with the apron of the canopy extending toward the foot of the crib. The zippered side openings permit nursing care.
3. Fill the ice chamber at the back of the tent with ice for cooling the tent. (The croupette is occasionally operated without ice if the child's temperature is below normal.)
4. Fill with distilled water the jar through which oxygen or air passes.
5. Connect the designated tubing to an oxygen wall outlet or a tank, or to the air compressor motor.
6. Allow humidified oxygen or air to flow into the tent for a few minutes before placing the child in the tent.
7. Set the liter gauge at the prescribed pressure.
8. Place the child in the tent, explaining the procedure if he can understand it. Position the child on his side, with his head slightly elevated. This usually helps to alleviate respiratory distress.

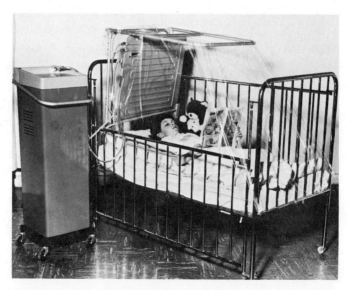

Fig. 8. A CAM tent, showing the refrigeration unit at the bedside and the CoolXChanger at the head of the bed.

9. Keep the distilled water jar filled. Clean it thoroughly when refilling.
10. When ice in the chamber has melted, the drainage tubing should be allowed to drain into a basin, and the chamber should be refilled.
11. After the child is removed from the croupette, wash all apparatus, and send the canopy to be autoclaved.

The Use of the Mistogen Tent Unit (CAM Tent)

This unit makes use of a small refrigeration unit placed at the bedside, which cools and circulates cool water through a panel (coolxchanger) inside the plastic canopy. No ice is needed.

Directions for setting up and for operating the CAM tent accompany the unit. After the unit is set up and the canopy is in place, a gallon of distilled water is placed in the tank of the refrigeration unit. The chilled water continually circulates through the CoolXChanger and returns for re-chilling. Water does not need replacing more often than every 30 days of continual use.

When not in use, the CAM tent can be taken down in a process that is the reverse of setting it up; the frame, the canopy, the CoolXChanger and the nebulizer may be washed, dried, and autoclaved if desired. All parts fold compactly and are hung from back of refrigeration unit for storage.

Fig. 8 (CAM tent)

METHODS FOR COMPUTING FRACTIONAL DOSES OF MEDICATIONS

When giving medications to infants and to children, it is often necessary to give a smaller dosage than that supplied by the drug company. It is therefore important that a pediatric nurse become proficient in computing fractional dosages. Two commonly used methods of computation are outlined here.

1. Fractional Method

In this method, the nurse merely considers the size of the desired dose to be a fraction of the dose supplied (on hand). The formula becomes: $\dfrac{\text{Desired Dose}}{\text{Dose on Hand}}$. Because children's medications are usually (fraction) (of) (quantity) given in liquid form, the formula becomes: $\dfrac{\text{Desired Dose}}{\text{Dose on Hand}} \times \text{diluent} =$ amount of medication to be given.

Example: doctor's order; give Tetracycline Suspension, 125 mg. q 4 hr. (Tetracycline Suspension comes as 250 mg. per 5 cc.)

$$\frac{\text{Desired Dose}}{\text{Dose on Hand}} = \frac{125 \text{ mg.}}{250 \text{ mg.}} \times \frac{5 \text{ cc.}}{1} = \frac{125}{250} \times 5 = 2.5 \text{ cc.}$$

Give 2.5 cc. of Tetracycline Suspension.

Example: doctor's order; give Demerol 30 mg. I.M., stat. (Demerol comes as 50 mg. per 1 cc.)

$$\frac{\text{Desired Dose}}{\text{Dose on Hand}} \times \text{diluent} = \frac{30 \text{ mg.}}{50 \text{ mg.}} \times \frac{1 \text{ cc.}}{1} = \frac{30}{50} \text{ or } 0.6 \text{ cc.} \text{ Give } 0.6 \text{ cc.}$$

of Demerol I.M. immediately.

Example: doctor's order; give atropine gr. $\frac{1}{500}$ I.M. pre-op. You may have on hand atropine gr. $\frac{1}{150}$ H.T. (hypodermic tablet).

$$\frac{\text{Desired Dose}}{\text{Dose on Hand}} = \frac{1/500}{1/150} = 1/500 \div 1/150 = 1/500 \times 150/1 = \frac{150}{500} = \frac{3}{10}.$$

Dissolve one tablet of atropine gr. 1/150 in 1 cc. of sterile water and give 0.3 cc. (5 minums). Discard 0.7 cc.

2. Formula for Proportion (Ratio) Method

Dose ordered: amount of solution needed::dose on hand: amount of solution on hand.

A. Example: Demerol 30 mg.:   X   L: 50 mg.   :   1 cc.
(Product of the means equal product of the extremes)   30:X::50:1

$$50X = 30 \quad X = \frac{30}{50} = 3/5 \quad \text{Give } 3/5 \ (0.6) \text{ cc. of Demerol.}$$

B. Example:

$$\left(\begin{array}{c} \text{dose ordered} \\ \text{atropine gr. } 1/500 \end{array} \right) \text{ is to } \left(\begin{array}{c} \text{amount of solution needed} \\ X \end{array} \right) \text{ as}$$

$$\left(\begin{array}{c} \text{dose on hand} \\ \text{atropine gr. } 1/150 \end{array} \right) \text{ is to } \left(\begin{array}{c} \text{amount of solution on hand} \\ 1 \text{ cc.} \end{array} \right)$$

or

gr. 1/500 : X :: gr. 1/150 : 1 cc.

step 1: gr. $\frac{1}{150}$ X = gr. $\frac{1}{500}$

step 2: $X = \frac{1}{500} \div \frac{1}{150}$

step 3: $\frac{1}{500} \div \frac{1}{150} = \frac{1}{500} \times \frac{150}{1}$

step 4: $\frac{1}{500} \times \frac{150}{1} = \frac{150}{500}$

step 5: $\frac{150}{500} = \frac{3}{10}$ (0.3)

step 6:   X = 0.3 cc.

Dissolve one tablet of atropine gr. 1/150 in 1 cc. of sterile water. Give 0.3 cc. Discard 0.7 cc.

BURN BATH (TUB BATH WHEN ORDERED)

Equipment

Isolation gown; mask and cap if used.

Two sterile sheets, plastic or Koroseal.

Two pairs of sterile gloves (if dressings are to be used).

Ordered solution for bath (pHisoHex, Ivory Snow, saline, etc.).

A bath thermometer.

A waxed paper bag (for soiled dressings).

Procedure

1. Clean the tub thoroughly with pHisoHex or with hexachlorophene soap.
2. Fill the tub with enough water to cover the burned area.
3. Check the temperature of water (105° to 110°).
4. Add the desired solution or Ivory Snow (about 1½ oz.).
5. Put on a gown, a mask, and a cap (if one is to be used).
6. Cover a stretcher with a sterile sheet, place the child on the sheet and wrap it lightly around him.
7. Move the child to the bathroom. If the child has dressings, put on gloves and remove the outer layers. Remove your gloves.
8. Put on clean gloves, and place the child in the tub, lowering him very slowly and carefully. The child may be very frightened, and may need much emotional support.
9. Support child as necessary while he is in the tub. Never leave a child alone.
10. Leave the child in the tub for the designated time. (Not longer than 15 to 20 minutes.) His dressings will soak off.
11. Place on sterile plastic, cover with sterile sheet on stretcher and lift the child onto the stretcher, wrapping the sheet around him.
12. Return him to his room, place him on a clean, sterile sheet on his bed.
13. Apply dressings (if any are to be used) using sterile technique.
14. Record the type of bath, the condition of the burned areas, and the child's response to the treatment.

Burn Soaks or Wet Packs

Equipment

A sterile basin.

Solution as ordered.

Sterile gloves (2 pairs if dressing is to be changed).

A sterile bulb syringe.

An isolation gown. A mask and a cap (if they are to be used).

Sterile dressings (if the dressing is to be changed).

Procedure

1. Wash hands, and assemble the equipment.
2. Put on a gown (and a cap and a mask).
3. Open a sterile basin, and add the solution.
4. Unwrap a sterile bulb syringe (if the dressing is to be moistened but not changed).
5. Put on gloves. If the dressing is to be changed—
   a. remove the outer layers, and place them in a waxed bag,
   b. change gloves,
   c. soak gauze in the solution, and cover with dry, sterile dressings.
6. If the dressings are to be moistened only—
   a. put on gloves, fill a syringe with solution and moisten the dressing. Sterile plastic or Koroseal may be laid under area.
7. Record the time, the child's response to his treatment, and the condition of the burned area if the dressings were changed.

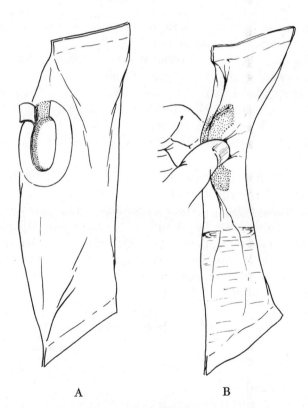

A   B

Fig. 9. Plastic urine collector:
a. soft sponge around opening.
b. Sides of opening pressed together makes the collector into a specimen container.

COLLECTION OF CLEAN URINE SPECIMEN

Equipment

A sterile basin containing cotton balls saturated with aqueous Zephiran 1:1000 or a soap solution.

A sterile specimen bottle.

A sterile potty, a bedpan, a urinal or a basin.

Procedure

1. Wash genitalia with soaked cotton balls using downward strokes. For girls, first separate the labia, wash, and discard the cotton ball. Wash the outer surface of the perineum and the anal region. Discard the cotton after each stroke.
2. A small child may sit on a potty chair and void into a sterile basin or into a potty. An older child may void into a sterile bedpan, a sterile urinal, or directly into a specimen bottle.
3. A midstream specimen is desirable, but difficult to obtain from small children. The child should start to void into an unsterile receptacle, stop the stream, and void into a sterile receptacle.
4. Pour the specimen into a sterile bottle, and cover it.
5. Label it and send it to the laboratory.
6. Record the time and other pertinent data.

For the collection of a urine specimen using a plastic urine collector, see Fig. 9.

ENEMA (CLEANSING)

Equipment

An irrigating can with clean tubing.

A rectal tube size 10 to 18, French.

Solution: isotonic saline (1 tsp. salt to 1 pint water) unless otherwise ordered. (Tap water should never be used for children unless specifically ordered.) Temperature 100° to 105°. Amount—infants 120 to 200 cc., children 200 to 300 cc.

A lubricant.

A bedpan.

Procedure

1. Remove the diaper or panties, and place the infant or small child on a small bedpan.
2. Insert a lubricated rectal tube into his rectum for a distance of two to three inches. (Less for an infant.)
3. Lift the can only enough to allow a flow. (Not above 18 inches.)
4. A small child will usually have better results if allowed to sit on a potty chair following the enema. Diapers should be fastened securely for an infant because returns may be delayed.

5. Clean the perineum, and replace the diaper or the panties.

6. Record the time, the amount and the kind of solution, and the results.

(Note: children with sluggish peristalsis may absorb tap water through the intestinal wall into the body tissues with a resultant water intoxication that may have serious consequences. This is particularly true in aganglionic megacolon.

Enema (Retention)

Equipment

A funnel and a small French catheter.

Oil as prescribed, usually 60 to 150 cc. at 100°.

Procedure

Give slowly into the rectum. Maintain pressure over the rectum after giving, or hold the buttocks together until the urge to defecate has passed. Instruct the child to retain the solution if possible. A cleansing enema (saline) may be given in about 30 minutes if the child has not defecated.

MEDICATION ADMINISTRATION FOR SMALL CHILDREN AND FOR INFANTS

Oral Medication

1. **Preparation**

    a. Compute a fractional dose if necessary; have the computation checked. (See Methods for Computing Fractional Doses.)

    b. Prepare according to the form of medication.

    1. *Tablet.* Crush it and dissolve it in a small amount of water or glucose water. If the tablet is bitter, crush it and mix it with honey or with corn syrup.

    2. *Suspension and syrup.* Shake well. Fruit flavored suspensions and syrups do not need dilution unless it is desired.

    3. *Elixir.* Alcohol base; these must always be diluted with an equal amount of water (or·more) to prevent aspiration.

    c. Heart medication. Check the apical beat before administration, and compare it with the previous reading for the rate, the quality, and the rhythm. Report any significant deviation.

2. **Administration (Infant)**

    a. Identify the infant.

    b. Pour the medication into a one-ounce disposable bottle. Raise the infant's head or hold him and allow him to suck. (Alternative.) Raise the infant's head, administer the medication with a plastic medicine dropper. Give it very slowly, and allow the infant to swallow before continuing.

c. Ascertain that the infant has swallowed all the medication before leaving. Look in his mouth.

d. Place the infant on his side to prevent aspiration.

3. Administration (Child)

a. Crush the tablet and dissolve it in water (for a small child) or give it in corn syrup or honey.

b. Identify the child.

c. Hold the child in an upright position. Allow the child to hold medicine cup if he wants. Give it slowly.

d. If the child resists, use firmness but do not force. Never hold the child's nose to force him to swallow.

e. Allow the child to swallow before continuing.

f. Check his mouth to ascertain that the medication has been swallowed before leaving.

g. If the child vomits, estimate the amount of emesis and report it. Do not repeat the medciation unless so ordered.

4. Recording

Record the time, the dosage, the route (p.o.), and the child's reaction, if it is unusual.

Intramuscular Injections

Principles

The point of the injection must be as far away as possible from the major nerves to avoid a serious injury to the system. (Note: a serious injury to the sciatic nerve, resulting in paralysis, has occurred following improperly placed injections in the buttocks.)

The nurse giving intramuscular injections should have a basic knowledge of anatomy, particularly about nerve pathways and muscle placement. For example, the gluteal area actually extends to the anterior superior iliac spine—which should be taken into account when measuring the buttock for an injection site.

The muscular area chosen should be sufficiently developed to tolerate the injection. (Note: infants under the age of six months have poorly developed gluteal muscles. The lateral aspect of the midanterior thigh is the preferred site for infants. (Some pediatricians prefer this site for young children as well.)

The needle should be long enough to penetrate well within the muscle before depositing the medication. The plunger of the syringe should not be depressed until the needle is well within the muscle.

Equipment

A sterile syringe. A 2 cc. Luer syringe; or a 2½ cc. disposable syringe;

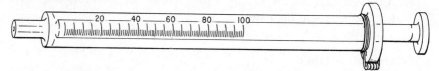

Fig. 10. A tuberculin, or one cc. syringe. These syringes are calibrated in one-hundredths of one cc.

or a 1 cc. tuberculin syringe for a fractional dosage computed in one-hundreth of one cc.

A sterile injection needle 20 to 22 gauge, 1 inch in length.
A sterile container with skin preparation material.
Bandaids.

Procedure

1. Prepare the medication under sterile conditions and take it to the bedside.
2. Identify the patient from his identi-band.
3. Explain the procedure to the child.

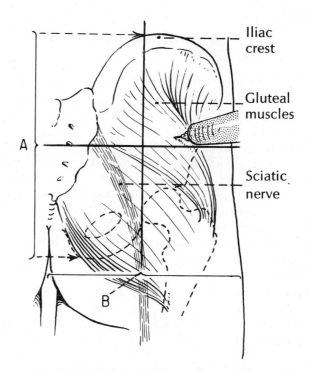

Fig. 11. Site for an intramuscular injection into the upper outer quadrant of the gluteal muscle.

4. Select the proper site and give the injection deep into the muscle. Withdraw the plunger slightly to check for blood in the syringe before injecting the medication.
5. Apply pressure over the site with sterile cotton, and withdraw the needle. Apply pressure and gentle massage. (Massage may be contraindicated if giving medication such as Imferon.)
6. Apply a Bandaid if there is any oozing.

Selection of the Site

A. Gluteal Area

Muscle: gluteus maximus. Area—upper outer quadrant of the gluteal area.

METHOD OF SELECTION

1. Place the patient on his abdomen with his toes turned in.
2. Using your thumb, define the anterior superior iliac spine. Fig. 11 (Site for I.M. injection into the gluteal muscle)
3. Place your index finger on the head of the trocanter.

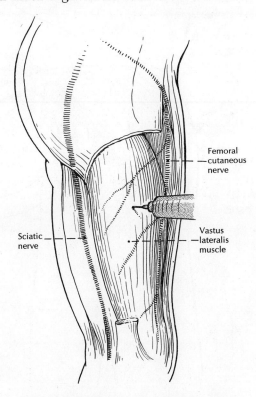

Femoral
—cutaneous
nerve

Vastus
—lateralis
muscle

Sciatic
nerve

Fig. 12. Site for an intramuscular injection into the anterior lateral aspect of the thigh.

4. Define the quadrants of the gluteal mass.
5. Select the inner angle of the upper outer quadrant.
6. Inspect the area for induration and for trauma from previous injections. Rotate the sites as indicated.
   Note: if a suitable site cannot be found within acceptable boundaries, report this and seek instruction before giving, or use the anterior lateral aspect of thigh (or the deltoid, if approved).
7. A second person should be present to assist when giving intramuscular injections to children. The assistant should help position the child, and can restrain and divert him.
   Note: explain to child that you are helping him hold still, not punishing him.
8. Give the injection as explained in procedure.
9. Comfort the child. Apply a Bandaid as a comfort measure. The

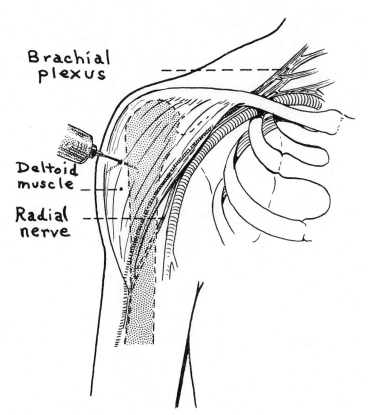

Fig. 13. Appropriate site for an intramuscular injection into the deltoid muscle.

child may hold the Bandaid until ready. Allow the child to give an injection to a stuffed toy animal or a doll if he wishes.

B. Area of Anterior Lateral Aspect of the Thigh
1. Place the infant on his back.
2. Measure the area from the greater trocanter to the patella. Select a site midway between the knee and the hip joint, using the lateral aspect of the thigh.

Fig. 12 (I.M. into thigh muscle)
3. Give the injection as explained in procedure.
4. One nurse alone may give this injection to a small infant. Two nurses are preferable for an older infant.
5. Hold and comfort the infant following the injection.

C. Deltoid Muscle

The use of this area is limited because of the small space available, the undeveloped muscle in young children and painfulness of the procedure. It may be useful for older children, particularly for those who have limited availability for other sites.

Only a small area between the upper and the lower portions of the deltoid muscle may be used in order to avoid the radial nerve. Fig. 13 (I.M. into deltoid muscle). Injections should not be made into the middle or the lower third of the upper arm. Permission should be obtained before using the deltoid area in children.

INSTILLATION OF EAR DROPS

Procedure

1. Turn the child's head with the affected ear uppermost.
2. Straighten the ear canal by pulling the pinna slightly down and straight back. For an older child (over three years) pull the pinna up and back as for an adult.
3. Drop warm drops into the external ear canal and hold him in position for few minutes to allow the drops to run onto the ear drum.

INSTILLATION OF NOSE DROPS

Procedure

1. Place a small pillow or a folded blanket under the child's shoulders to allow his head to drop back, or hold the child in your lap with his head lowered.
2. Instill the prescribed drops, using a plastic dropper in order to prevent injury should the child jerk his head.
3. Keep the child's head below the level of his shoulders for one or two minutes. Note: oily nose drops are not used for infants and children because of possibility of causing lipid pneumonia.

RECTAL MEDICATIONS (SUPPOSITORIES)

Procedure

1. Turn the child on his side or, for an infant, raise his buttocks as for taking a rectal temperature.
2. Insert the lubricated suppository with a finger covered with a finger cot or a glove.
3. Apply pressure to the rectum, or hold the buttocks together for a few minutes to prevent expulsion of suppository.
4. Explain to the child, if he can understand, the importance of retaining the suppository.

PROCEDURE FOR THE USE OF THE Z TRACT METHOD IN THE ADMINISTRATION OF IRON DEXTRAN (IMFERON)*

Iron dextran is recommended for use solely in the treatment of iron deficiency anemia—situations in which the oral administration of iron is unsatisfactory or impossible. Imferon is absorbed rapidly from the muscle, but slowly from the subcutaneous tissue. Injected into, or leaking into, subcutaneous tissue, it is broken down and stored as hemosiderin. Use of the Z tract method of injection is of great importance to prevent leakage.

Technique

1. Use one needle to withdraw Imferon from the ampul, and another needle for the injection.

* This information is from the brochure of distributors of IMFERON (Lakeside Laboratories) and from private correspondence with them.

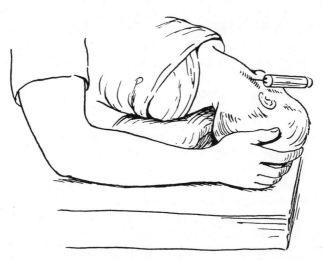

Fig. 14. Positioning a child for jugular vein puncture.

2. A needle long enough to insure injection into the muscle tissue must be used.
3. Use a gauge 19 or 20 needle for the injection.
4. Allow enough air to remain in syringe to void the syringe and the needle completely of any iron dextran so that there is no tissue staining when the needle is withdrawn. The use of 0.5 cc. of air is recommended for an adult. Less air should be necessary when given to an infant.
5. Inject iron dextran only into the upper outer quadrant of the buttock, never into the arm or some other exposed area.
6. Before injecting the needle, retract the skin laterally, displacing it firmly to one side. The skin should be held in this position until after the injection.
7. Insert the needle and withdraw the plunger to check against entry into a blood vessel.
8. Inject the medication and a small amount of air from the syringe.

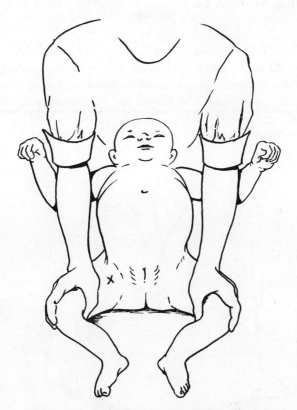

Fig. 15. Positioning a child for a femoral venipuncture.

9. After the injection, wait 10 seconds before withdrawing the needle or releasing skin.
10. Withdraw the needle, and release the skin.
11. Rotate sides, using opposite buttocks.

POSITIONING AN INFANT OR A CHILD FOR TREATMENT

1. Positioning for Venipuncture

A. Scalp vein technique.
   1. Apply mummy restraint.
   2. Standing at the foot of the table, immobilize the infant's trunk with your forearms.
   3. Turn the infant's head to one side, place your hands over the occiput and over the face, holding his head firmly.
B. Jugular vein venipuncture. (Fig. 14)
   1. Apply mummy restraint.
   2. Lower the child's head over the top of the examining table.
   3. Hold his head in the manner described for a scalp vein procedure.
C. Femoral venipuncture. (Fig. 15)
   1. Place the infant on his back on the examining table.
   2. Stand above the infant's head, with his arms outstretched at his sides. Restrain his arms and his trunk with your forearms. The child's legs should be flexed and held in an abducted position by your hands. (An older infant may need a clove hitch restraint for his hands.)

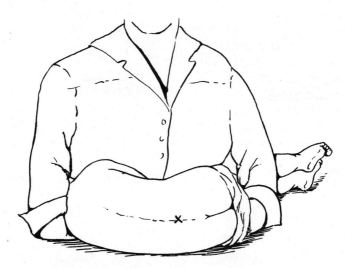

Fig. 16. Positioning a child for a lumbar puncture.

2. Positioning for Lumbar Puncture. Fig. 16

1. Place the child on his side with the lumbar region at the edge of the examining table.
2. Restrain his legs by wrapping them in a sheet if necessary.
3. Flex the child's knees and bend his head forward.
4. Hold the child's head within a circle of your arm and with your other arm under his flexed knees.

TEPID SPONGE BATH (TO REDUCE FEVER)

Equipment

A basin containing tepid water.
A bath blanket (two for an older child).
A wash cloth.
Isopropyl alcohol 35 per cent (only if ordered).

Technique

1. Take the child's temperature and record it.
2. Wash your hands, and assemble the equipment.
3. Undress the child, and place a bath blanket under the child (to absorb moisture and to prevent undue chilling).
4. Cover an older child with a second bath blanket.
5. Expose his arms and his chest. Wring wash cloth lightly from tepid water, sponge gently, making long, even strokes. Apply gentle friction with your hands, following the sponge. Repeat 2 or 3 times, giving attention to the axillary area.
6. Sponge the abdomen, the legs and the feet in the same manner.
7. Turn the child on his abdomen and sponge his back.
8. Sponge the inner surface of the groin and the perineal region. (Sponge the anal region last.)
9. Do not continue longer than 15 or 20 minutes.
10. Take the child's temperature every half-hour until it is reduced to an acceptable level. Note: the child's temperature may continue to fall after sponging. Wait for 30 minutes before resuming the sponge bath. The child may be left uncovered following the sponge bath if his temperature remains elevated.

Index

Abandoned child, in primitive
  societies, 5
    institutional care of, development
      of, 12
Abbreviations, common, 511
Abdomen, irradiation of, in preg-
  nancy, 61
Accidents, 218. *See also*
  Emergencies; Injuries.
    burns, 241
    guilt and, 302
    in home, 220
    poisoning, 222
Acetylsalicylic acid. *See* Aspirin.
Acidosis, diabetic, 390
Acne vulgaris, 467
Activities, extracurricular,
  convalescence and, 329
    in adolescence, 474
    physical. *See* Physical activity.
    play. *See* Play activities; Toys.
    quiet, bed rest and, 328
Addis sediment count, 515
Adenoidectomy, 263
Adenoids, 263
Adolescence, defined, 457
Adolescent, 455-475
  activities for, 474
  antisocial behavior of, 471
  clinics for, 462
  developmental tasks of, 459
  diabetes mellitus in, 399
  emotional development of, 460,
    467-475
  emotional problems of, 470
  employment for, 474
  growth and development of,
    457-475
  handicapped, 469
  hospitalization of, 461
  illegitimacy and, 472
  personality development of, 460
  physical development of, 458
  pregnant, care of, 473
    diet of, 62
  sexual relationships of, 472
Adolescent wards, 461, 464, 465

Adoption, 486
  intercountry, 499
  of illegitimate child, 473
Aerosol treatments in cystic fibrosis,
  278
Age. *See* Newborn; Infant; Premature
  infant; Toddler; Preschool child;
  School age child; Adolescent.
AHG deficiency, 344
Albumin, in urine, test for, 517
Allergic reaction, glomerulonephritis
  as, 368
    malnutrition and, 178
Ambulation, early, 25
Ancient civilizations, child care in, 5
Anemia(s), 337
  iron dextran administration in, 552
  Mediterranean, 340
  sickle cell, 339
Angiocardiography, 408
Anomalies, congenital. *See* Congenital
  defects.
Anoxia, in tetralogy of Fallot, 418
Antibody, defined, 354
Anticonvulsant therapy, 364
Antidote, universal, 227
Antigen, defined, 354
Antitoxin, defined, 354
  diphtheria, 355
Anxiety. *See* Emotional support;
  Fear.
Aorta, coarctation of, 412, 413
    case history of, 414
    overriding, in tetralogy of Fallot,
      417
    transposition of, 420
Apgar scoring chart, 72, 73
Appetite. *See also* Diet; Food;
  Nutrition.
    observation of, 50
    of infant, 119, 130
    of newborn, 80
    of school age child, 377
    of toddler, 207
    restricted diet and, 326
Aqueduct of Sylvius, atresia of, 156
Arnold-Chiari malformation, 156

557

Arthritis, migratory, in rheumatic
    fever, 423
Ascorbic acid. *See* Vitamin C.
Aseptic technique, 523-530.
    See also Isolation.
Aspirin, dosage of, 225
    in rheumatic fever, 426
    poisoning from, 225, 264, 426
Astigmatism, 442
Asylums. *See* Institutional care.
Athetosis, 447, 450
Audiogram, 434, 435, 436
Audiometry testing, 437
Auditory disorders, 433
Autograft, in burns, 251

"Baby-farming," 9
Back rest, homemade, 328
Bathing, burns and, 251, 543, 555
    hydrocephalus and, 160
    of infant, 136, 137, 139
    of newborn, 75
    of premature infant, 91
Battered-child syndrome, 236
    legal action in, 240
Bed rest, complete, defined, 35
    play program in, 34
    home care and, 327
    in rheumatic fever, 427
    simple, play activities in, 37
Behavior. *See also* Discipline;
    Emotional development;
    Emotional support; Social
    development.
    adaptive, norms of, 306
    antisocial, of adolescent, 471
    in burns, 254
    case history of, 255
    observation of, 48, 49
    of newborn, reflexes and, 70
    pain and, 50
Birth, circulatory adjustments at, 66
    trauma of, 64
Birth defects. *See* Congenital defects.
Bladder, extrophy of, 106
Bladder control, 200
    hospitalization and, 210
Blalock-Taussig operation, 418, 420
Blindness, 441
    defined, 441
    gonorrheal infection and, 282
    retrolental fibroplasia and, 282
    temporary, eye surgery and, 285

Blood circulation. *See* Circulation.
Blood dyscrasias, 337
Blood pressures, average, 520
    readings, 519
Blood test for phenylketonuria, 109
Blood values, average, normal, 512
Blood, vessels, great, transposition of,
    420
Body temperature, Fahrenheit,
    conversion to Centigrade, 513
    of newborn, 74
    of premature infant, 89
Bones, skull, of newborn, 71
Books, children's collection of, 43
Bottle feeding, 79, 81
Bowel, intussusception of, 169
Bowel control, 200
    hospitalization and, 210
Braces, in cerebral palsy, 452
Brain, of newborn, 67
Brain damage. *See also* Mental
    retardation.
    from injuries, 233
    in battered-child syndrome, 237
    in phenylketonuria, 321
Breast feeding, 77
Breathing, mouth-to-mouth, 521
    of newborn, 65
    of premature infant, 90
Bronchi, infections of, 268
    suctioning of, 532
Bronchiolitis, acute, 182
    hospitalization in, case history of,
    181
Bronchitis, acute, 183
Bronchopneumonia, 184
Bryant's traction, 234, 235
*Bulletin of the World Health
    Organization*, 498
Burn unit, supplies stocked in, 245
Burns, 241
    bathing and, 251, 543, 555
    causes of, 242
    complications in, 253
    débridement in, 251
    electrical, 242
    emotional support and, 248, 249
    equipment and, 246
    esophageal, 224
    fire or heat, 242
    fluid balance in, 244, 246
    check sheet for, 247
    infections in, 250, 252

Burns (*Continued*)
  nutrition in, 252
  physical therapy in, 254, 256
  physiological manifestations, 244
  play therapy in, case history of, 33
  prevention of, 243
  procedure tray and, 246
  rehabilitation from, 254
  "rule of nines" in, 244
  scalds, 242
  second degree, 243, 244
  septicemia in, 252
  skin grafts and, 251
  soaks or wet packs, 543
  superficial, 243
  third degree, 243, 244
  urinary output and, 247
  vital signs in, 248

CAM tent, 279, 540, 541
Camp nursing, 504
Carbohydrate metabolism test, 515
Cardiac. *See also* Heart.
Cardiac arrest, emergency treatment
  for, 520
Cardiac catherization, 407
Cardiovascular defects, congenital.
  See Heart defects, congenital.
Carditis in rheumatic fever, 424. *See
  also* Illness, chronic.
Caries, dental. *See* Dental caries.
Carrier, defined, 354
Carrier state, defined, 354
Cast, frog leg, 192, 193
  in clubfoot, 188, 190
Cataracts, 283
Catheterization, cardiac, 407
Celiac disease, 272
Celiac syndrome, 271
Centigrade temperature, conversion to
  Fahrenheit, 513
Cerebral palsy, 445
  braces in, 452
  case histories of, 447
  home appliances in, 452
  physical therapy in, 452
Cerebrospinal fluid, hydrocephalus
  and, 155
Chest drainage, water seal suction for,
  406, 533
Chickenpox, 359

Child. *See also* Newborn; Infant;
  Premature infant; Toddler;
  Preschool child; School age child;
  Adolescent.
Child care, history of, 3-11
  in hospitals, *See* Hospital care.
  nursing plan for, 47
Child care centers, 485
Child health conference, 505
Child labor, 9, 10, 482
Children, 481
Children's Bureau, 479
  publications of, 481
Chorea, in rheumatic fever, 424
    play program and, 35
Christmas disease, 345
Cinefluorography, 408
Circulation, of fetus, 66
  of newborn, 66, 67
Clavicle, fracture of, 232, 233
Cleft lip, 95
Cleft palate, 100
  home care in, 261
  repair of, 260
Clinics, adolescent, 462
  prenatal, 62
  specialized, 487
Clinitest, 518
Clot formation, mechanism of, 344
Clubfoot, congenital, 188
"Code 99" in cardiac arrest, 520
Cold, common, 258
    tonsillectomy and, 263
Coma, diabetic, 395
Communicable diseases, 353
  isolation procedures in, 361, 523-530
  of world, 496
Communicating with patients, 51
Congenital defects, 95, 155
  cataracts, 283
  cleft lip, 95
  esophageal atresia with fistula, 101
  genetic factors in, 61
  glaucoma, 283
  heart. *See* Heart defects, congenital.
  hydrocephalus, 155
  in primitive societies, 4
  intussusception, 169
  mental retardation. *See* Mental
    retardation and Mentally retarded
    child.
  metabolic, 107. *See also*
    Metabolism, inborn errors of.

Congenital defects (*Continued*)
  mongolism, 317
  of central nervous system, 155, 163
  of hip, dislocation, 191
  of nasolacrimal duct, impatency, 282
  orthopedic, 188
  pyloric stenosis, 173
  rubella and, 110
    cataracts in, 283
  spina bifida, 163
  superstitions and, 58
Conjunctivitis, bacterial, acute, 284
Convalescence. *See* Home care;
  Illness, chronic.
Convalescent hospitals, 429
Convulsions, epileptic, 364
  febrile, 363
  in diabetes mellitus, 395
Corticosteroids in rheumatic fever, 426
Cough, whooping, 356
Counseling. *See also* Teaching.
  genetic, 61
  of family. *See* Family counseling.
  of unwed mothers, 473
Coxsackie viral infection in pregnancy,
  61
Cradle-cap, 71
Crippling from hemophilic
  arthropathies, 351
Croup, spasmodic, 267
Croupette, 185, 539, 540
Curling's ulcer, 253
Cyanosis in congenital heart defects,
  409, 416
Cystic fibrosis. *See* Fibrosis, cystic.

Day care homes, 135
Deafness, 437
  causes of, 433
  education in, 440
Death, attitude toward, 334
Death rate, in accidents, 218
  in foundling homes, 13
  in institutions, 12
  infant, 480
  neonatal, 86
Defects, metabolic. *See* Metabolism,
  inborn errors of.
  physical. *See* Congenital defects;
  Handicapped child.
DeLee mucus trap, 531
Delinquency, juvenile, 471
Denis Browne splint, 189

Dental care. *See* Teeth.
Dental caries, 375
Dependence vs. independence in
  toddler, 202
Deprivation, 383
  eye surgery and, 285, 286
  from isolation, 14
  maternal, 18
    malnutrition and, 178
  mental retardation and, 307
  of American Indians, 489
  physical abuse and, 236
Development. *See also* Growth and
    development; Emotional develop-
    ment; Physical development;
    Social development.
  periods of, classified, 57
Diabetes insipidus, 389
Diabetes mellitus, 389-401
  acidosis in, 390
  camp nursing and, 504
  defined, 389
  detection of, 390
  diet in, 392
  etiology of, 389
  glucagon in, 399
  home care in, 397
  in adolescence, 399
  in pregnancy, 400
  incidence of, 389
  insulin injections in, types and
    methods of, 394
  physical activities in, 398
  prognosis in, 400
  urine reduction in, 393
Dialysis, peritoneal, 536, 537
Diaper folding, 140, 141, 142
Diarrhea, 361
  in institutions, history of, 14
  isolation in, 361
  malnutrition from, 178
Diet. *See also* Appetite; Food;
    Nutrition.
  diarrhea and, 361
  gluten-free, in celiac disease, 272
  in burns, 252
  in cystic fibrosis, 277
  in diabetes mellitus, 392
  in galactosemia, 109
  in metabolic disorders, 326
  in obesity, 469
  in phenylketonuria, 108, 321, 322
  iron deficiency anemia and, 338

Diet (*Continued*)
    protein malnutrition and, 175, 494
    protein-rich, foods in, 495
    restricted, home care and, 326
Diphtheria, 354
    antitoxin, 355
    toxoid, 131
Discipline, defined, 386
    for mentally retarded child, 314
    in hemophilia, 349
    in home care, 330
    in hygiene, 378
    of school age child, 386
    of toddler, 204
Diseases, virus. *See* Virus disease(s).
Dosage. *See* Medicine, doses of.
Down's syndrome, 317
Drug. *See* Medication; Medicine.
Drug toxicity in pregnancy, 61
Ductus arteriosus, patent, 412
Duodenal aspiration, 516
Doudenum, ulcer of, in burns, 253
Dyspnea, paroxysmal, in tetralogy of
    Fallot, 418

Ear, middle, inflammation of, 434
Ear drops, instillation of, 551
Echo viral infection in pregnancy, 61
Edema, nephrosis and, 370
Education. *See also* Counseling;
    Teaching.
    deafness and, 440
    for parenthood, 62
    of American Indians, 490
    of nurse, play experience in, 32
    sex, 382
    visual defects and, 444
Educational personnel in hospital, 26
Ego development of school age child,
    380, 381
Eisenmenger's syndrome, 416
Elbow, fracture of, 233
Elbow restraints in cleft lip, 97
Electrical burns, 220, 242
Electrocardiography, 407
Emergencies. *See also* Accidents;
    Injuries.
    cardiac arrest, 520
    emotional support in, 301
    intussusception, 169
    poisoning. *See* Poisoning.
    regression and, 303

Emergencies (*Continued*)
    tracheotomy, in laryngotracheo-
      bronchitis, 269
Emotional deprivation. *See*
    Deprivation.
Emotional development, immobili-
    zation and, 235
    of adolescent, 460, 467-475
    of infant, 120, 132
    of school age child, 380, 381
Emotional support, burns and, 248,
    249
    for infant, 151
    in emergencies, 301
    in eye surgery, 285, 286
    in fatal illness, 331, 334
    in heart surgery, 404
    in hemophilia, 349
    in hydrocephalus, 160
    in leukemia, 343
    in modern hospital, 15
    in painful treatments, 214
    injections and, 214, 299
    of infant, 151
    of parents, hydrocephalus and, 162
    of premature infant, 94
    of school age child, 380
    of toddler, 204
    trust and, 299
Employment, adolescent, 474
    child, 9, 10, 482
Enanthem, defined, 354
Endemic, defined, 354
Enema, cleansing, 545
    retention, 546
Enteropathy, gluten-induced, 272
Environment, home, of newborn, 76
    hospital, modern, 15
    of mentally retarded child, 313
    of premature infant, 89
    prenatal, 58
Enzymes, pancreatic, in cystic fibrosis,
    276
Epidemic, defined, 354
Epilepsy, marriage and, 368
    mental retardation and, 367
    schooling and, 365
    seizures in, 364
Epistaxis, 259
Erythema, defined, 354
Erythema marginatum in rheumatic
    fever, 424
Erythrocyte sedimentation rate, 425

Esophagus, atresia of, 101
  burns of, 224
Esotropia, 283
Exanthem, defined, 354
Exercise. *See* Physical activity.
Exotropia, 283
Eye, cataracts of, 283
  conditions of, 281
  coordination, of infant, 120, 121
  fibroplasia of, 282
  foreign objects in, 284
  infections of, 284
    gonorrheal, in newborn, 281
  injuries, 284
    cataracts and, 283
    glaucoma and, 283
  of newborn, 74
  pink, 284
  surgery, 282
    home visit and, 287
    nursing care study of, 286
    sensory deprivation in, 285

Fahrenheit temperature, conversion to
    Centigrade, 513
Family, foster, 484
  of mentally retarded child, 315
Family counseling, in diabetes
    mellitus, 391
  in mental retardation, 308
Farsightedness, 442
Fear. *See also* Emotional support.
  eye surgery and, 285
  in adolescence, 462
  of death, 334
  of needles, 214, 299
  of separation, 335
Feeding. *See also* Appetite; Diet;
    Food; Nutrition.
  gastrostomy, in esophageal atresia,
    104, 105
  in cleft lip, 97, 99
  in hydrocephalus, 160
  in malnutrition, 179
  in pyloric stenosis, 174
  of infant, 127, 144
  of premature infant, 91
Feeding equipment, ancient and
    modern, 8
Feeding tube, 535
Femoral venipuncture, positioning for,
    553
Femur, fracture of, 233

Fetus, circulation of, 66
  drug toxicity and, 61
  environment of, 58
  factors affecting, 58
  physical development of, 60
    hazards to, 60
  syphilitic infection of, 61
  viral infections affecting, 60
Fever, convulsions in, 363
  reduction of, tepid bath for, 555
  rheumatic, 423-432. *See also*
    Rheumatic fever.
  scarlet, 358
  typhoid, 358
Fibroplasia, retrolental, 282
Fibrosis, cystic, 273, 274
  camp nursing and, 504
  diagrammatic review of, 277
  diet in, 277
  home care in, 281
  postural drainage in, 280
  test for, 516
Fire, burns from, 242
Fluid(s), cerebrospinal, hydro-
    cephalus and, 155
  force, 211
  intravenous, types of, 148
Fluoridation, 84, 198
Fontanelles, 71
Food. *See also* Appetite; Diet;
    Nutrition.
  favorite, 209
  finger, 208
  solid, introduction of, 125, 126
Foot, talipes equinovarus of, 188
Foramina of Luschka and Magendie,
    atresia of, 156
Foreign bodies, aspiration of, 229
  in eye, 284
  in nose, 260
Formulas, 81
  preparation of, 83
Foster homes, 484
  for infants, 135
Foundling homes, mortality and, 13.
    See also Institutional care.
Fractures, 230
  causes of, 230
  in battered-child syndrome, 237
  in newborn, 232
  of clavicle, 232, 233
  of elbow, 233
  of femur, 233

Fractures (*Continued*)
  of humerus, 233, 234
  of skull, 233
  types of, 232
Fredet-Ramstedt operation, 174
Frejka splint, 192, 193

Galactosemia, 109
Gastrostomy feedings, in esophageal
    atresia, 104, 105
Gavage, 91, 535
Genetic counseling, 61
German measles. *See* Rubella.
Gestation period, defined, 60
Glaucoma, 283
Glomerulonephritis, acute, 368
Glucagon, 399
Glucose tolerance test, 515
Growth and development. *See also*
    Emotional development;
    Physical development;
    Social development.
  card index file of, 46
  immobilization and, 235
  intrauterine, mental retardation and,
    307
  neonatal, 64-85
  of adolescent, 457-475
  of fetus, 60
  of infant, 117
  of preschool child, 293-304
  of school age child, 375-388
  of toddler, 197-217
  periods of, classified, 57
Guilt, accidents and, 302
Guthrie inhibition assay test, 109

Hand coordination of infant, 121
Handicapped child, 433-454
  camps for, 504
  mentally. *See* Mental retardation.
Head injuries, 233
  in battered-child syndrome, 237
Head measurement in hydrocephalus,
    161
Health. *See* Growth and development.
Health education, in hospital,
    opportunity for, 24
  in Project Head Start, 505
Hearing loss, symptomatic behavior of,
    435
  types of, 433

Hearing problems, 433
  language development and, 437,
    438, 439
Heart. *See also* Cardiac.
  catheterization of, 407
  defects. *See* Heart defects.
  inflammation of, in rheumatic fever,
    424
  roentgenography of, 408
Heart defects, congenital, atrial septal,
    410, 411
  cyanotic, 409, 416
  diagnostic tests of, 407
  patent ductus arteriosus, 412
  tetralogy of Fallot, 417
  ventricular septal, 409, 416, 417
Heart disease, acyanotic, 409
  congenital, 402-422
  types of, 408
Heart failure, congestive, 403
Heart murmur, 403
Heart surgery, 405
  Baffes procedure in, 421
  chest drainage apparatus and, 406
  Hanlon-Blalock procedure in, 421
  in atrial septal defect, 411
  in patent ductus arteriosus, 413
  in tetralogy of Fallot, 420
  in transposition of great vessels, 420
  in ventricular septal defect, 410
  Mustard procedure in, 421
  preparation for, home care and, 404
    in hospital, 385, 404
  Senning procedure in, 421
Heartbeat of newborn, 65
Height, conversion to metric
    equivalents, 514
  of infant, 117
  of toddler, 197
Hemoglobin, abnormal, sickle cell
    disease and, 339
Hemophilia, 343
  bleeding into joint cavities in,
    347, 348
  dental care in, 347
  discipline in, 349
  emotional support in, 349
  home care in, 350
  isolation in, 348
  nosebleeds in, 347
  parental anxiety in, 350
  rehabilitation in, 351
  schoolwork in, 350

Hemophilia (*Continued*)
  transfusions in, 346
  types of, 344
Herpes zoster, 359
Hip, dislocation of, congenital, 191
Home accidents, 220
Home care, bed rest and, 327
  in chronic illness, 326
    discipline and, 330
  in cleft palate, 261
  in clubfoot, 191
  in cystic fibrosis, 281
  in diabetes mellitus, 397
  in hemophilia, 350
  in iron deficiency anemia, 339
  in leukemia, 342
  in mental retardation, vs.
    institutional care, 315
  in metabolic disorder, 326
  in nephrosis, 371
  in rheumatic fever, 428
  of newborn, 76
  schoolwork and, 329
Homemaker service, 136, 486
  battered-child syndrome and, 241
Hordeolum, external, 284
Hospital care, emotional support in.
    See Emotional support.
  mothers in, 23, 153, 205
  of infant, 137
    parent-nurse relationship in, 153
  of preschool child, 297
  of school age child, 383
    discipline in, 386
  of toddler, 203
    mother in, 205
  present day concepts of, 20-27
Hospitalism, defined, 13
Hospitalization. *See also* Hospital care.
  emotional support in, 15
  long-term, visiting and, 25
  of adolescent, 461
  of infant, 151
  of preschool child, 297
  of school age child, 383
  of toddler, 203
  parental anxiety toward, 297
  procedures, preparation for, 385
Host, defined, 354
Humerus, fracture of, 233, 234
Humidifiers, 185, 186
  in cystic fibrosis, 278, 279

Hydrocephalus, 155
  emotional support in, 160
  surgery in, 157
Hygiene, discipline in, 378
  hospital care and, 24
  in acne vulgaris, 468
Hyperopia, 442
Hypertension, pulmonary, ventricular
    septal defect and, 416

Ileoureterostomy, cutaneous, in spina
    bifida, 167
Ileus, meconium, in cystic fibrosis, 274
Illegitimacy, 472
  adoption and, 473
Illness, chronic, 325
    daily care in, 327
    extracurricular activities and, 329
    hemophilia, 343
    home care in, 326
      discipline in, 330
    nephrosis, 370
    parental adjustment to, 330
    resistance to infection in, 329
    schoolwork in, 329
  fatal, 331
    counseling in, 333
    emotional support in, of child, 334
      of parents, 332
    leukemia, 341
Imferon, 339
  administration of, 552
Immaturity, defined, 88
Immunity, defined, 354
Immunization. *See also* Vaccination.
  cystic fibrosis and, 279
  diphtheria toxoid, 355
  in infancy, 130
    schedule for, 130
  rubella, 61
Incubation period, defined, 354
Incubator for premature infant, 93
Independence vs. dependence in
    toddler, 202
Indians, American, 489, 504
Industrial revolution, child care and, 9
Infant, 115-194. *See also* Premature
    infant.
  appetite of, 119
  behavior of, bizarre, 50
    observation of, 49
    pain and, 50
  body proportions of, 68

Infant (*Continued*)
  clothing for, 142
  congenital anomalies of, 155.
    See also Congenital defects.
  emotional development of, 120, 132
  eye coordination of, 120, 121
  growth and development of, 117
  height of, 117
    chart of, 118
  hospital care of, 137
  hydrocephalus in, 155
  illness in, physical signs of, 50
  maturation of, 119
  medication administration for, 546
  mortality rates of, 480
    American Indians and, 489
  motor coordination of, 120
  muscular state of, 49
  nutrition of, 125
  orthopedic conditions of, 188-194
  play program for, 39
  skin of, observation of, 50
  social development of, 120, 124
  toys for, 42
  weight of, 117
    chart of, 118
Infant Care, 481
Infantile paralysis, 356
Infections. *See also* Communicable
    diseases.
  acute, convulsions in, 363
  cross, protection from, 362
  diarrheal, 361
  diphtheritic, 354
  eye, 284
    gonorrheal, of newborn, 281
  in burns, 250, 252
  in pregnancy, hazards of, 60
  inapparent, defined, 354
  laryngeal, 267, 268
  mental retardation and, 307
  middle ear, 433
  mumps, 355
  of adenoids, 263
  of bronchi, 268
  of tonsils, 263
  prenatal, mental retardation and,
    307
  resistance to, in chronic illness, 329
  respiratory, in toddler, 258
  streptococcal. *See also* Illness,
    chronic.
    glomerulonephritis and, 368

Infections, streptococcal (*Continued*)
    rheumatic fever, 423-432. *See
    also* Rheumatic fever.
    scarlet fever, 358
    virus. *See* Virus disease(s).
Inflammation, of heart in rheumatic
    fever, 424
  of middle ear, 434
Infusion, intravenous, 146
  scalp vein, 146, 147
Inhalation treatment in cystic fibrosis,
    278
Injections, insulin, type and method of,
    394
  intramuscular, 144, 145, 146, 547
    fear of, 214, 299
    sites for, 547, 548, 549, 550
  iron dextran, 552
Injuries. *See also* Accidents;
    Emergencies; Fractures.
  eye, 284
    cataracts from, 283
    glaucoma and, 283
  head, 233
  in battered-child syndrome, 236, 237
Inoculations. *See* Immunization;
    Vaccination.
Institutional care, 483
  asepsis and, 14
  death rate and, 12
  development of, 12
  diarrhea and, history of, 14
  emotional deprivation and, 14
  employed mother and, 135
  of healthy child, 483
  of mentally retarded child, vs.
    home care, 315
Instruction. *See* Counseling; Teaching.
Insulin, injection of, types and
    method of, 394
  reactions to, 395
Insulin shock, 394, 395, 399
Intelligence, measurement of, 305
International Social Service, 499
Intestine, celiac disease of, 271, 272
  disorders, drinking water and, 496
  of newborn, 67
Intravenous cut-down, 147
Intravenous flow, regulation of, 147,
    149
Intravenous fluids, types of, 148
Intravenous therapy, 146
Intussusception, 168, 169

Iron, newborn and, 84
Iron deficiency anemia, 337
Iron dextran, administration of, 552
Irradiations, abdominal, in pregnancy,
  61
Isolation, 361
  emotional care and, 153
  in congenital rubella, 110
  in hemophilia, 348
  of premature infant, 92
  procedures of, 523-530
  protective technique of, 362, 529
  termination of, 528
Isolette, 92, 93

Jacket restraint, 231, 232
Jugular vein puncture, positioning for,
  552
Juvenile delinquency, 471

Kerosene poisoning, 228
Kidney, of newborn, 67
Kidney disease, glomerulonephritis,
  368
  nephrosis, 370
Kidney function test, 515
Kwashiorkor, 493

Labor laws, child employment and, 482
  reform and, 10
Laboratory tests. *See* Test.
Language development, 122, 124
  hearing problems and, 437, 438, 439
  in toddler, 199
Laryngitis, spasmodic, 267
Laryngospasm, 267
Laryngotracheobronchitis, acute, 268
  tracheotomy in, 269
Larynx, spasm of, 267
Leukemia, 341. *See also* Illness,
  chronic.
  drugs in, 342
Leukocytosis in rheumatic fever, 426
Library, children's, 43
Lip, cleft, 95
Lofenalac, 322
Lumbar puncture, positioning for,
  554, 555
Lungs. *See also* Pulmonary;
    Respiratory.
  cystic fibrosis of, 273
  irritation of, by petroleum
    distillages, 225

Macule, defined, 354
Maladie de Roger, 410
Malformations. *See* Congenital
  defects.
Malnutrition, 175
  in battered-child syndrome, 238, 239
  in rickets, 176
  in world population, 493
  protein-calorie, 493
Marasmus, malnutrition in, 178
Marriage, epilepsy and, 368
Measles, 357
  German. *See* Rubella.
Meconium, 67
Meconium ileus, 274
Medical emergencies. *See* Accidents;
  Emergencies; Poisoning.
Medication, 212. *See also* Medicine.
  aerosol, in cystic fibrosis, 278
  errors in, 145, 212, 228
  in burns, 248
  intramuscular. *See* Injections,
    intramuscular.
  methods for, 212
  oral, 546
    for infant, 144
  penicillin, in rheumatic fever,
    427, 428
  rectal, 552
  steroid, in nephrosis, 370
Medicines, accidental poisoning from,
  222
  anticonvulsant, 364
  doses of, fractional, computing, 541
    metric, apothecary equivalents
      and, 514
  in home, safety measures, 223
  in leukemia, 342
Menarche, 457, 458
Meningitis, isolation and, 361
Meningomyelocele, 163
Menstruation, 458
Mental retardation, 305-324
  acquired, 307
  congenital metabolic defects and,
    107
  defined, 305
  dependence in, 306
  deprivation and, 307
  discipline in, 314
  dressing skills in, 311
  environment and, 313
  epilepsy and, 367

Mental retardation (*Continued*)
etiological factors in, 307
family and, 315
hearing problems and, 433
home care of vs. institutionalized
care, 316
mental development in, 309
mongolism and, 317
motor skills in, 312
needs in, 308
perinatal causes, 307
phenylketonuria and, 108, 320
play program in, 39, 313
prenatal causes, 307
rejection in, 308
self-help and, 310
toilet training in, 310
toys in, 313
Metabolic disorder, celiac syndrome
and, 271
galactosemia, 109
home care in, 326
case history of, 326
in toddler, 271
malnutrition and, 176
Metabolism, carbohydrate, test of, 515
inborn errors of, 107
galactosemia, 109
hemophilia and, 344
mental retardation and, 307
phenylketonuria, 108, 320
Migrant workers, children of, 488
Milk, breast, 78
cow's, 78, 81
allergy to, 178
Minerals, daily allowances of, 181
sources of, 180
Mist tent, in cystic fibrosis, 278, 279
therapy, 539
Mistifier, 186
Mistogen tent unit, 540, 541
Molars, six year, 375
Mongolism, 317
clinical manifestations of, 319
Moro reflex, 70
Mortality. *See* Death rate.
Mother, day care, 135
employed, infant's needs and, 135
in hospital care, 23, 153, 205
infant's relationship to, 134
teenage, unmarried, 472
volunteer, 26
Motor coordination, of infant, 120

Motor skills, norms for, 312
Mucoviscidosis, 273
test for, 516
Mummy restraint, 148
Mumps, 355
Muscles, development of, in newborn,
68
Myelomeningocele, 163
Myopia, 442

Nap time, 303
Nasolacrimal duct, impatency of,
congenital, 282
Nasopharyngeal suction, 530
Nasopharyngitis, acute, 258
Nearsightedness, 442
Needles, fear of, 214, 299
Neighborhood Youth Corps, 474
Neonatal. *See also* Newborn.
Neonatal period, death rate during, 86
growth and development during,
64-85
Nephrosis, 370. *See also* Illness,
chronic.
home care in, 371
steroid therapy in, 370
Nephrotic syndrome, 370
Nervous system, central, anomaly of,
155, 163
Newborn, 64-113
breathing of, 65
circulation of, 66, 67
cleft lip in, 95
congenital defects of. *See*
Congenital defects.
developmental tasks of, 71
esophageal atresia in, 101
eyes, gonorrheal infection of, 281
prophylactic treatment of, 281
fontanelles of, 71
galactosemia in, 109
heartbeat of, 65
home care of, 76
fractures in, 232
hazards to, 86
hospital care of, 72
identification of, 74
immaturity of. *See* Premature
infant.
intestinal tract of, 67
kidneys of, 67
metabolic defects of, 107. *See also*
Metabolism, inborn errors of.

Newborn (*Continued*)
  mortality rate of, 86
  muscular development of, 68, 71
  needs of, 69
  nutrition of, 77
  of diabetic mother, 400
  phenylketonuria in, 108
  physical development of, 67
  reflexes of, 79
  respiration of, 65, 72
  rooming-in of, 75
  rubella in, 110
  skull of, 71
  temperature of, 74
Newborn nursery, 74
Nose, foreign bodies in, 260
Nose drops, instillation of, 551
Nosebleeds, 259
  in hemophilia, 347
Nursery day, 485
  newborn, 74
Nutrients, daily allowances of, 181
  sources of, 180
Nutrition. *See also* Appetite; Diet;
    Food.
  disturbances of. *See* Nutritional
    disturbances.
  in burns, 252
  in pregnancy, 62
  of infant, 125
  of newborn, 77
  of school age child, 377
Nutritional disturbances. *See also*
    Malnutrition.
  obesity, 469
  protein malnutrition, 494
  rickets, 176
  vitamin A deficiency, 178, 495
  vitamin C deficiency, 177
  vitamin D deficiency, 176

Obesity, 469
Observation, of behavior, 49
  of premature infant, 90
Obstetrics. *See* Newborn; Pregnancy;
    Prenatal.
Occupational therapy, 40
  in burns, 254
Operation. *See* Surgery.
Ophthalmia, sympathetic, 284
Ophthalmia neonatorum, gonococcal,
    281
Organogenesis, 60

Orphanages, 483
Orthodontic treatment, in cleft palate,
    262
Orthopedic conditions of infancy,
    188-194
Otitis media, 433
Oxygen administration to premature
    infant, 90
Oxygen inhalation by newborn, 73

Pain, behavior indicating, 50
  in treatments, emotional support in,
    214
Palate, cleft, 100, 260
Palsy, cerebral, 445. *See also* Illness,
    chronic.
Pancreas, cystic fibrosis of, 273, 274
Papule, defined, 354
Paralysis, infantile, 356
Parenthood, education for, 62
Parents. *See also* Family.
  anxiety of, hemophilia and, 350
    hospitalization and, 297
  battered-child syndrome and, 236
  emotional support of. *See* Emotional
    support, of parents.
  of premature infant, emotional
    support for, 94
  specialized services for, 487
Parotitis, infectious, 355
Patient. *See* Newborn; Infant;
    Premature infant; Toddler;
    Preschool child; School age child;
    Adolescent.
Pediatric Urine Collector, 150
Penicillin in rheumatic fever, 427, 428
Peritoneal dialysis, apparatus for,
    536, 537
Personality development, of adolescent,
    460
  of school age child, 380, 381
  of toddler, 202
Pertussis, 356
Phenylalanine, 108
Phenylketonuria, 108, 320
  prevention of, 322
  test for, 518
Physical activity, diabetic and, 397,
    398
  hemophilia and, 350
  in cystic fibrosis, 281
  in rheumatic fever, 429
  in tetralogy of Fallot, 418

Physical activity (*Continued*)
  of newborn, 71
  of premature infant, 91
Physical deformity, parental adjustment to, 330
Physical development. *See also* Growth and development.
  of adolescent, 458
  of fetus, 60
  of infant, 117
  of newborn, 67
  of toddler, 197
Physical examination, school preparation and, 380
Physical therapy, in burns, 254, 256
  in cerebral palsy, 452
Pink eye, 284
PKU. *See* Phenylketonuria.
Play activities, as therapy, 32, 33, 40
  bed rest and, 35
  hospital environment and, 15
  isolation and, 38
  restrictions and, 387
  suggestions for, 35
  surgical preparation and, 298
  toy construction as, 30
Play program, 28-44
  bed rest and, 37
  for infant, 39
  in mental retardation, 39, 313
  in rheumatic fever, 34
Play supplies, homemade, recipes for, 43
Play therapy, 32, 33, 40
Playroom in hospital, 29
Pleasure principle vs. reality principle, 133
Pleural cavity, water seal suction of, 533
Pneumonia, 184
Pneumonitis, from petroleum distillates, 225
  interstitial, acute, 182
Poison Control Center, 227
Poisoning, accidental, 222
  antidote in, 227
  aspirin, 225, 264, 426
  emergency measures in, 225
  kerosene, 228
  mental retardation and, 307
  oxygen, retrolental fibroplasia and, 282
Polio vaccine, 131

Poliomyelitis, 356
Polyarthritis in rheumatic fever, 423
Postoperative care. *See* Surgery.
Postural drainage in cystic fibrosis, 279, 280
Potts operation in tetralogy of Fallot, 419, 420
Pregnancy, attitude toward, 59
  diabetes in, 400
  in adolescence, 473
  infections in, hazards of, 60
  instruction during, 62
  iron deficiency anemia in, 337
  irradiations in, abdominal, 61
  nutrition in, 62
  rubella in, 111
    prevention of, 111
  syphilis in, 61
Premature infant, 87
  appearance of, 89
  bathing of, 91
  body temperature of, 89
  environment for, 89
  feeding patterns of, 91
  handling of, 91
  observation of, 90
  parents of, emotional support for, 94
  physical activity of, 91
  respiratory system of, 90
  weighing of, 92
Prematurity, causes of, 88
  defined, 88
  prevention of, 88
Prenatal. *See also* Fetus; Pregnancy.
Prenatal clinic, 62
Prenatal environment, 58
Prenatal period, 57-63
  adolescent and, 473
  infection in, mental retardation and, 307
  physical development in, 60
Preoperative care. *See* Surgery.
Preschool child, 291-372
  deaf, classes for, 440
  growth and development of, 293-304
  hospitalization of, 297
  toys for, 42
Preventive health services, rheumatic fever and, 430
Primitive societies, child care in, 4
Project Head Start, 505
Protein, C-reactive, 426
  malnutrition and, 494

Psychological support. *See* Emotional support.
PTC deficiency, 345
Puberty. *See also* Adolescent.
  defined, 457
Pubescent period, defined, 457
Pulmonary. *See also* Lungs; Respiratory.
Pulmonary hypertension, ventricular sepal defect and, 416
Pulmonary stenosis in tetralogy of Fallot, 417
Pulse rate, average, 512
Puppet play, surgery and, 298
Pustule, defined, 354
Pyloric stenosis, hypertrophic, congenital, 173

Reality principle vs. pleasure principle, 133
Recreation. *See* Play activities; Play program.
Rectal medications, 552
Reflex(es), of newborn, 79
  tonic neck, 70
Regression, 303
Religions, child care and, 6
Renal function test, 515
Respiration, of newborn, 65
Respiratory. *See also* Lungs; Pulmonary.
Respiratory disorders, Croupette in, 185
Respiratory infections, 258
  adenoidectomy and, 263
  in cystic fibrosis, 274
  in toddler, 258
  prevention of, 258
  tonsillectomy and, 263
Respiratory rate, average, 513
Respiratory system of premature infant, 90
Respiratory tract, disorders of, 180
Restraint, clove-hitch, 148, 149
  elbow, cleft lip and, 97
  emotional care and, 152
  eye surgery and, 285
  in scalp vein infusion, 148
  jacket, 231, 232
  mummy, 148
Restrictions. *See* Discipline.
Resuscitation, cardiopulmonary, closed-chest, 522

Resuscitation (*Continued*)
  mouth-to-mouth, 521
  of newborn, 72
    apparatus for, 73
Retardation, mental. *See* Mental retardation.
Retinoblastoma, 282
Rheumatic fever, 423-432. *See also* Illness, chronic.
  bed rest in, 427
  carditis in, 424
  case history of, 430
  chorea in, 424
  convalescent hospital and, 429
  diagnosis of, Jones criteria in, 425
  etiology of, 423
  home care in, 428
  medications in, 426
  play program and, 34
  polyarthritis in, 423
  preventive health services and, 430
  recurrences of, 427
Rickets, malnutrition and, 176
Ritualism of toddler, 203
Roentgenography of heart, 408
Rooming-in of newborn, 75
  of parents in hospital, 24
Rubella, 357
  congenital, 110
  in pregnancy, 60
  prevention of, 111
Rubeola, 357
Russell's traction, 234

Safety, home medicines and, 223
  on toddler ward, 231
  school preparation and, 380
Salicylates in rheumatic fever, 426
Scalds, 242
Scalp vein, infusion of, 146, 147
  puncture of, positioning for, 554
Scarlet fever, 358
Scarletina, 358
School, readiness for, 379
School age child, 373-454
  characteristics by age, 378
  deaf, education for, 440
  deprivation and, 383
  discipline of, 386
  emotional support for, 380
  growth and development of, 375-388
  health of, 375
  hospitalization of, 383

School age child (*Continued*)
  nutrition of, 377
  of migrant workers, 488
  preventive health services for,
    rheumatic fever and, 430
  toys for, 42
School nurse, 503
Schoolwork, home care and, 329
  in epilepsy, 365
  in hemophilia, 350
  in hospital, 26
  in rheumatic fever, 429
Scurvy, 177
Seizures, convulsive, 363
  epileptic, 364
Septicemia in burns, 252
Sex characteristics, secondary, 457
Sex education, 382
  school nurse in, 503
Sexual relationships in adolescence,
  472
Shock, insulin, 394, 395, 399
Siblings, of newborn, attitude of, 77
Sickle cell disease, 339
Skin, acne vulgaris of, 467
  grafts, burns and, 251
  of infant, care of, 139
    observation of, 50
Skull, fracture of, 233
  injuries, in battered-child syndrome,
    237
  of newborn, 71
Smallpox, 353, 360
  vaccination, 360
    contraindications to, 132
Snellen chart, 443
Snellen test, 442
Social development, immobilization
    and, 235
  in hydrocephalus, 161
  of infant, 120, 124
Speech development. *See* Language
  development.
Speech therapy, in cleft palate, 263
Spina bifida, 163
Splint, Denis Browne, 189
  Frejka, 192
Staphylococcal pneumonia, 184
Startle reflex, 70
Stenosis, pulmonary, in tetralogy of
  Fallot, 417
Sterilization of formulas, 83
Steroid therapy in nephrosis, 370

Stomach, ulcer of, in burns, 253
Stool, examination, cystic fibrosis and,
  276
  of newborn, 67
Strabismus, 283
Streptococcus infections. *See*
  Infections, streptococcus.
Streptomycin in rheumatic fever, 427
Sty, 284
Sulfadiazine in rheumatic fever, 428
Support, emotional. *See* Emotional
  support.
Suppositories, rectal, 552
Surgery, adenoidectomy, 263
  emotional support in. *See* Emotional
    support.
  explanation of, puppet play and, 298
  eye, 282
  in cleft lip, 96
  in cleft palate, 100, 260
  in clubfoot, 190
  in coarctation of aorta, 414
  in esophageal atresia, 101, 102, 104
  in hydrocephalus, 157
  in intussusception, 170
  in pyloric stenosis, 174
  in spina bifida, 164
  of heart. *See* Heart surgery.
  tonsillectomy, 263, 264
  tracheotomy, in laryngotracheo-
    bronchitis, 269
Swaddling, 7
Sweat test, for cystic fibrosis, 275
Sydenham's chorea, 424
  play program and, 35
Syphilis, in pregnancy, 61

Talipes equinovarus, congenital, 188
Tantrums, temper, 203
Teaching. *See also* Counseling.
  puppet play in, 298
  self-help, mental retardation and,
    310
Tear duct, impatency of, 282
Teenager. *See* Adolescent.
Teeth, care of, hemophilia and, 347
  deciduous, eruption of, 123, 125,
    197
    loss of, 375
  extraction, hemophilia and, 347
  permanent, eruption of, 375, 376
Temper tantrums, 203

Temperature. *See* Body temperature.
  Fahrenheit, conversion to
    Centigrade, 513
Temperature taking, 143
Teratogenic agents, 307
Test, Addis sediment count, 369, 515
  audiometry, 437
  carbohydrate metabolism, 515
  C-reactive protein, 426
  erythrocyte sedimentation rate, 425
  for diabetes mellitus, 391
  for phenylketonuria, 108
  galactose tolerance, 109
  glucose tolerance, 515
  Guthrie inhibition assay, 109
  hearing, 437
  laboratory, preparation for, 515
  mucoviscidosis, 516
  of duodenal fluid for tryptic activity,
    276
  phenylketonuria, 518
  pilocarpine iontophoresis, for cystic
    fibrosis, 275
  renal function, 515
  Snellen, 442
  sweat, for cystic fibrosis, 275
  tryptic activity in duodenal fluid,
    516
  tuberculin, 131
  urine, 517
    ferric chloride, 518
    for albumin, 517
    for phenylketonuria, 108, 320
    in diabetes mellitus, 393
    pH, 518
    protein in glomerulonephritis, 369
    specific gravity, 517, 518
    sugar, 518
  visual, 442
Tetanus toxoid, 131
Tetralogy of Fallot, 417
  surgery in, 418, 419, 420
Thalassemia, 340
Toddler, 195-290
  growth and development of, 197-217
  hospitalization of, 203
  personality development of, 202
  toys for, 39, 42
Toilet training, 200
  hospitalization and, 210
  of mentally retarded child, 310
Tonsillectomy, 263, 264
  case history of, 266

Tonsillitis, acute, 264
Toothbrushing, 197
Toxicity. *See* Poisoning.
Toxin, defined, 354
Toxoid, defined, 354
  diphtheria, 355
Toys. *See also* Play activities.
  collection of, 43
  for age groups, 42
  for mentally retarded child, 313
  homemade, constuction of, 30, 41
  in hemophilia, 348
Tracheotomy care, 531
Tracheotomy tube, 270, 532
  care of, 533
  suctioning of, 270, 271, 531
Traction, Bryant's, 234, 235
  Russell's, 234
Transfusions, in hemophilia, 346
Trauma, emotional. *See also*
    Emotional support.
  physical. *See* Injuries.
Tub bath for infant, 136, 137
Tube feeding, 535
Tuberculin testing, 131
Tumor of retina, malignant, 282
Typhoid fever, 358

Ulcer, Curling's, 253
Umbilical cord, care of, 73
United Nations International Chil-
    dren's Emergency Fund, 498
Urinary incontinence, in spina bifida,
    166
Urine collection, 149, 544, 545
  continuous, 150
Urine collectors, 150, 151, 544
  application of, 150
Urine excretion, average normal, 512
Urine test. *See* Test, urine.
Urinometer, 517

Vaccination, *See also* Immunization.
  in infancy, schedule for, 131
  smallpox, 360
    contraindications to, 360
Vaccine, defined, 354
  measles, 357
  mumps, 355
  pertussis, 356
  poliomyelitis, 356
Varicella, 359
Variola, 360

Vein puncture, femoral, 553, 554
  jugular, 552, 554
Ventricular hypertrophy in tetralogy
  of Fallot, 417
Ventricular septal defect, 409
Ventriculoauricular shunt in hydrocephalus, 157, 158
Ventriculoauriculostomy, 159
Ventriculoureterostomy, 158
Virus disease(s), bronchiolitis, acute,
    182
  chickenpox, 359
  Coxsackie, in pregnancy, 61
  diarrheal, 361
  Echo, in pregnancy, 61
  herpes zoster, 359
  measles, 357
  mumps, 355
  pneumonia, 184
  poliomyelitis, 356
  respiratory. *See* Respiratory
    infections.
  rubella, 357
    congenital, 110
    in pregnancy, 61
  smallpox, 353, 360
Visiting hours, 21, 25
Visual defects, 441
  education and, 444
  in strabismus, 283
  long term planning and, 444
  surgery and, 285, 286
Visual loss, symptomatic behavior of,
    442
Visual testing, 442

Vitamin(s), daily allowances of, 181
  sources of, 180
Vitamin A, deficiency of, 178, 495
Vitamin C, 126
  deficiency of, 177
  for newborn, 83
Vitamin D, deficiency of, 176
  for newborn, 83
Von Willebrand's syndrome, 345

Wastebasket, aseptic technique and,
    527
Weighing, aseptic technique of, 525
  of infant, 142, 143
  of premature infant, 92
Weight, body, avoirdupois, conversion
    to metric equivalents, 513
  in metric and apothecary scales, 514
  low-birth-, 88. *See also* Premature
    infant.
  of infant, 117
  of toddler, 197
Well Child Conference, 505
Wet nurse, 7
White House Conference, 481
  on Children and Youth, pledge of,
    490
WHO Chronicle, 498
Whooping cough, 356
World Health Organization, 497

Xerophthalmia, 495
X-ray. *See also* Irradiation.

Yaws, 496